Preparing for Doctoral Study in Nursing

MAKING THE MOST OF THE YEAR BEFORE YOU BEGIN

Laura A. Taylor, PhD, RN, ANEF, FAAN
Owner
GuIDE to Degree, LLC
Ellicott City, Maryland

Mary F. Terhaar, RN, PhD, ANEF, FAAN
Professor & Associate Dean for Graduate Programs
Fitzpatrick College of Nursing
Villanova University
Villanova, Pennsylvania

ELSEVIER

Elsevier
3251 Riverport Lane
St. Louis, Missouri 63043

PREPARING FOR DOCTORAL STUDY IN NURSING:
MAKING THE MOST OF THE YEAR BEFORE YOU BEGIN   ISBN: 978-0-323-87589-9

Notice

Practitioners and researchers must always rely on their own experience and knowledge in evaluating
and using any information, methods, compounds or experiments described herein. Because of rapid
advances in the medical sciences, in particular, independent verification of diagnoses and drug
dosages should be made. To the fullest extent of the law, no responsibility is assumed by Elsevier,
authors, editors or contributors for any injury and/or damage to persons or property as a matter of
products liability, negligence or otherwise, or from any use or operation of any methods, products,
instructions, or ideas contained in the material herein.

Executive Content Strategist: Lee Henderson
Senior Content Development Manager: Meghan Andress
Content Development Specialist: Deborah Poulson
Publishing Services Manager: Deepthi Unni
Project Manager: Nayagi Anandan
Design Direction: Renee Duenow

Printed in India

Last digit is the print number: 9   8   7   6   5   4   3   2   1

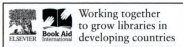

Working together
to grow libraries in
developing countries

www.elsevier.com • www.bookaid.org

*We are particularly proud of the extensive
collaboration and diverse contributors who have
brought this text to life, and so we dedicate this book
to strong partners everywhere who make nursing
and healthcare better every day!*

CONTRIBUTORS

Jonathan Hubert Aebischer, DNP, FNP
PhD student
School of Nursing
Oregon Health and Science University
Portland, Oregon

Paula Alexander-Delpech, BSN, MSN, PhD, PMHNP-BC
Associate Professor
Psychiatric Mental Health
Frontier Nursing University
Versailles, Kentucky

Taura L. Barr, PhD, RN, NC-BC
Associate Professor
College of Nursing
The Ohio State University
Columbus, Ohio

Amy Bieda, PhD, APRN, PCPNP-BC, NNP-BC
Associate Professor
Nursing
Temple University
Philadelphia, Pennsylvania

Mary L. Blankson, DNP, APRN, FNP-C, FAAN
Chief Nursing Officer
Nursing
Community Health Center, Inc.
Middletown, Connecticut

Lt Col David Bradley, DNP, APRN, AGCNS-BC, CNOR
Assistant Professor
Daniel K. Inouye Graduate School of Nursing
Uniformed Services University of the Health Sciences
Bethesda, Maryland

Latina M. Brooks, PhD, CNP, FAANP
Director, MSN and DNP Programs
Frances Payne Bolton School of Nursing
Case Western Reserve University
Cleveland, Ohio

Jennifer M. Brown, DNP, MSN, RN, APN
Assistant Professor
College of Public Health
Department of Nursing
Temple University
Philadelphia, Pennsylvania

Kim Curry, PhD, FNP-C, FAANP
Editor in Chief
Journal of the American Association of Nurse Practitioners
American Association of Nurse Practitioners
Tampa, Florida

Katherine Dudding, PhD, RN, RN-NIC, CNE
Assistant Professor
Family, Community, and Health Systems
University of Alabama at Birmingham
Birmingham, Alabama

Mary Anne Dumas, PhD, FNP-BC, GNP-BC, FAANP, FAAN, FNAP
Consultant
Stony Brook University
Huntington, New York

Cheryl Lynn Fattibene, DNP, MSN, MPH, FNP-BC
Associate Professor
Thomas Jefferson College of Nursing
Philadelphia, Pennsylvania

Nicole Angelique Gonzaga Gomez, DNP, CRNA, APRN, CHSE
Associate Program Director—DNP Nurse Anesthesia Program
School of Nursing and Health Studies
University of Miami
Coral Gables, Florida

Bethany Hall-Long, PhD, MSN, BSN
LT Governor, State of Delaware
Professor of Nursing
Associate Policy Scientist
University of Delaware
Newark, Delaware

Stacia Marie Hays, DNP, APRN, CPNP-PC, CNE, CCTC, FAANP
Clinical Associate Professor
Nursing
Baylor University, Louise Herrington School of Nursing
Dallas, Texas

Ronald Lee Hickman, Jr., PhD, RN, ACNP-BC, FNAP, FAAN
The Ruth M. Anderson Endowed Professor
   & Associate Dean for Research
Frances Payne Bolton School of Nursing
Case Western Reserve University
Cleveland, Ohio

Cassandre Jean-Antoine, PhD, RN, NEA-BC
Nursing Leadership
Nursing
Howard University
Washington, DC

Versie Johnson-Mallard, PhD
Dean and Endowed Professor
Nursing
Kent State University
Kent, Ohio

Kim Dupree Jones, PhD, FNP, FAAN
Professor and Associate Dean for Academic
   Advancement
The Nell Hodgson Woodruff School of
   Nursing
Emory University
Atlanta Georgia

Sunghee Kim, DNP, ANP-BC, NP-C
Emergency Department
Loma Linda University Medical Center
Loma Linda, California

Shanina C. Knighton, PhD, RN, CIC
Associate Professor
School of Nursing
Case Western Reserve University
Cleveland, Ohio

Jennifer A. Korkosz, DNP, WHNP-BC, APRN
Associate Professor
School of Nursing
University of Delaware
Newark, Delaware

Khalilah McCants, DNP, MSN, RN-BC
Associate Professor
Daniel K. Inouye Graduate School of Nursing
Uniformed Services University of the Health
   Sciences
Bethesda, Maryland

Kathleen McGrow, DNP, MS, RN, PMP
Chief Nursing Information Officer
Health and Life Sciences
Microsoft
Redmond, Washington

Tiffany Monique Montgomery, PhD, MSHP, RNC-OB
Coordinator, Women's Services
Medical City
Las Colinas, Texas

Susan Painter, DNP, APRN, PMHCNS-BC
Lead Faculty, Frances Payne Bolton School
   of Nursing
Family Systems Psychiatric Nurse
   Practitioner Program
Case Western Reserve University
Cleveland, Ohio

Marcia Parker, EdD
EdD Alumna
Educational Leadership for Social Justice
Loyola Marymount University
Los Angeles, California

Jose A. Rodriguez, DNP, JM, RN, APRN, CCNS, CNOR
Assistant Professor
Daniel K. Inouye Graduate School of
   Nursing
Uniformed Services University of the Health
   Sciences
Bethesda, Maryland

Lydia D. Rotondo, DNP, RN, CNS, FNAP
Professor of Clinical Nursing and Associate
   Dean for Education and Student Affairs
University of Rochester School of Nursing
Rochester, New York

Nancy Rudner, DrPH, MPH, MSN, APRN
Associate Professor
School of Nursing
University of Alabama at Birmingham
Birmingham, Alabama

Carolyn Morcom Rutledge, PhD, FNP-BC, FAAN
Professor, Associate Chair
Nursing
Old Dominion University
Virginia Beach, Virginia

Krista Schroeder, PhD, RN
Assistant Professor
Nursing
Temple University College of Public Health
Philadelphia, Pennsylvania

Diane Siebert, PhD, APRN, FAANP, FAAN
Professor and Associate Dean for Academic
Affairs
Daniel K. Inouye Graduate School of Nursing
Uniformed Services University of the Health
Sciences
Bethesda, Maryland

Laura Sinko, PhD, MSHP, RN, CCTS-I
Assistant Professor
Nursing
Temple University College of Public Health
Philadelphia, Pennsylvania

Laura A. Taylor, PhD, RN, ANEF, FAAN
Owner
GuIDE to Degree, LLC
Ellicott City, Maryland

Mary F. Terhaar, RN, PhD, ANEF, FAAN
Professor & Associate Dean for Graduate
Programs
Fitzpatrick College of Nursing
Villanova University
Villanova, Pennsylvania

Vanessa Velez, DNP, RN
Director, Graduate Nursing Programs and
Chief Nurse Administrator
School of Nursing and Health Professions
Stevenson University
Owings Mills, Maryland

Angelo Venditti, DNP, MBA, RN, FACHE, NEA-BC
Senior Vice President, Strategic Workforce
Solutions
AMN Healthcare
Irving Texas

Marisa L. Wilson, DNSc, MHSc, MHSc, RN-BC, CPHIMS, FAMIA, FIAHSI, FAAN
Associate Professor and Director, Nursing
Health Services Leadership Pathways
Coordinator, Specialty Track Nursing
Informatics
Family, Community, and Health Systems
School of Nursing
University of Alabama at Birmingham
Birmingham, Alabama

I am delighted to have the opportunity to write the foreword for this much-needed and important resource book by Drs. Laura A. Taylor and Mary F. Terhaar on preparing for doctoral study in nursing. The United States and the world need many more nurses prepared at the doctoral level to advance nursing science and practice, and to use those advancements to influence, lead, educate, and mentor future generations of nurses and advanced practice nurses. We also need many more nurses from historically excluded and underrepresented groups, to join and help lead in efforts to combat racism and achieve health equity, as well as to continue to advance our efforts to transform healthcare and achieve culturally sensitive care. As with all professions, career advancement in nursing is linked with advanced degree preparation. Choosing and earning the highest degree preparation, a doctorate, needs to be intentional and must be planned. Terminal degree achievement opens career opportunities and paths for individual nurses and ensures high-level preparation for the profession, health and health policy, and healthcare. Nurses need and deserve to be guided and to have accurate information and support as they decide on the degree pathway that aligns with their career goals and aspirations.

While nurses may obtain doctorates outside of nursing, the discipline of nursing has two doctoral pathways: the Doctor of Philosophy (PhD) degree, which prepares nurse scientists and discipline leaders; and the Doctor of Nursing Practice (DNP) degree, which prepares advanced practice nurses and discipline leaders. Knowing and understanding the opportunities afforded through both degrees are important for the discipline. Some nurses will choose one or the other degree, some will choose both, and the profession needs both PhD- and DNP-prepared nurses. Nurse scientists with PhD preparation are particularly in high demand due to stagnant enrollments for at least the past decade and retirements. The need for advanced practice nurses for patient care, education, and quality improvement science is expected to continue to grow significantly. This book provides accurate information and lived experience "narratives," providing the reader with knowledge and personal examples to inform and relate to with regard to considering and choosing the degree path best aligned with one's goals.

Nurses are at every point of care, as Registered and Advanced Practice Nurses, a reality that became highly visible during the COVID pandemic when the demand for nurses and nursing care needed to save lives headlined national news reports. The pandemic dramatically accelerated and exacerbated a workforce supply/demand mismatch at all levels of nursing preparation, including the doctoral level. The need to educate and mentor large numbers of nurses will require many more nurses with doctoral preparation, for practice, research, education, and health policy. Nurse scientists will be critical for conducting the research and defining the science that will underpin nursing practice for the future. Doctorally prepared nurses are also needed to influence and lead the major changes required to address population health, social determinants of health, healthcare delivery, and health disparities.[1]

Nurses have maintained their position as the most trusted profession due to honesty and ethics for more than two decades,[2] and nursing remains the profession having the most direct contact with patients across systems of healthcare. Evidence-based nursing care must continue to evolve through science to meet needs across the full continuum of health and healthcare, from the high-technology and high-acuity needs of hospital care, to the complex care needs of those with chronic and serious illnesses, to care coordination and transitional care needs, population health and public health, and health and wellness care. This requires high-level and high-quality prepared nurses, for patient care, discovery and translational science, quality/improvement science, and health policy.

Drs. Taylor and Terhaar have produced a well-thought-out and instructive book that provides the big picture of nurses prepared at the doctoral level, including demand and a view into the future, guidance in choosing one's path, deciding on the degree and developing a plan, voices of lived experience from PhD- and DNP-prepared nurses, and a toolkit for preparing for doctoral study. Necessary considerations such as financing one's education, choosing and applying to a program, and getting past barriers are some of the important areas of focus that Drs. Taylor and Terhaar have included, based on their collective experience with the GuIDE to Degree program, Guiding Initiatives for Doctoral Education. They developed GuIDE to support nurses in the important process of deciding on an advanced degree path, providing information and support sessions as well as follow through to help nurses successfully apply and enroll in PhD and DNP programs.

Advising and mentoring from early in a nurse's educational path influence career choices and interest in seeking advanced degrees. Students often seek faculty members' advisement as they consider their future. I recommend this book for adoption by nurse faculty, especially for prelicensure students, as a resource and foundation for dialog, to benefit our future nurses and our profession.

Susan Bakewell-Sachs, PhD, RN, FAAN
Vice President for Nursing Affairs, Professor, and Dean
Oregon Health & Science University School of Nursing, Portland, Oregon

References

1. National Academies of Sciences, Engineering, and Medicine. *The Future of Nursing 2020–2030: Charting the Path to Achieve Health Equity.* Washington, DC: The National Academies Press; 2021. https://doi.org/10.17226/25982.
2. https://news.gallup.com/poll/388649/military-brass-judges-among-professions-new-image-lows.aspx January 12, 2022, retrieved July 8, 2022.

PREFACE

Doctoral students face many of the same challenges, discouragements, and overwhelming emotions that nurses have encountered for many years. As nurses with doctorates ourselves, we understand the kinds of information most valuable to prospective students. Our search for a resource to support and assist other nurses considering pursuit of a doctorate fell short.

Thus, we reached out to esteemed colleagues to expand the notion of what is possible in a nursing career. We asked them to help us open the eyes of rising nurses to the incredible opportunities available within their careers and to provide reliable information and resources to help these nurses take their crucial first steps. Together we outline strategies that will promote successful scholarship, program completion, and professional contribution; and we tell a few inspirational stories of doctoral-prepared nurses shaping the future of nursing and the science of healthcare. Our purpose is to facilitate smooth progression toward a rewarding and impactful career as a nurse who practices at the highest level. We want to provide nurses considering a doctoral degree with a comprehensive yet practical resource to effectively guide you during the year before you begin a doctoral program.

Authors selected to contribute chapters have successfully navigated the doctoral journey. They are nurse scientists, scholars, educators, and leaders in their field. All currently serve in higher education institutions, service areas, industry, and professional organizations across gender, race, specialty, and accomplishment disciplines. In writing the text this way, we showcase exemplars of doctoral nurses who continue to figure out how to take on and conquer doctoral education.

The book is organized into four sections: **Section 1** describes the social mandate for nurses, the history of doctoral nursing and education, and available options for doctoral education in nursing. **Section 2** presents a plan for the year leading up to doctoral study. It details how to select a degree and program, submit your most effective application, and organize your commitments and priorities to promote success. **Section 3** tells the stories of nurses who have earned one of the many doctoral degrees available and have linked their career trajectories and education for effect and satisfaction. **Section 4** provides a set of tools that can be used in preparation for and for completion of a doctoral degree.

Each chapter explores a discrete component that educators and nursing leaders have encountered as they began their journey. We dug in hard to find the building blocks to elevate your ability to get accepted into your program of choice, persevere from beginning to end, and offer strategies for skillfully pivoting capabilities to address challenges and roadblocks (because there will be roadblocks).

Section 1: The Big Picture of Nurses Educated at the Highest Level

CHAPTER 1: THE DEMAND FOR THE DOCTORALLY PREPARED NURSE

This chapter describes the critical position papers, workforce studies, professional nursing associations, and national policy statements that establish the demand for doctorally prepared nurses. Your understanding of the impact of the professional organizations' influence on the health and well-being of our society will be the target.

CHAPTER 2: THE STORY OF THE DOCTORALLY PREPARED NURSE

This chapter presents the history of the doctorally prepared nurse. It describes the contribution of doctoral nurses toward improving the quality and safety of healthcare and the rigor and effectiveness of nursing education and leadership needed to make change happen. The chapter connects doctoral education to the quality of care and the public's health. We present overviews of remarkable nursing careers spanning the first earned doctorates in the 1950s through the 21st century. We connect doctoral education to the development of nursing theory, research, education, and leadership to the substantial impact on the public's health quality and safety, the broad range of public policy, and the implications for global health.

CHAPTER 3: LOOKING TO THE FUTURE OF THE DOCTORALLY PREPARED NURSE

This chapter looks ahead to the future of professional nursing. It forecasts high-need areas for the scholarship, research, practice, and education. These areas include informatics, health policy, population health, telehealth, public health, tech development, industry services, and entrepreneurial endeavors.

CHAPTER 4: REFLECTION ON CHALLENGES

This chapter provides an overview of nursing workforce shortages, the critical need for diversity, and the vital importance of retaining talent. We present the case for our position that the current process leading to doctoral study is ineffective in meeting present and future challenges, and we lay the foundation for the three remaining parts of the book, which seek to correct the problems we identify.

Section 2: Choosing Your Path, Making Your Decision and Developing Your Plan

CHAPTER 5: CLARIFYING YOUR OPTIONS

This chapter introduces the different options for doctoral study and links each to the career trajectory they support. Each degree option is linked to a career story written by a nurse who has earned that credential and pursued a related career (Part 3 of this book).

CHAPTER 6: CLARIFYING YOUR ASPIRATIONS

This chapter presents approaches to focus your efforts and obtain the information you need to begin.

CHAPTER 7: COMMON IMPEDIMENTS TO SUCCESS

This chapter presents a set of barriers to successful entry to and progress through doctoral education. The chapters that follow introduce a set of evidence-based strategies to manage them, and Part 4 provides tools to help readers track progress goals.

CHAPTER 8: MENTORS

This chapter introduces mentoring—what it is and how it works. Securing a mentor *before* beginning a doctoral program is encouraged to increase success in preparation, application, progress through, and completion of doctoral study. Seeking, finding, securing, and working with a mentor is unfamiliar to many nurses. This chapter describes the characteristics of a successful mentoring relationship.

CHAPTER 9: UNDERSTANDING AND MANAGING EXPENSES

This chapter presents the business case for doctoral education. It describes important financial considerations reported by students across the United States. Resources and processes to address the financial burden of doctoral education are offered. Tactical approaches to assessing, planning for, managing, and monitoring financial challenges are described to support informed decision-making and effective financial planning.

CHAPTER 10: PRESENTING A STRONG AND AUTHENTIC APPLICATION

This chapter outlines the process and components of the application. Attention to detail across the process and emotional intelligence have proven to result in more successful admissions experiences.

CHAPTER 11: USING TIME WISELY AND WELL

This chapter describes strategies to manage daily distractions and to optimize working to your strengths in conquering perceived time barriers as you prepare for and progress through doctoral education. It helps align abilities, goals, and priorities and offers evidence-based actions to empower you to move forward through each day with greater confidence. The resources offered are linked with tools presented in Part 4 of this text.

CHAPTER 12: BECOMING A WRITER

This chapter describes basic practices to help improve writing quality, clarity, and precision. It focuses on finding one's voice, telling one's story, and connecting with the reader in ways that advance one's goals.

CHAPTER 13: DETERMINING GOOD FIT

This chapter identifies points to consider when selecting the program that best fits your goals and aspirations.

CHAPTER 14: THE FIRST STEP AND BEYOND

This chapter offers strategies to keep the drive alive. The evidence shows that taking on doctoral work demands positivism and attitudes of "can-do" confidence and competence.

Section 3: Shared Experiences of Doctorally Prepared Nurses on the Edge of Tomorrow

Section 3 presents narratives of doctorally prepared nurses around the world. It highlights expansive knowledge and expertise across realms of clinical practice, academia, the armed forces, industry, entrepreneurialism, business ownership, leadership in both small and large healthcare systems, and national and global health policy.

Section 4: ToolKit

Section 4 is a compendium of tools that will be useful from the point one begins to contemplate doctoral study through the application process, on make this onto course work and completion of the program, and well into professional life as a doctorally prepared nurse. These tools are presented in sets according to their utility and focus.

Evolve Resources

In addition to the text, resources including podcasts with contributors from Section 3 can be found on the accompanying Evolve site (http://evolve.elsevier.com/Taylor/doctoralstudy/).

Make It Your Reality

We hope you enjoy using this text as much as we enjoyed building it—a text that leaves you with a sense of strength, possibility, and a spirit of confidence to face a fear, tackle a challenge, and successfully conquer your doctoral educational journey. We wish to catapult you on your way to transforming nursing and the healthcare system of tomorrow!

Laura A. Taylor
Mary F. Terhaar

CONTENTS

SECTION 3 *Shared Experiences of Doctorally Prepared Nurses on the Edge of Tomorrow* 231

The Big Picture of Nurses Educated at the Highest Level

CHAPTER 1

The Demand for the Doctorally Prepared Nurse

Laura A. Taylor, PhD, RN, ANEF, FAAN ■ Mary F. Terhaar, RN, PhD, ANEF, FAAN

A nation cannot fully thrive until everyone—no matter who they are, where they live, or how much money they make—can live their healthiest possible life, and helping people live their healthiest life is and has always been the essential role of nurses. Nurses have a critical role to play in achieving the goal of health equity, but they need robust education, supportive work environments, and autonomy. Accordingly, at the request of the Robert Wood Johnson Foundation, on behalf of the National Academy of Medicine, an ad hoc committee under the auspices of the National Academies of Sciences, Engineering, and Medicine conducted a study aimed at envisioning and charting a path forward for the nursing profession to help reduce inequities in people's ability to achieve their full health potential. The ultimate goal is the achievement of health equity in the United States built on strengthened nursing capacity and expertise.

—National Academy of Science (2021)

Nursing is an essential presence globally. We comprise the largest segment of the healthcare workforce with more than 3.8 million nurses around the world and are consistently recognized among the most trusted of all disciplines (Saad, 2020). By virtue of our numbers, education, experience, and the incredible sustained public trust we have earned and continue to enjoy, nursing will increasingly be asked to lead in healthcare, industry, public health, administration, education, research, policy, and advocacy. Nurses must be ready to respond to these requests. We must be prepared to maximize our contributions to the health of society. We must be poised to rise to a broad range of challenges brought on by the complexities of the systems in which care is provided and the brisk pace at which science, interventions, and therapeutics advance. Doctoral education positions nurses to improve outcomes, lead systems and communities, advance science, apply evidence to transform care, innovate, collaborate, influence, and inform. These are the contributions of doctorally prepared nurses who are greatly needed now and in the future, locally and around the globe.

This chapter describes the demand for doctorally prepared nurses, introduces a set of position papers and policy statements that explain the conditions that create and sustain this demand, and outlines strategies that will help meet the need.

The Challenge Before Us

Many conditions globally demand advances in nursing practice, science, and education. These include:

1. tremendous advances in health promotion and preventive care,
2. prevalence of chronic conditions, such as obesity and diabetes,
3. new and reemerging infectious diseases,
4. aging of baby boomers,
5. lengthier and more vibrant lives,
6. overwhelming calls for team science and interdisciplinary research, and
7. burgeoning knowledge of basic and applied sciences in healthcare.

Nurses and nursing will continue to be indispensable contributors to achieving and expanding a more healthful populace (AACN, 2020; Drennan & Ross, 2019; NLN, 2021).

KEY POSITION PAPERS AND POLICY STATEMENTS

At the beginning of the second decade of the 2000s, two pivotal documents were generated in the United States: *The Patient Protection and Affordable Care Act* and *The Future of Nursing: Leading Change, Advancing Health.* Together, they significantly altered the landscape for nursing practice and for healthcare. Both serve to challenge the status quo of education and practice with the intent to achieve the highest level of health for our country. The components and recommendations of each are essential to understand. A decade after their release, their impact on nursing education and practice is relevant as you move ahead in your professional career.

PATIENT PROTECTION AND AFFORDABLE CARE ACT

In March 2010, the *Patient Protection and Affordable Care Act (ACA)* became law. Commonly referred to as Obamacare, this landmark healthcare law has three primary goals:

- Make affordable health insurance available to more people. The law provides consumers with subsidies ("premium tax credits") that lower costs for households with incomes between 100% and 400% of the federal poverty level (FPL). **Note:** If income is above 400% FPL, you may still qualify for the premium tax credit in 2021.

- Expand the Medicaid program to cover all adults with income below 138% of the FPL. (Not all states have expanded their Medicaid programs.)
- Support innovative medical care delivery methods designed to lower health-care costs.

(https://www.healthcare.gov/glossary/affordable-care-act/; 2021)

Its implementation has been bumpy. Regardless, the ACA represents a paradigm shift in policy that has had a significant impact on access to healthcare, especially primary care, as well as the health and quality of life for many who previously were unable to receive care. This was an important initial step toward overcoming health disparities.

INSTITUTE OF MEDICINE AND ROBERT WOOD JOHNSON FOUNDATION: FUTURE OF NURSING REPORT

The Future of Nursing: Leading Change, Advancing Health white paper was released as a part of a collaboration between the Institute of Medicine (IOM—now the National Academy of Sciences—NAS) and the Robert Wood Johnson Foundation (RWJ) in 2010. It asserts that nurses will be more essential than ever before in the care delivery, design, and evaluation of healthcare systems innovation that lies ahead. It makes a strong and data-driven case for society to ensure that nurses are able to practice at the highest level of their education (doctoral degrees). According to the Report, nursing has excellent potential to monumentally impact the future healthcare landscape

> *by virtue of their regular, close proximity to patients and their scientific understanding of care processes across the continuum of care, nurses have a considerable opportunity to act as full partners with other health professionals and to lead in the improvement and redesign of the health care system and its practice environment.*

> IOM (2011, p. 23)

It further asserts that regulations need to unencumber the practice of nurses and enable them to practice in ways that apply their competencies, knowledge, and experience to the service of those in need.

The Report offers five recommendations for nursing and healthcare delivery:

1. Build common ground around the scope of practice and other issues in both scope and practice,
2. Increase the percentage of baccalaureate nurses in the workforce to 80% by 2020,
3. Provide a transition to practice residencies to reduce attrition,

4. Promote nurses' pursuit of doctoral degrees to double the number of doctorally prepared nurses by 2020, and

5. Promote interprofessional and lifelong learning (Tables 1.1 and 1.2).

The Report states no preference for the type of doctorate (Doctor of Nursing Practice—DNP; Doctor of Philosophy—PhD in nursing or another field) and does not set numerical targets for each degree. More importantly, it sets ambitious goals for the profession to prepare a larger percentage of its members to bring elevated knowledge and skill to bear on the healthcare needs of society. The text you are reading is explicitly intended to address recommendation #4, *promoting the doctoral degree*'s pursuit. Still, the aggregate impact of the five recommendations is important to appreciate. Throughout this and subsequent chapters, we will highlight the relevance and connection between the *Future of Nursing Report* and the goal of preparing a cadre of nurse leaders for the future. As future nurse leaders, you will promote nurse-led science and discovery, advance the application of evidence to improve outcomes, and develop more nurses to be faculty to educate the next generation of nurses.

Together, the ACA and IOM/RWJ sharpened the focus of the nursing profession in the provision of patient-centered, accessible, and affordable care as well as the development of the professionals in the broad range of roles required to accomplish ambitious yet logical objectives. Today's graduates enter nursing or advance in our ranks in the context of demographic and economic forces that have given rise to an urgent national need for access to safe, high-quality, cost-effective care. The opportunities are simply endless and include developing and implementing innovations in nursing science, education, practice, theory, leadership, advocacy, informatics, and more. However, be-fore we explore all the fantastic options open to you, we intend to brief you on the most immediate challenges facing nurses today and prepare you to navigate those features on the healthcare horizon.

Text continued on page 11

TABLE 1.1 ■ **Deadlines for the Practice Doctorate**

Entity	Deadline
ANA	Now
NLN	2020 double the number of doctorates
AANA	2025
ACM	Demands impact evidence
AANP	Demands impact evidence
NONPF	2025
NACNS	2030
AACN	2025

TABLE 1.2 ■ Key Recommendations From the Future of Nursing: Leading Change, Advancing Health Report

Original Recommendations and Scope	Assessing Progress Report
1. Remove scope-of-practice barriers.	Continued work is needed to remove scope-of-practice barriers. The policy and practice context has shifted since *The Future of Nursing* report was released. This shift has created an opportunity for nurses, physicians, and other providers to work together to find common ground in the new context of healthcare, and to devise solutions that work for all professions and patients. RECOMMENDATION Recommendation 1: Build Common Ground Around Scope of Practice and Other Issues in Policy and Practice. The Future of Nursing: Campaign for Action (the Campaign) should broaden its coalition to include more diverse stakeholders. The Campaign should build on its successes and work with other health professions groups, policymakers, and the community to build common ground around removing scope-of-practice restrictions, increasing interprofessional collaboration, and addressing other issues to improve healthcare practice in the interest of patients.
2. Expand opportunities for nurses to lead and diffuse collaborative improvement efforts.	Recommendation 2: Expand opportunities for nurses to lead and diffuse collaborative improvement efforts. Private and public funders, healthcare organizations, nursing education programs, and nursing associations should expand opportunities for nurses to lead and manage collaborative efforts with physicians and other members of the healthcare team to conduct research and to redesign and improve practice environments and health systems. These entities should also provide opportunities for nurses to diffuse successful practices. To this end: • The Center for Medicare and Medicaid Innovation should support the development and evaluation of models of payment and care delivery that use nurses in an expanded leadership capacity to improve health outcomes and reduce costs. Performance measures should be developed and implemented expeditiously where best practices are evident to reflect the contributions of nurses and ensure better-quality care. • Private and public funders should collaborate, and when possible pool funds, to advance research on models of care and innovative solutions, that will enable nurses to contribute to improved health and healthcare. • Healthcare organizations should support and help nurses in taking the lead in developing and adopting innovative, patient-centered care models. • Healthcare organizations should engage nurses and other front-line staff to work with developers and manufacturers in the design, development, purchase, implementation, and evaluation of medical and health devices and health information technology products. • Nursing education programs and nursing associations should provide entrepreneurial professional development that will enable nurses to initiate programs and businesses that will contribute to improved health and healthcare.

| 3. Implement nurse residency programs. | The following actions should be taken to implement and support nurse residency programs:
• State boards of nursing, in collaboration with accrediting bodies such as the Joint Commission and the Community Health Accreditation Program, should support nurses' completion of a residency program after they have completed a prelicensure or advanced practice degree program or when they are transitioning into new clinical practice areas.
• The Secretary of Health and Human Services should redirect all graduate medical education funding from diploma nursing programs to support the implementation of nurse residency programs in rural and critical access areas.
• Healthcare organizations, the Health Resources and Services Administration and Centers for Medicare & Medicaid Services, and philanthropic organizations should fund the development and implementation of nurse residency programs across all practice settings.
• Healthcare organizations that offer nurse residency programs and foundations should evaluate the effectiveness of the residency programs in improving the retention of nurses, expanding competencies, and improving patient outcomes |
| 4. Increase the proportion of nurses with a baccalaureate degree to 80% by 2020. | Academic nurse leaders across all schools of nursing should work together to increase the proportion of nurses with a baccalaureate degree from 50% to ~80% by 2020. These leaders should partner with education accrediting bodies, private and public funders, and employers to ensure funding, monitor progress, and increase the diversity of students to create a workforce prepared to meet the demands of diverse populations across the lifespan.
• The Commission on Collegiate Nursing Education, working in collaboration with the National League for Nursing Accrediting Commission, should require all nursing schools to offer defined academic pathways, beyond articulation agreements, that promote seamless access for nurses to higher levels of education.
• Healthcare organizations should encourage nurses with associate's and diploma degrees to enter baccalaureate nursing programs within 5 years of graduation by offering tuition reimbursement, creating a culture that fosters continuing education, and providing a salary differential and promotion.
• Private and public funders should collaborate, and when possible pool funds, to expand baccalaureate programs to enroll more students by offering scholarships and loan forgiveness, hiring more faculty, expanding clinical instruction through new clinical partnerships, and using technology to augment instruction. These efforts should take into consideration strategies to increase the diversity of the nursing workforce in terms of race/ethnicity, gender, and geographic distribution.
• The U.S. Secretary of Education, other federal agencies, including the Health Resources and Services Administration, and state and private funders should expand loans and grants for second-degree nursing students.
• Schools of nursing, in collaboration with other health professional schools, should design and implement early and continuous interprofessional collaboration through joint classroom and clinical training opportunities.
• Academic nurse leaders should partner with healthcare organizations, leaders from primary and secondary school systems, and other community organizations to recruit and advance diverse nursing students |

Continued

TABLE 1.2 ■ Key Recommendations From the Future of Nursing: Leading Change, Advancing Health Report—cont'd

Original Recommendations and Scope	Assessing Progress Report
	Indicator: 　Percentage of employed nurses with a baccalaureate degree in nursing or higher degree Supplemental indicators: 　● New RN graduates by degree type, by race/ethnicity 　● New RN graduates by degree type, by gender 　● Number and percent of U.S.-educated, first-time NCLEX-takers with a BSN 　● Percent of hospitals that have new RN graduate residencies 　● Percentage of hospital employers that offer RNs tuition reimbursement 　● Number of RN-to-BSN graduates annually
5. Double the number of nurses with a doctorate by 2020.	Schools of nursing, with support from private and public funders, academic administrators and university trustees, and accrediting bodies, should double the number of nurses with a doctorate by 2020 to add to the cadre of nurse faculty and researchers, with attention to increasing diversity. 　● The Commission on Collegiate Nursing Education and the National League for Nursing Accrediting Commission should monitor the progress of each accredited nursing school to ensure that at least 10% of all baccalaureate graduates matriculate into a master's or doctoral program within 5 years of graduation. 　● Private and public funders, including the Health Resources and Services Administration and the Department of Labor, should expand funding for programs offering accelerated graduate degrees for nurses to increase the production of master's and doctoral nurse graduates and to increase the diversity of nurse faculty and researchers. 　● Academic administrators and university trustees should create salary and benefit packages that are market competitive to recruit and retain highly qualified academic and clinical nurse faculty. Indicator: 　Total enrollment in nursing doctorate programs Supplemental indicators: 　● Number of employed nurses with a doctoral degree 　● Number of people receiving nursing doctoral degrees annually 　● Diversity of nursing doctorate graduates by race/ethnicity 　● Diversity of nursing doctorate graduates by gender

6. Ensure that nurses engage in lifelong learning.	Accrediting bodies, schools of nursing, healthcare organizations, and continuing competency educators from multiple health professions should collaborate to ensure that nurses and nursing students and faculty continue their education and engage in lifelong learning to gain the competencies needed to provide care for diverse populations across the lifespan. • Faculty should partner with healthcare organizations to develop and prioritize competencies so curricula can be updated regularly to ensure that graduates at all levels are prepared to meet the current and future health needs of the population. • The Commission on Collegiate Nursing Education and the National League for Nursing Accrediting Commission should require that all nursing students demonstrate a comprehensive set of clinical performance competencies that encompass the knowledge and skills needed to provide care across settings and the lifespan. • Academic administrators should require all faculty to participate in continuing professional development and to perform with cutting-edge competence in practice, teaching, and research. • All healthcare organizations and schools of nursing should foster a culture of lifelong learning and provide resources for interprofessional continuing competency programs. • Healthcare organizations and other organizations that offer continuing competency programs should regularly evaluate their programs for adaptability, flexibility, accessibility, and impact on clinical outcomes and update the programs accordingly.
7. Prepare and enable nurses to lead change to advance health	Nurses, nursing education programs, and nursing associations should prepare the nursing workforce to assume leadership positions across all levels, while public, private, and governmental healthcare decision-makers should ensure that leadership positions are available to and filled by nurses. • Nurses should take responsibility for their personal and professional growth by continuing their education and seeking opportunities to develop and exercise their leadership skills. • Nursing associations should provide leadership development, mentoring programs, and opportunities to lead for all their members. • Nursing education programs should integrate leadership theory and business practices across the curriculum, including clinical practice. • Public, private, and governmental healthcare decision-makers should include representation from nursing on boards, on executive management teams, and in other key leadership positions.

Continued

TABLE 1.2 ■ Key Recommendations From the Future of Nursing: Leading Change, Advancing Health Repor—cont'd

Original Recommendations and Scope	Assessing Progress Report
8. Build an infrastructure for the collection and analysis of interprofessional healthcare workforce data.	Build an infrastructure for the collection and analysis of interprofessional healthcare workforce data. The National Health Care Workforce Commission, with oversight from the Government Accountability Office and the Health Resources and Services Administration, should lead a collaborative effort to improve research and the collection and analysis of data on healthcare workforce requirements. The Workforce Commission and the Health Resources and Services Administration should collaborate with state licensing boards, state nursing workforce centers, and the Department of Labor in this effort to ensure that the data are timely and publicly accessible.
	• The Workforce Commission and the Health Resources and Services Administration should coordinate with state licensing boards, including those for nursing, medicine, dentistry, and pharmacy, to develop and promulgate a standardized minimum data set across states and professions that can be used to assess healthcare workforce needs by demographics, numbers, skill mix, and geographic distribution.
	• The Workforce Commission and the Health Resources and Services Administration should set standards for the collection of the minimum data set by state licensing boards; oversee, coordinate, and house the data; and make the data publicly accessible.
	• The Workforce Commission and the Health Resources and Services Administration should retain, but bolster, the Health Resources and Services Administration's registered nurse sample survey by increasing the sample size, fielding the survey every other year, expanding the data collected on advanced practice registered nurses, and releasing survey results more quickly.
	• The Workforce Commission and the Health Resources and Services Administration should establish a monitoring system that uses the most current analytic approaches and data from the minimum data set to systematically measure and project nursing workforce requirements by role, skill mix, region, and demographics.
	• The Workforce Commission and the Health Resources and Services Administration should coordinate workforce research efforts with the Department of Labor, state and regional educators, employers, and state nursing workforce centers to identify regional healthcare workforce needs and establish regional targets and plans for appropriately increasing the supply of health professionals.
	• The Government Accountability Office should ensure that the Workforce Commission membership includes adequate nursing expertise.

DOUBLE THE NUMBER OF DOCTORAL PREPARED NURSES

Within the RWJ/IOM report, recommendation #4 calls for our discipline to *promote nurses' pursuit of doctoral degrees to double the number of doctoral prepared nurses by 2020*. This closely aligns with recommendation #2, which calls for *nursing to Increase Baccalaureate Nurses' numbers to 80% of the workforce by 2020*. Although the discipline will be unable to increase the number of doctorally prepared nurses without increasing the number of entry-to-practice nurses, the purpose of this text is to address the former, and we will address the latter in other forums. Fig. 1.1 illustrates the interconnectivity of RWJ/IOM objectives as well as concerns and consequences related to the current nursing shortage.

Good News Ahead: Earning a doctoral degree in nursing expands your career options and influence. This education activates your potential and increases your impact on health. It helps level the playing field by providing you with tools on par with colleagues in other disciplines who increasingly enter practice with doctoral degrees. Doctorally prepared nurses bring powerful skills, understanding, and experience to the healthcare workforce, improving patient and population outcomes. These same skills will be useful and help you navigate an increasingly complex healthcare system (Rhoades, 2011).

Today, doctoral nurses are doing the extraordinary. They lead science, practice, education, and theory development in ways never imagined even 40 years ago. It is a wonderful time to consider your doctoral journey because of the many career opportunities and educational opportunities open to you.

DNP programs have increased to over 400, with enrollments reaching 36,069 in 2019. DNP-prepared nurses have increased by 800% since ACA was enacted in 2010. At the same time, the number of PhD programs has increased to 135, with enrollments reaching 5290 in 2021, which is a 15% increase over 5 years (AACN, 2021). Yet, the Campaign for Action Resource estimates nursing has only achieved a 20% cumulative increase in doctorally prepared nurses between 2015 and 2021, which falls far short of the goal of doubling the number of doctoral prepared nurses. As a result, nurses with terminal degrees increased from 1.1% to 1.3% (https://www.doctorsofnursingpractice.org/dnp-survey-results/, September 2021). Although these data document significant progress, they also spotlight continued demand and a great need to redouble efforts in this area.

Let us consider the number of doctorally prepared nurses first. The numbers reported above reveal that we have made progress and that there is still much to achieve. As you approach your decision, keep in mind that the call to double the number of nurses with a doctorate by 2020 does not prefer one doctorate over the other. It advocates for a better-educated nursing workforce overall that will tackle the challenges in healthcare on the near and far horizon. We intend to help you make informed decisions that advantage you in relation to your career goals and position you to meet the needs of individuals, families, and communities in your care (https://campaignforaction.org/resource/number-people-receiving-nursing-doctoral-degrees-annually/).

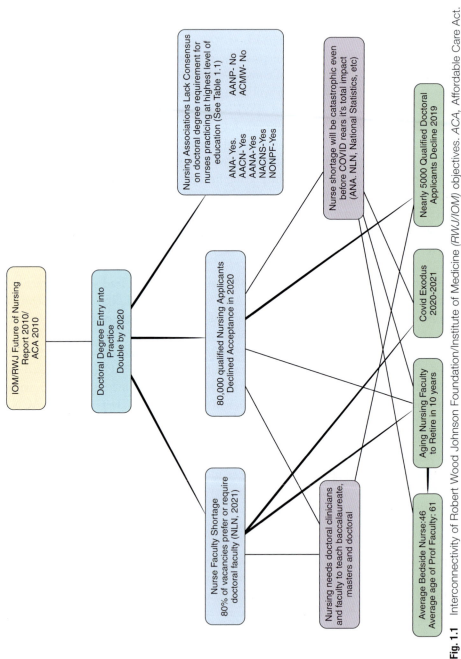

Fig. 1.1 Interconnectivity of Robert Wood Johnson Foundation/Institute of Medicine (RWJ/IOM) objectives. ACA, Affordable Care Act.

Let us also consider our diversity. We have made progress toward expanding the diversity of our doctorally prepared nursing workforce, and still we have far to go. The number of PhD nursing students from underrepresented groups has increased by 56%, from 1141 in 2009 to 1781 in 2019 (AACN, 2020). The *Future of Nursing Report* charges today's nurse leaders to press on and design avenues to expand the doctorally prepared nursing workforce in both number and diversity. The challenge is to achieve meaningful inclusivity in academia and in practice. This requires attention to structures and processes. It requires making diversity in the faculty a priority and ensuring mentors can guide and support all students to inclusion, belonging, success, and impact (Institute of Medicine, 2019).

Throughout this text, the authors will introduce you to nurse leaders, educators, clinicians, and researchers who have in the past or are now marching the profession toward greater diversity, equity, inclusivity, and excellence. Our goal is to capture your interest, remove barriers to your advancement, and promote your success.

Turning to Our Professional Associations for Leadership and Direction

As the largest segment of the professional healthcare workforce, nurses' contribution to care is witnessed (archived?) through our professional associations. These same entities offer guidance and support as you return to school. They provide a strong and clear voice for nursing as we transform the care paradigm moving through the 21st century. Both nationally and internationally, these organizations assert that a capable and nimble workforce, doctorally educated, will be key to achieving the potential of science and navigating the challenges ahead.

Professional nursing organizations are dedicated to advancing the progress of our discipline, promoting our nation's health, leading collaboration and innovation, and transforming care. They carry the voice of nursing to inform and improve policy on the local, state, national, and international levels. For 130 years, professional national and international associations have informed and empowered nurses and helped us keep abreast of best practices, research, and innovation (Box 1.1).

BOX 1.1 ■ Chronology of Major Nursing Organizations

- National League for Nursing (est. 1893)
- The American Nurses Association (est.1896)
- American Association of Nurse Anesthesia (est.1931)
- American College of Nurse-Midwives (est. 1962)
- American Association of Colleges in Nursing (est. 1969)
- American Association of Nurse Practitioners (est. 1970)
- National Organization of Nurse Practitioner Faculty (est.1980)
- National Association of Clinical Nurse Specialists (est. 1995)

Nursing associations are organizations devoted to the professional and personal development of members and the general advancement of the profession. Joining a professional nursing association is essential due to the ever-changing field of nursing. https://nurse.org/articles/benefits-of-nursing-organizations/

Each prominent nursing association has issued a position statement regarding *The Future of Nursing Report*, the call for nurses to practice at the top of their license and for more nurses to practice at the highest level of education: the doctoral degree. Six of the eight professional organizations have called for doctoral-level preparation for nurses in education, leadership, and advanced practice by 2030, if not sooner. These position statements are presented in Table 1.3.

Taking the Doctoral Challenge: Your Turn!

Assuredly, pursuing doctoral education will be a challenge. Rising to challenges is at the heart of nursing, and it is essential to providing quality healthcare for all. Recently policies have been promulgated and resources dedicated to helping nurses who choose to pursue their terminal degree and become tomorrow's nursing leaders. Leaders across many nursing organizations, institutions of higher education, and leadership think-tanks are building, shaping, and executing policies that will support your doctoral education journey. These policies will help mitigate the impact of common critical impediments nurses have faced for nearly 75 years of pursuing doctorates.

RESETTING GRADUATE-DOCTORAL EDUCATION TIMELINES

As a whole, the nursing workforce is aging, approaching retirement, and leaving significant vacancies in practice and academia. The average age of academic professors is in the late 50s to early 60s, and data project that one-third will retire within the next 5 years (2021, October 22; Scott, NPR). The forecasted need for nurses with doctorates to fill these faculty positions is sobering and will be compounded by persistent capacity issues in the educational programs that prepare them (Berlin and Sechrist, 2002; Melnyk et al., 2010; NCSBN, 2015). Let's consider the data for each doctorate separately.

RESEARCH DOCTORATES: THE DOCTOR OF PHILOSOPHY

The 1% of nurses prepared with research doctorates is approaching retirement quickly. The average age at which nurses earn their PhD today in the US is 46, which is fully 13 years later than PhD earners in other fields (Campaign for Action, 2019). CCNE and NLNAC encourage monitoring graduate progression into master's or doctoral programs within 5 years of graduation for all accredited

Text continued on page 20

TABLE 1.3 ■ **Statements of Nursing Organizations on Pursuit of the Doctoral Degree**

Year Established # Members	Mission, Vision, Values	Position Statement on Terminal Degrees in Nursing
American Nurses Association—ANA ***https://www.nursingworld.org/ana/*** 1896—Nurses Associated Alumnae 1911—American Nurses Association *Represents the interests of nearly 4 million nurses*	The ANA is a professional organization that represents registered nurses (RNs) across the United States through its 54 constituent member associations Three subsidiary organizations: (1) **American Academy of Nursing** serves the public and nursing profession by advancing health policy and practice through the generation, synthesis, and dissemination of nursing knowledge. (2) **American Nurses Foundation** is the charitable and philanthropic arm of the ANA (3) **American Nurses Credentialing Center** supports excellence in practice by credentialing nurses in their specialty and credentialing facilities that exhibit nursing excellence (https://en.wikipedia.org/wiki/American_Nurses_Association#cite_note-17).	Practice Doctorate ANA supports the Doctor of Nursing Practice as a terminal practice-focused degree in nursing offered to educate RNs in advanced levels of clinical judgment, systems thinking, and leadership to the profession of nursing. The Doctor of Nursing Practice graduate provides leadership, mentorship, and support to colleagues to improve patient outcomes and achieve excellence in nursing practice. (2011 Position Statement) The EdD is considered a terminal practice degree designed for those desiring to be experts and lead change in nursing education as they seek preparation for faculty and/or educator roles. The role of the EdD is to lead change in nursing education. Research Doctorate ANA supports the PhD as the terminal degree for nurse scientists. Position Statements: https://www.nursingworld.org/practice-policy/nursing-excellence/official-position-statements

Continued

TABLE 1.3 ■ Statements of Nursing Organizations on Pursuit of the Doctoral Degree—cont'd

Year Established # Members	Mission, Vision, Values	Position Statement on Terminal Degrees in Nursing
American Association of Colleges in Nursing—AACN acnnursing.org/		
1969 *825 member schools*	Vision: Nurses are transforming healthcare and improving health. Mission: As the collective voice for academic nursing, AACN serves as the catalyst for excellence and innovation in nursing education, research, and practice (AACN, 2006a; AACN, 2006b). Values: Leadership, innovation, diversity and inclusion, and integrity.	Practice Doctorate In 2004, AACN adopted the position that all advanced practice nurses, including nurse anesthetists, earn a DNP. As part of its initiative, AACN developed a document containing "essential" elements of a DNP curriculum and influenced programs offering a Nursing Doctor (ND) to transition to providing DNP education. Research Doctorate
National League for Nursing—NLN http://www.nln.org/		
1893—American Society of Superintendents of Training Schools of Nurses. *40,000 individual members & 1,200 institutional member*	The NLN promotes excellence in nursing education to build a strong and diverse nursing workforce to advance the health of our nation and the global community. Premier organization for nurse faculty and leaders in nursing education.	Set goal to double the number of faculty with doctoral preparation in nursing education by 2020. (NLN The Vision Series, 2013, 2017) Supports the inclusion of formal academic preparation for the nurse educator and/or faculty role in doctoral program curricula. Seeks to maximize program capacity by establishing partnerships or consortia between schools of nursing with doctoral programs offering nurse educator preparation courses and/or faculty role preparation courses, and those lacking such programs. Seeks to facilitate doctoral student progression with effective curriculum sequencing and support (e.g., learning activities designed to contribute to the final scholarly product; structured faculty and peer mentoring; use of student cohorts; flexible pre-requisite requirements).

Continued

American Association of Nurse Practitioners—AANP
https://www.aanp.org/

2013
Over 119,000 members

AANP represents the interests of nurse practitioners licensed to practice nursing, not medicine, in the U.S. Continually advocates at local, state, and federal levels for the recognition of nurse practitioners as providers of high-quality, cost-effective, and midlevel personalized healthcare.

Nurse Practitioner DNP Education, Certification and Titling Statement 2008.

Evidence is inconclusive that the DNP degree directly influences care quality or that it is contributing to improved quality indicators and patient outcomes. It is expensive to seek doctoral education. No requirement for DNP as APRN entry into practice degree has been set.

Advocates that the evolution of master's programs to practice doctoral programs can add strength to both academic programs and nurse practitioner (NP) practice as well as increase recognition for NPs in the healthcare arena.

Development of DNP programs must be conducted in a manner that allows for a smooth transition and supports further development of DNP NP educational programs in the future.

National Organization of Nurse Practitioner Faculties—NONPF
https://www.nonpf.org/

1980
As of 2021, 90% of all US NP programs participate

Mission: to be the leader in quality nurse practitioner education.

Vision: to be the preeminent global leader in providing timely and critical resources for NP educators. We advance innovative models that support NP educational programs to meet the highest quality standards. We unite and lead NP educators in transforming healthcare.

Committed in 2018 to move all entry-level NP education to the DNP degree by 2025.

Has led more than 300 DNP programs throughout the United States (US) to transition NP educational preparation to the DNP degree (NONPF, 2015).

Maintains dedication to all currently credentialed NPs and faculty members while recognizing that the healthcare delivery system has grown increasingly complex and the role of NPs has evolved. The DNP reflects the rigorous education that NPs receive to lead and deliver quality healthcare.

TABLE 1.3 ■ Statements of Nursing Organizations on Pursuit of the Doctoral Degree—cont'd

Year Established # Members	Mission, Vision, Values	Position Statement on Terminal Degrees in Nursing
National Association of Clinical Nurse Specialties—NACNS https://nacns.org/		
1995 *1,600 members*	Mission: to advance the unique expertise and value the clinical nurse specialist contributes to healthcare. Goals: to • Increase awareness of the value and differentiated skills of the CNS • Enable excellence in the CNS profession by providing high-quality educational resources and programs and fostering the creation of CNS curricula in nursing programs nationwide • Position CNS' to practice at the top of their scope of practice	The NACNS Board a 15-year transition to the DNP as entry level for the CNS believing that this timeline enables schools, universities, and individuals to plan for implementation of the DNP as entry level for CNS practice. Individuals currently in practice with a master's degree as a clinical nurse specialist should be considered eligible to practice as long as they comply with the regulatory requirements of their state. NACNS strongly supports grandfathering for these individuals when the 2030 implementation date is reached. The NACNS Board believes that no individual should be disenfranchised by this change to DNP as entry level for CNS practice in 2030. The NACNS Board differentiates between the DNP as a terminal degree for practice and the PhD a terminal degree that is focused on nursing research. The nursing profession needs nurses prepared with both types of degrees with their respective different skill sets and encourages CNSs to critically identify which professional track is most interesting to them. The CNS DNP student should be prepared to meet the requirements for certification in a population and then seek certification within their specialty if available.

American College of Nurse Midwives—ACNM
https://www.midwife.org

1962—Certified Nurse Midwives CNMS

1994—Certified Midwives

6,500 Members

Vision: Midwifery for every community.
Mission: to support midwives, advance the practice of midwifery, and achieve optimal, equitable health outcomes for the people and communities midwives serve through inclusion, advocacy, education, leadership development, and research.

The value of graduate degree preparation in midwifery, nursing, public health, and other related fields is widely recognized. However, the Doctor of Nursing Practice (DNP) degree will not be a requirement for entry to practice for CNMs or CMs.[1]

American Association of Nurse Anesthesia—AANA
Council on Accreditation of Nurse Anesthesia Educational Programs (COA)
https://www.aana.com/about-us/who-we-are

AANA—1931; 59,000 members
COA—1998

Vision: the transformative leader driving innovation and patient-centered excellence in anesthesia and healthcare (Hawkins & Nezat, 2009).
Mission: to advance patient safety and our profession through excellence in practice and service to members.

In 2007, the chartered Task Force on Doctoral Preparation of Nurse Anesthetists (DTF) and the Board of Directors moved forward unanimously with the adoption of the position for supporting doctoral education for entry into nurse anesthesia practice by 2025. The DTF report, including the AANA position statement, is available on the AANA website at www.aana.com.

baccalaureate nursing programs. This will help evaluate the impact of efforts to streamline education progression and strengthen current accreditation standards to support the goals of *The Future of Nursing goals Report*. So let us look at who is looking at the research doctorate.

The AACN Task Force on the Research-Focused Doctorate in Nursing (2020) identifies strategies to increase the number of research doctorates (PhD) by facilitating earlier entry to PhD programs, increasing retention and graduation, and promoting student success. The Report outlines what must be done to increase the number of nurse scientists correct the historical trend and lead nurses to pursue doctoral education so much earlier in their careers. This would increase the years during which nurses can contribute at the highest level and achieve the most significant impact. The Task Force report is available online: https://www. aacnnursing.org/News-Information/Position-Statements-White-Papers/ Nursing-Research.

The Future of Nursing: Campaign for Action 2010, which is a joint statement taken by The American Association of Retired Persons (AARP) and Robert Wood Johnson RWJ, emphasizes the vital importance of creating an exceptionally diverse cadre of nurses who have earned research doctorates. This younger and more diverse group will serve as faculty and accelerate the capacity of our discipline to educate PhD-prepared nurses earlier in their careers, and provide the education, opportunity, support, experiences, and mentorship necessary to accomplish this goal. The Report offers the following suggestions to achieve the goal of preparing a highly educated nursing workforce:

- Identify those nurses who have a proclivity to research.
- Create strong peer connections and real mentorship experiences.
- Create opportunities for early exposure to research and develop a curriculum that reflects modernization in science.
- Develop consortia between academic institutions to support the science. Create a culture of accountability in which all parties shape nursing science and the research brand.
- Consider purposeful recruitment strategies. Maximize external partners (e.g., industry, community) to demonstrate the impact of nursing science (National Academy of Science, 2021).

PRACTICE DOCTORATES: THE DOCTOR OF NURSING PRACTICE

Higher levels of nursing education are associated with better patient outcomes (Aiken et al., 2003, 2009, 2014; McHugh et al., 2020). Other health disciplines, including Medicine (MD), Dentistry (DDS), Pharmacy (PharmD), Psychology (PsyD), Physical Therapy (DPT), and Audiology (AudD), have all come to the same conclusion and all offer practice doctorates. This evidence led to the development of the DNP.

Today nursing programs graduate five DNPs for every one PhD (McCauley et al., 2020). This trend may speak as much to the popularity of the degree as to the attention paid by DNP programs to offering a pedagogy and program structure that is responsive to the needs of learners. Interestingly, DNPs have added to the ranks of faculties even more than they have increased the number of clinicians (McCauley et al., 2020). This trend may speak to the age and career stage of early adopters, the availability of funding for those who would join faculties, or the fact that expert clinicians make inspiring teachers.

Now that entry to DNP programs is being encouraged for younger nurses, and now that more programs are designing pedagogies to meet the needs of less experienced learners, more DNP graduates are being counted as APRNs, are penetrating the workforce providing direct care, and are preparing to test the impact of the original design of the DNP, which was to bring greater knowledge, skill, and evidence to direct care for populations in need.

A predominant number of faculty positions prefer a doctoral degree with the PhD best suited to the research mission and the DNP particularly valuable for the teaching mission.

FINANCIAL CONSIDERATIONS

Earning a doctoral degree is expensive, and you will not be alone in seeking financial support. It is important to have your career goals in mind as you approach the decision to return to school. Take time to reflect on your personal mission and career aspirations. Do you intend to conduct research? Provide direct care? Lead nursing practice? Teach nurses for the future? Your answer to these questions and prioritization of these different contributions will point the way to both the degree you choose and the funding available to you.

For those who prioritize practice, three funding options are available. First, many DNP students continue to work in clinical practice and use employer-sponsored tuition benefits, which are offered as a retention strategy to pay for their education. This approach can enable the new DNP to graduate with minimal debt and valuable clinical experience. Second, gifts from alumni and generous friends of nursing programs and universities may be available to you. Third, as a practicing nurse, there may be scholarship funds available from your specialty organization, your local or state government, or any organization that advances the health of the population you serve (American Heart Association, March of Dimes, Alzheimer's Association, and many more). Although these pools of funds are likely to be modest, they certainly should be explored and tapped if your goals and those of the organization align. It is always important to ask what kinds of funding options exist in the program you are considering.

For those who prioritize research, funds may be available in the form of gifts from alumni and generous friends of nursing programs and universities. Research assistant (RA) positions, teaching assistant (TA) positions, NIH-funded opportunities, and other extramural funding may be available to support your education. Funding from specialty organizations and health-related interest groups may also be available. Again, it is always important to ask about funding support in any program you consider. ■

For those who prioritize education, funds may be available in the form of gifts from alumni and generous friends of nursing programs and universities. TA positions and other extramural funding may be available to support your education.

Regardless of the terminal degree you seek, Nurse Faculty Loan Program funding may also be available. This program targets preparing faculty to teach in nursing programs and enables the doctoral student to incur debt across the program of study, which is canceled by years of teaching 1 year of service for one year of the loan. Once again, it is always important to ask about funding support in any program you are considering.

Data from 2018 reveal that 44% of all graduate and doctoral students receive financial assistance (Douglas-Gabriel, 2018). The American Hospital Association is offering scholarships, loan repayment, increasing wages compensation, and designing recruitment strategies to retain the loyal and skilled nurse workforce (Van den Heede et al, 2013). Health Resources Service Administration Division of Nursing is a larger driver of federal funding encouraging baccalaureate and doctoral nursing. Other national policies and financial programs are answering the call for economic reform regarding providing monetary support to adequately move the nursing workforce toward their highest level of practice. Nurses especially report finding it difficult to pay for a doctoral degree.

Private and public sources offer a wide array of funding support that promises to increase the number of master's or doctoral nurse graduates and do so in ways that promote diversity among students, faculty, and researchers (IOM, 2011). A summary of select federal and private resources to support the attainment of your terminal degrees for nurses is presented in Table 1.4.

Questions Remain

The purpose of this chapter is to make a case for the need for more doctorally prepared nurses using position statements and policies from the public and private sector,

TABLE 1.4 ■ **Federal and Private Resources for Nurses Seeking Terminal Degrees**

Organizations	Doctoral Education Supportive Action
The American Hospital Association www.aha.org	Institutions are offering scholarships, loan repayment, increasing wages compensation, and designing recruitment strategies to retain the loyal and skilled nurse workforce they currently have and attract the newest members of the nursing workforce.

TABLE 1.4 ■ **Federal and Private Resources for Nurses Seeking Terminal Degrees—cont'd**

Organizations	Doctoral Education Supportive Action
Title VIII Programs **Health Resources Service Administration Division of Nursing (HRSA)** hrsa.gov	Mitigate the financial barriers for nurses to pursue graduate studies and careers in nursing. A significant source of federal funding encouraging more students to seek baccalaureate degrees
American Association of Retired Persons (AARP) and Robert Wood Johnson RWJ: *The Future of Nursing: Campaign for Action 2010* https://campaignforaction.org/resources/future-of-nursing-2030-action-hub/	This partnership is dedicated to emphasizing the power of transdisciplinary research, clinical, and educational teams to effectively shape the interprofessional care delivery culture. Driven to create a large and diverse cadre of PhD-prepared nurses; to develop a model that supports a 3-year PhD program and shift the paradigm in PhD education while expanding mentorship and resources.
Jonas Center for Nursing and Veterans Healthcare and The Rita & Alex Hillman Foundation https://jonasphilanthropies.org/nursing-and-veterans-healthcare/	Spearheading programs to fund nurse-led approaches to transforming the cost and delivery of care. Encouraging nurses to pursue a doctorate earlier in their career and increasing the number of nurses with research-focused PhDs in nursing.
The Interdisciplinary Nursing Quality Research Initiative (INQRI) https://www.rwjf.org/en/library/research/2013/04/the-interdisciplinary-nursing-quality-research-initiative.html	Est. 2005—research conducted by interdisciplinary teams that address gaps in knowledge relating to nursing and healthcare delivery and care quality, efficiency, and cost-effectiveness
American Association of Colleges in Nursing *Task Force on the Research-Focused Doctorate in Nursing* (2020)	Identifies strategies to increase the number of research doctorates (PhD) by facilitating earlier entry to PhD programs, increasing retention and graduation, and promoting student success.
Nurse Faculty Loan Repayment Program (NFLP) An HRSA resource: https://www.hrsa.gov/grants/find-funding/hrsa-20-004	This 1-year funding opportunity aims to increase the number of qualified nursing faculty. We seek to accomplish this by providing funding to accredited schools of nursing to offer loans to students enrolled in advanced education nursing degree programs who are committed to becoming nurse faculty. In exchange for full-time post-graduation employment as nurse faculty, the program authorizes the cancelation of up to 85% of any such loan (plus interest thereon).
American Nurses Association (ANA): https://www.nursingworld.org/	ANA and its educational partners with colleges and universities across the country. The Tuition Discount Program gives ANA members access to a variety of educational programs across the country. These programs help nurses enhance their knowledge and advance their careers.

professional organizations, and government entities. Still, it is true that progress is not tidy, and action suspended until irrefutable proof is available can devolve into no action at all. This is certainly true for the profession of nursing and progress in nursing education.

The DNP was implemented as a work in progress. It grows stronger as graduates enter the workplace and the community fully describes what it needs. It grows stronger as outcomes data become available and the prospective students vote with their choices and tuition dollars. It grows stronger as criticism and praise drive rapid cycles of improvement.

The PhD is the most familiar doctoral degree. It grows stronger as it challenges long-standing practices and observes the kinds of pedagogies being rolled out across higher education. It grows stronger as it embraces team science and innovation. It grows stronger as it emphasizes its fidelity to the demands of science and the needs of the communities its discoveries serve.

Some may argue that the evidence relating the level of educational preparation to higher-quality care and improved patient outcomes, although intuitively appealing, remains inconclusive (AANP, 2020). Others strongly disagree (Aiken et al., 2003, 2009, 2014; McHugh et al., 2020). Because many who earn doctorates in any profession go on to teach, and because nursing salaries, especially for those in service-side leadership positions, are attractive, many ask, *"Why earn a doctorate only to earn less as a faculty member than nurses can earn as APRNs or bedside nurses?"* (Noguchi, 2021; Deitrow & Yoguchi, 2021; Farmer, 2021). The answer to this question will clarify your personal mission and professional goals. The decision rather than the conclusion about the benefit of investing your time and resources in doctoral education lies with you, and the drive to move ahead will be personal. We hope we have helped point out the many factors to consider as you make your choice.

Summary

Rapid advancements in science, nursing practice, healthcare, and education are creating an urgent need for nurse scientists, clinicians, leaders, and educators prepared at the highest level of education. The world needs you to develop your clinical reasoning, refine your skills, raise your expectations, and expand your potential to deliver more effective evidence-based care, achieve optimal health, maximize effectiveness, generate much needed science, and create exceptional quality.

The future of healthcare calls for nurses to be agile, nimble, and responsive. Stepping up to the challenge of being a nurse leader will be attended by high expectations for creativity, forward-thinking, and boldness tempered by reason and discipline. Earning a doctorate will equip you for these challenges. As a doctorally prepared nurse, you will qualify for positions of influence in our profession and in the larger healthcare and social arena. You and the network and skills you build will find solutions yet to be conceived. You are much needed.

The workforce of tomorrow is YOU!

Bibliography

Aiken LH, Cheung RB, Olds DM. Education policy initiatives to address the nurse shortage in the United States. *Health Affairs*. 2009;28(4):w646-w656. doi:10.1377.hlthaff.28.4.w646.

Aiken LH, Clarke SP, Cheung RB, et al. Educational levels of hospital nurses and surgical patient mortality. *JAMA*. 2003;290(12):1617-1623. doi:10.1001/jama.290.12.1617.

Aiken LH, Sloane DM, Bruyneel L, et al. Nurse staffing and education and hospital mortality in nine European countries: a retrospective observational study. *Lancet*. 2014;383(9931):1824-1830. doi:10.1016/S0140-6736(13)62631-8.

American Association of Colleges of Nursing. *DNP essentials*. 2006a. https://www.aacnnursing.org/DNP/DNP-Essentials.

American Association of Colleges of Nursing. *The Essentials of Doctoral Education for Advanced Practice Nurses*. 2006. https://www.aacnnursing.org/DNP/DNP-Essentials#

American Association of Colleges of Nursing. *The PhD Pathway in Nursing: Sustaining the Science*. August 22, 2018. Available at: https://www.aacnnursing.org/Portals/42/news/surveys-data/PhD-Pathway.pdf.

American Association of Colleges of Nursing. *Fact Sheet: Nursing Shortage*. 2020. Available at: https://www.aacnnursing.org/Portals/42/News/Factsheets/Nursing-Shortage-Factsheet.pdf.

American Association of Colleges of Nursing. *Student Enrollment Surged in U.S. Schools of Nursing in 2020 Despite Challenges Presented by the Pandemic*. 2021. Available at: https://www.aacnnursing.org/NewsInformation/Press-Releases/View/ArticleId/24802/2020-survey-data-student-enrollment%20%20%20%20%20.

American Association of Nurse Practitioners. *Discussion Paper: Doctor of Nursing Practice*. (2005, Revised 2008, 2010, 2013). Available at: https://storage.aanp.org/www/documents/advocacy/position-papers/DoctorOfNursingPracitice.pdf.

Berlin LE, Sechrist KR The shortage of doctoral prepared nursing faculty: a dire situation. *Nurs Outlook*. 2002;50:50–56. doi:10.1067/mno.2002.124270.

Cathro H. Pursuing graduate studies in nursing education: driving and restraining forces. *Online J Issues Nurs*. 2011;16(3):7. doi:10.3912/OJIN.Vol16No03PPT02.

Detrow S, Noguchi Y. *Just When More Nurses Are Needed, It's More Difficult to Get into Nursing School*. NPR; 2021. Available at: https://www.npr.org/2021/10/22/1048289060/just-when-more-nurses-are-needed-its-more-difficult-to-get-into-nursing-school.

Douglas-Gabriel D. *Use of financial aid continues to grow, though fewer students are borrowing for college*. 2018. Available at: https://www.washingtonpost.com/news/grade-point/wp/2018/01/30/use-of-financial-aid-continues-to-grow-though-fewer-students-are-borrowing-for-college/.

Drennan VM, Ross F. Global nurse shortages-the facts, the impact and action for change. *Br Med Bull*. 2019;130(1):25-37. doi:10.1093/bmb/ldz014.

Farmer B. *Worn-Out Nurses Hit the Road for Better Pay Stressing Hospital Budgets—and Morale*. NPR, Health News from NPR; 2021. Available at: https://www.npr.org/sections/health-shots/2021/10/20/1046131313/worn-out-nurses-hit-the-road-for-better-pay-stressing-hospital-budgets-and-moral.

Hawkins R, Nezat G. *Doctoral Education: Which Degree to Pursue?* Education News; 2009. Available at: https://www.aana.com/docs/default-source/aana-journal-web-documents-1/educnews_0409_p92-96.pdf?sfvrsn=e24c5ab1_6.

Institute of Medicine (US) Committee on the Robert Wood Johnson Foundation Initiative on the Future of Nursing, at the Institute of Medicine. *The Future of Nursing: Leading Change, Advancing Health*. Washington, DC: National Academies Press; 2011. doi:10.17226/12956.

McCauley LA, Broome ME, Frazier L, et al. Doctor of nursing practice (DNP) degree in the United States: reflecting, readjusting, and getting back on track. *Nurs Outlook*. 2020;68(4):494–503. doi:10.1016/j.outlook.2020.03.008.

Marć M, Bartosiewicz A, Burzyńska J, et al. A nursing shortage—a prospect of global and local policies. *Int Nurs Rev*. 2019;66(1):9-16. doi:10.1111/inr.12473.

McHugh MD, Aiken LH, Windsor C, et al. Case for hospital nurse-to-patient ratio legislation in Queensland, Australia, hospitals: an observational study. *BMJ Open*. 2020;10:e036264. doi:10.1136/bmjopen-2019-036264.

Melnyk BM, Fineout-Overholt E, Stillwell SB, Williamson KM Evidence-based practice: step by step: the seven steps of evidence-based practice. *Am J Nurs*. 2010;110(1):51–53. doi:10.1097/01.NAJ.0000366056.06605.d2.

National Academies of Science. *Consensus Report: The Future of Nursing 2020–2030: Charting a Path to Achieve Health Equity*. 2021. Available at: https://nap.nationalacademies.org/resource/25982/Highlights_Future%20of%20Nursing_4.30.21_final.pdf.

National Academies of Sciences, Engineering, and Medicine. *Assessing Progress on the Institute of Medicine Report the Future of Nursing*. Washington, DC: The National Academies Press; 2016. Available at: https://doi.org/10.17226/21838.

National Council State Board of Nursing (NCSBN) Annual Report. *Leadership, Vision, and Progress: A Year in Review*. 2015. Available at: https://ncsbn.org/public-files/NCSBN-2015-Annual-Report.pdf.

National League for Nursing. *A Vision for Doctoral Preparation for Nurse Educators*. https://www.nln.org/docs/default-source/uploadedfiles/about/nlnvision_6.pdf?sfvrsn=75163694_3, 2013.

National Task Force on Quality Nurse Practitioner Education. *Criteria for evaluation of nurse practitioner programs*. Washington, DC: National Organization of Nurse Practitioner Faculties; 2008.

Noguchi Y. *The U.S. needs more nurses, but nursing schools don't have enough slots*. 2021. Available at: https://www.npr.org/sections/health-shots/2021/10/25/1047290034/the-u-s-needs-more-nurses-but-nursing-schools-have-too-few-slots.

NONPF. *The Doctorate of Nursing Practice NP Preparation: NONPF Perspective*. 2015. Available at: https://cdn.ymaws.com/www.nonpf.org/resource/resmgr/DNP/NONPFDNPStatementSept2015.pdf.

Rhodes MK. Using effects-based reasoning to examine the DNP as the single entry degree for advanced practice nursing. *Online J Issues Nurs*. 2011;16(3):8. Available at: https://ojin.nursingworld.org/MainMenuCategories/ANAMarketplace/ANAPeriodicals/OJIN/TableofContents/Vol-16-2011/No3-Sept-2011/Articles-Previous-Topics/DNP-as-the-Single-Entry-Degree-for-Advanced-Practice-Nursing.html.

Robert Wood Johnson Foundation. *Robert Wood Johnson Foundation Announces $20 Million Grant to Support Nurse PhD Scientists*. 2013. Available at: https://www.rwjf.org/en/library/articles-and-news/2013/06/a-new-generation-of-nurse-scientists–educators–and-transformat.html.

Saad L. *U.S. Ethics Ratings Rise for Medical Workers and Teachers*. 2020. Available at: https://news.gallup.com/poll/328136/ethics-ratings-rise-medical-workers-teachers.aspx.

The Center to Champion Nursing in America (Campaign for Action). *Number of People Receiving Nursing Doctoral Degrees Annually*. 2019. Available at: https://campaignforaction.org/resource/number-people-receiving-nursing-doctoral-degrees-annually/.

Van den Heede K, Florquin M, Bruyneel L, et al. Effective strategies for nurse retention in acute hospitals: a mixed method study. *Int J Nurs Stud*. 2013;50(2):185-194. doi:10.1016/j.ijnurstu.2011.12.001.

CHAPTER 2

The Story of the Doctorally Prepared Nurse

Diane Seibert, PhD, APRN, FAANP, FAAN

If you are planning for a year, sow rice; if you are planning for a decade, plant trees; if you are planning for a lifetime, educate people.
—Chinese Proverb

Introduction

THE NURSES LEGENDS ARE MADE OF

At some point every nurse learns something about the nurses who shaped our profession, like Florence Nightingale, Clara Barton, Mary Breckenridge, Lillian Wald, Adelaide Nutting, and Walt Whitman. Many nurses and new graduates are not as familiar with the nurse leaders who are shaping the profession *today*, so in this chapter we share stories from some of the doctorally prepared nurses currently shaping the profession of nursing. These nursing leaders are working toward a common goal of improving care outcomes and healthcare systems, making them more effective, safer, and more cost effective.

A brief history of nursing provides some context for the environment in which today's nursing leaders work. Although humans have shared resources and cared for vulnerable or injured community members since the dawn of time, the nursing profession did not exist until the early 16th century. Another 300 years would pass before modern nursing was defined and described by Florence Nightingale (1947), when she outlined the profession's fundamental principles, including public health, nutrition, environmental health, and nursing leadership. Together these represent the defining characteristics of American nursing. In addition, nursing practice has and always will be closely tied to cultural and political events. The following few paragraphs will outline the significant interactions of political influence throughout the first half of the 20th century, which profoundly changed American nursing:

Tremendous expansion in understanding of human health and disease
Accelerations in scientific discoveries (human genome)

Global conflicts (World War I, World War II)
Financial crises (Great Depression)
Disease outbreaks (e.g., malaria, yellow fever, polio)
Industrialism
Advances in technology (automobiles, airplanes, and televisions)

UNDERGRADUATE/COMMUNITY COLLEGE EDUCATION

Before World War II, almost all nurses were trained in hospital-based programs that were focused on learning by doing and in-house hospital residences (Stanhope and Lancaster, 2022). Recognizing that the scope of nursing practice was expanding, leaders instigated a valiant effort to transition entry-level hospital-prepared nursing education toward university learning. This educational shift impacted nursing faculty and students; faculty became university (not hospital) employees, and students had to meet college admissions and graduation requirements. Graduates from these new university-level nursing programs were better prepared to assume clinical and leadership roles in the rapidly changing and evolving practice environment. The shift from hospital to 4-year university/college program-based education also added a year of training to basic nursing education, while a simultaneous boom in hospital construction increased the demand for nurses. By the mid-1950s, the US healthcare system experienced the first of many severe nursing shortages.

This chronic nursing shortage problem spawned some very innovative ideas, and today's multiple paths to a nursing license can be traced directly back to decisions made about increasing the nursing workforce in the early 1960s. In 1959, Mildred Montag proposed that an abbreviated (2 years) nursing program delivered by junior (or community) colleges could help address the nursing shortage (Montag & Gotkin, 1959). The Associate Degree in Nursing (ADN) curriculum would provide learners with basic and laboratory sciences and clinical nursing experiences that prepared them to pass the nursing licensure exam (Montag & Gotkin, 1959). However, in her model, the ADN-prepared nurse would be focused on providing direct patient care, whereas nurses with university/college degrees would provide leadership, orchestrate care teams, or care for acutely ill or highly complex patients. The ADN still exists today, as do three other paths to a nursing license: the 3-year hospital-based diploma program, the 4-year baccalaureate (Bachelor of Science in Nursing [BSN]) program, and the entry-level master's degree (Ervin, 2015; AACN 2021b). (See Table 2.1 for a list of postnominals and credentials.)

GRADUATE EDUCATION

Graduate education in nursing has an equally fascinating and complex history. Like the transitions in basic preparation, the stimulus for change did not come

TABLE 2.1 ■ **Post Nominals and Credentials**

Post Nominals	Credentials of Our Nurse Leaders
APRN	Advanced Practice Registered Nurse
BSN	Bachelor of Science in Nursing
CNP	Certified Nurse Practitioner
CRNP	Certified Registered Nurse Practitioner
DNP	Doctor of Nursing Practice
FRCN	Fellow, Royal College of Nursing
MPA	Master in Public Administration
MSN	Master of Science in Nursing
NEA-BC	Nurse Executive Advanced-Board Certified
PhD	Doctor of Philosophy
RN	Registered Nurse

from nurse educators but rather from the broader healthcare community. As more nurses earned undergraduate degrees, the demand for graduate programs grew (Harker, 2017), but in the early 1950s there were few options for nurses to choose from, and the curriculum was highly diverse. For example, one program might be advertised as a 12-month curriculum, but it might take three semesters to complete the required prerequisite courses (Ervin, 2015). Despite the diversity, credit burden, and lack of a standardized curriculum, enrollment in graduate nursing programs doubled between 1951 and 1962. One primary driver was the need to grow nursing faculty to support expanding university nursing programs. Over the next 60 years, nurses continued to earn graduate degrees in nursing, education, health policy, public health, informatics, and healthcare administration.

DOCTORAL EDUCATION

Doctoral education in nursing occurred in four waves over the past century. Nurses began earning doctoral degrees in education (the EdD or similar) early in the 20th century to prepare them for faculty roles. Then in the years leading up to and following World War II, nurses earned doctoral degrees in basic or social sciences to keep pace with a rapidly evolving scientific and technologic healthcare industry. Midcentury nurses were attracted to graduate programs that combined social or basic sciences with a concentration in nursing. These finally evolved into research doctorates in nursing (Langevin, 2021).

Recently, nursing, like many other healthcare disciplines (Olubadewo, 2012), has embraced the Doctor of Nursing Practice (DNP) degree, a clinical doctorate in nursing. The idea of launching the DNP had been discussed for several years by nursing leaders, and the degree was endorsed by the American Association of Colleges of Nursing (AACN) in 2004 as the preferred terminal degree for advanced practice nurses (nurse practitioners, nurse anesthetists, nurse midwives, and clinical nurse specialists). The stunning growth in both the number of DNP programs and enrollment in those programs is an echo of what occurred in the discipline of pharmacy a decade earlier (AACN, 2021a; Olubadewo, 2012). The DNP and Doctor of Philosophy (PhD) degrees are considered equivalent terminal degrees, and both prepare nurses to make important contributions to nursing science, to clinical care, and to improving healthcare systems. Nurses with doctoral degrees have made important contributions to every aspect of healthcare in the United States. Some focus on improving the quality of care and care delivery; others commit their lives to improving health outcomes for populations or communities; others choose to serve by leading healthcare systems; and others conduct research to find answers to questions that will improve nursing and patient outcomes. The following are descriptions of a *few* of today's most prominent nursing voices and leaders sorted approximately into eight categories: theorists, researchers, educators, healthcare systems leaders, public health, public policy, military, and global. As you read and review the multiple hyperlinks to key contributions of these nursing leaders in Table 2.2, perhaps one (or more) of these specialty areas might intrigue you enough to learn more about that person or that particular area. As you will see, nursing can be a very rich platform from which to change the world.

Nursing Leadership in Theory Development

Advances in any discipline begin with a theory that identifies and defines constructs and frameworks for examining the discipline-specific phenomenon. Nursing theories identify nursing constructs, identify and describe nursing tasks, explain what nurses do for patients, and explore nursing roles within the healthcare system. Theories help nurses articulate the reasons they do the things they do. After selecting an appropriate theory, researchers design studies, evaluate results in the context of that theory, and provide support for or against relationships and constructs in that theory. Research is an iterative process that continually refines and develops the discipline of nursing. As elements and relationships become clear, nurses work on policy efforts at the national, state, and local levels and focus their messages and actions. Nursing executives restructure healthcare processes and environments, and educators better align curricula to guide the profession's future. Nursing theories are generally sorted into one of three categories (Table 2.3).

Martha Alligood's book *Nursing Theorists and Their Work*, 8th Edition (2017), is an excellent resource to learn more about these nursing theories and the nurses who created them.

TABLE 2.2 ■ **Supplemental Content Links**

Research	<ul><li>Number of nursing journals</li><li>Dr. Hinshaw</li><li>Dr. Melnyk</li><li>National Academy of Medicine (NAM)</li><li>United States Preventive Services Task Force</li><li>National Consortium for Building Healthy Academic Communities</li></ul>
Education	<ul><li>Dr. Malone</li><li>National League for Nursing (NLN)</li><li>Future of Nursing</li><li>Minority Health Federal Advisory Committee</li><li>Dr. Begley</li><li>American Organization for Nursing Leadership</li><li>American Hospital Association</li><li>Dr. Grant</li><li>American Nurses Association</li></ul>
Genomics	<ul><li>International Society for Nurses in Genomics (ISONG)<ul><li>Genetic Information Nondiscrimination Act (GINA)</li><li>Dr. Calzone</li></ul></li><li>Global Genomics Nursing Alliance</li><li>Genomic Nurse State of the Science Advisory Panel</li><li>Genetics/Genomics Competency Center for Education for Genetic Counselors, Nurses, and Physician Assistants (G2C2)</li><li>Global Genetics/Genomics Community case studies (G3C)</li><li>Dr. Williams</li><li>Clinical Genetics Nursing Research Postdoctoral Fellowship Program</li><li>Institute of Medicine's Roundtable on Genomics and Precision Health</li><li>Dr. Seibert</li><li>Essential Genetic and Genomic Competencies for Nurses with Graduate Degrees</li></ul>
Quality, Safety & Public Health	<ul><li>Susan Hassmiller</li><li>Future of Nursing: Campaign for Action</li><li>World Health Organization Quality of Care</li><li>Dr. Hassmiller Staff Bio</li><li>National Board of Governors for the American Red Cross</li><li>Homeland Security Disaster and Chapter Services Committee</li><li>Immigration and Customs 9/11 recovery program</li><li>Peter Buerhaus</li><li>Center for Interdisciplinary Health Workforce Studies</li><li>National Health Care Workforce Commission</li><li>NAM Committee on the Future of Nursing, 2020–2030</li><li>Loretta Ford</li></ul>
Public Policy	<ul><li>Dr. Wakefield</li><li>World Health Organization (WHO)'s Global Program on Acquired Immunodeficiency Syndrome (AIDS)</li><li>To Err is Human and Crossing the Quality Chasm</li><li>Health Professions Education a Bridge to Quality</li><li>Quality Through Collaboration: Health Care in Rural America</li><li>Medicare Payment Advisory Commission</li><li>National Advisory Council for the Agency for Healthcare Research and Quality</li></ul>

Continued

TABLE 2.2 ■ **Supplemental Content Links—cont'd**

	• Advisory Commission on Consumer Protection and Quality in the Health Care Industry • National Advisory Committee to Health Resources and Services Administration (HRSA)'s Office of Rural Health Policy and the Commonwealth Fund's Commission to Create a High Performing Health System • Dr. Aiken • Center for Health Outcomes and Policy Research Director • Senior Fellow of the Leonard Davis Institute for Health Economics
Military	• Rear Admiral (Ret) CAROL ROMANO, PhD, RN, FAAN
Global	• Dr. MacIntyre • American Red Cross • Academic Service-Learning • Dr. Meleis • Carnegie Great Immigrants Award • Dr. Stillwell

Nursing Leadership in Research

The trajectory of nursing research has not been a straight line. Florence Nightingale was one of the first nurse researchers to describe the practice and impact of nursing care, but it took a century for nursing research to come into its own. One of the biggest challenges for nurse researchers has been identifying areas of research that are "nursing sensitive" or "nursing specific." Over the years, nursing research has been centered around developing new knowledge about how to maintain human health, and nurse researchers often explore ways to improve quality of life and healthcare outcomes for individuals and communities. However, that does not mean that nurses do not conduct basic science (animal or genetic research), but these research questions eventually tie back to answering questions in areas that are nursing sensitive. Because nursing is a very broad field, nurse researchers often collaborate with colleagues in disciplines such as neuroscience, social networking, and infectious disease.

Over the decades, nurses have secured sources of research support focused on answering nursing questions, and more journals have emerged offering nurses more opportunities to disseminate their findings. Currently, more than 250 nursing journals and hundreds of conferences are dedicated to disseminating nursing scholarship. The following are several stories of nurses who are making significant impacts in nursing research.

ADA SUE HINSHAW, PhD, RN, FAAN

Dr. Hinshaw has had a significant impact on human health through her efforts to expand nursing research. She was the first director of the National Institute of

TABLE 2.3 ■ Grand, Middle-Range, and Practice Level Nursing Theories

Grand Theories	Grand theories are broad, abstract, and highly complex, containing constructs like "people" or "human health," and as a result, constructs within grand theories are difficult to test or measure. These theories do provide a scaffold from which researchers can examine concepts broadly applicable to human health. Some of the more well-known grand theories include: • **Nursing as Caring** (Dr. Anne Boykin and Dr. Savina Schoenherr) • **Transitions Theory** (Dr. Afaf Melis) • **Health Promotion** (Dr. Nola Pender) • **Theory of Culture Care Diversity and Universality** (Dr. Madeline Leninger) • **Health as Expanding Consciousness** (Dr. Margaret Newman) • **Human Becoming** (Dr. Rosemarie Rizzo Parse) • **Modeling & Role Modeling** (Dr. Helen Erickson, Dr. Evelyn Tomlin, and Dr. Mary Ann Swain) • **Symphonological Bioethical Theory** (Dr. Gladys Husted and James Husted)
Middle-Range Theories	Mid-range theories are more concrete than grand ones, focusing on specific areas of nursing practice or phenomena that can often be translated more directly into an intervention or therapy. Nursing theories considered midrange theories include • **Maternal Role Attainment** (Dr. Romana Mercer) • **Uncertainty in Illness Theory** (Dr. Merle Mishel) • **Self-Transcendence Theory** (Dr. Pamela Reed) • **Theory of Illness Trajectory** (Dr. Carolyn Weiner and Marilyn Dodd) • **Theory of Chronic Sorrow** (Dr. Georgene Eakes, Dr. Mary Burke, and Dr. Margaret Hainsworth) • **The Tidal Model of Mental Health Recovery** (Dr. Phil Barker) • **Theory of Comfort** (Dr. Katharine Kolcaba) • **Postpartum Depression Theory** (Dr. Cheryl Beck) • **Theory of Caring** (Dr. Kristen Swanson) • **Peaceful End of Life Theory** (Dr. Cornelia Ruland and Dr. Shirley Moore)
Practice-Level Theories	Practice-level theories are practice oriented and focus on understanding and explaining concepts concerning a population of patients (or individuals) at a specific time in their health journey. Practice-level theories are much more likely to result in an outcome that directly impacts patients than the other two types of theories. Nursing theories amenable to being directly applied in a clinical setting include • **Conservation Model** (Dr. Myra Levine) • **Unitary Human Beings** (Dr. Martha Rogers) • **The Self-Care Deficit Theory** (Dr. Dorthea Orem) • **The Theory of Goal Attainment** (Dr. Imogene King) • **The Systems Model** (Dr. Betty Newman) • **The Adaptation Model (**Dr. Sister Callista Roy) • **The Behavioral System Model** (Dorothy Johnson) • **The Novice to Expert Model** (Dr. Patricia Benner)

Nursing Research (NINR) at the National Institutes of Health (NIH), was selected to serve as a Distinguished Nurse Scholar-in-Residence at the Institute of Medicine (IOM) in Washington, DC, and served as President of the American Academy of Nursing. Her personal research focused on disease prevention and health promotion.

BERNADETTE MAZUREK MELNYK, PhD, APRN-CNP, FAANP, FNAP, FAAN

Dr. Melnyk is the Vice President for Health Promotion, University Chief Wellness Officer, Dean, and Professor at The Ohio State University College of Nursing. She is a Professor of Pediatrics and Psychiatry at The Ohio State University College of Medicine, serves as Executive Director of The Helene Fuld Health Trust National Institute for Evidence-Based Practice, and is the editor of *Worldviews on Evidence-Based Nursing*. Her work spans evidence-based practice, intervention research, health and wellness, and child and adolescent mental health, and she is recognized nationally and internationally for her innovative approaches to a wide range of healthcare challenges. A frequent keynote speaker at national and international conferences, Dr. Melnyk has consulted with hundreds of healthcare systems and colleges worldwide on improving the quality of care and patient outcomes by implementing and sustaining evidence-based practice. Elected to the IOM (now the National Academy of Medicine) in 2013, Dr. Melnyk served a 4-year term on the US Preventive Services Task Force, which makes evidence-based recommendations about clinical preventive services such as screenings, counseling services, or preventive medications. In 2012, she founded the National Interprofessional Education and Practice Collaborative to advance the US Department of Health and Human Services (HHS) Million Hearts initiative to prevent one million heart attacks and strokes by 2017. She also founded the National Consortium for Building Healthy Academic Communities, a collaborative organization to improve population health in the nation's institutions of higher learning.

Nursing Leadership in Education

Nursing education shapes how nurses think and act, but it also impacts the structure of American healthcare. As providing care for the sick and infirm gradually shifted from home to hospitals, nursing leadership became increasingly important. Leaders in hospital systems expect new nurses to have been trained to a certain level of clinical as well as leadership competency. Leadership is a key component in nursing and nurses' function in leadership roles that span the gambit from leading teams at the bedside, to leading units, clinical sections, or nursing departments, or being responsible for the care provided across a multihospital system. Preparing nurses to function as both safe clinicians and systems leaders in such a rapidly evolving healthcare environment is challenging. The following is a brief description of just some of the people who are shaping the future of nursing education.

BEVERLY MALONE, PhD, RN, FAAN

Dr. Malone is the Chief Executive Officer of the National League for Nursing (NLN). She promotes collaboration among stakeholders, increased nursing and nursing education diversity, and advanced excellence in patient care. Over her career, she has served in various policy, education, administration, and clinical practice roles, including Deputy Assistant Secretary for Health under President Bill Clinton and as a member of his Advisory Commission on Consumer Protection and Quality in the Healthcare Industry. She served as a reviewer of the IOM's *The Future of Nursing: Leading Change, Advancing Health* report and served on the Minority Health Federal Advisory Committee, a federal panel established to advise the US Secretary of Health and Human Services (HHS). She has served on the Kaiser Family Foundation Board of Directors and the Board of Directors for the Institute for Healthcare Improvement. In the 1980s, she was Dean of the School of Nursing at North Carolina Agricultural and Technical State University. In the late 1990s, she was elected to two terms as President of the American Nurses Association (ANA), representing more than 180,000 American nurses. Congressional leaders and policymakers frequently call on Dr. Malone to offer her perspective and public testimony on nursing workforce development and education for nurses to address the persistent shortage of nurses.

Dr. Malone has been active in the global nursing community and serves as the Royal College of Nursing (RCN) general secretary and as a member of the UK delegation to the World Health Assembly.

ROBYN BEGLEY, DNP, RNN, NEA-BC

Dr. Begley is the Chief Executive Officer (CEO) of the American Organization for Nursing Leadership (AONL) and Senior Vice President and Chief Nursing Officer of the American Hospital Association. As the AONL CEO, she is responsible for leading an organization of more than 10,000 nurse leaders focused on excellence in nursing leadership. She oversees critical initiatives involving workforce, quality and safety, and future care delivery models. These two roles are synergistic in that she can collaborate with the AHA to ensure the perspective and needs of nurse leaders are heard and addressed in public policy issues related to nursing and patient care. Prior to assuming these responsibilities, Dr. Begley was Vice President of Nursing and chief nursing officer at AtlantiCare in Atlantic City, NJ, for 35 years in which the organization received the American Nurses Credentialing Center's Magnet designation four times. She actively promotes diversity in the nursing workforce by establishing a nursing fellowship and scholarship and a mentoring program for students by collaborating with the local National Association for the Advancement of Colored People (NAACP), Hispanic Alliance, and Pan Asian leaders.

ERNEST GRANT, PhD, RN, FAAN

Dr. Grant is the first man to be elected to President of the American Nursing Association (ANA) and is internationally recognized as a burn care and fire safety expert. As the burn outreach coordinator for the North Carolina Jaycee Burn Center at the University of North Carolina (UNC) Hospitals in Chapel Hill, he oversees burn education for physicians, nurses, and other allied healthcare personnel. He runs the center's nationally acclaimed burn prevention program, focusing on reducing burn-related injuries through public education and legislative processes. Frequently sought out for his expertise as a clinician and educator, Dr. Grant has designed and taught numerous burn education courses for the US military. President George W. Bush awarded him a Nurse of the Year Award for treating burn victims from the World Trade Center site following the 9/11 terrorist attacks. Dr. Grant is past chair of the National Fire Protection Association board of directors, served on the American Burn Association board of trustees, and was President of the North Carolina Nurses Association

Nursing Leadership in Genomics

Even before the NIH announced that the human genome had been sequenced, a small but committed group of nurses was working to ensure that the nursing community was at the table in this new space. They began by creating Genetic and Genomic Essentials for undergraduates and later for nurses prepared at the graduate level. They formed the International Society for Nurses in Genomics (ISONG), created genomics certifications for undergraduate and graduate nurses, collaborated to develop new policies (Genetic Information Nondiscrimination Act [GINA]), and created research agendas. Because of the innovative nurse leaders showcased in the following paragraphs, nurses globally are more prepared to address genetic needs.

KATHLEEN CALZONE, PhD, RN, FAAN

Dr. Calzone is a research geneticist in the Genetics Branch of the Center for Cancer Research (CCR) at the National Cancer Institute (NCI). She serves as the CCR Genomic Program Administrator to implement the NIH Genomic Data Sharing Policy. Board-certified in genetics by the American Nursing Credentialing Commission, she is a founder of the Global Genomics Nursing Alliance. As President of ISONG, Dr. Calzone co-chaired the Essentials of Genomic and Genomic Nursing: Competencies, Curricula Guidelines, and Outcome Indicators taskforce. As the senior nurse specialist, she further leads the Genomic Nursing Science Blueprint development as part of the Genomic Nurse State of the Science Advisory Panel that is actively dedicated to translating genomics into research, practice, and education. She guides the design and development of the Genetics/Genomics Competency Center (G2C2) for Education for Genetic Counselors, Nurses, and Physician Assistants and the Global Genetics/Genomics Community (G3C) case studies and provides significant guidance and recommendations for researchers as part of the NINR's Genomic State of the Science Advisory Group.

JANET WILLIAMS, PhD, RN, FAAN

Dr. Williams is a genetics nurse specialist, a genetic counselor, and Professor and Chair of the University of Iowa Behavioral and Social Science Institutional Review Board. Her current work is building and directing the Clinical Genetics Nursing Research Postdoctoral Fellowship Program, funded by the NINR. She is the Director of the Enrichment Core of the Center for Advancing Multimorbidity Science (CAMS) and is the American Academy of Nursing's representative at the IOM's Roundtable on Genomics and Precision Health. Dr. William's research explores the day-to-day functionality in individuals with prodromal Huntington disease, family caregiving by adults and adolescents for Huntington disease, and ethical issues in disclosing secondary findings from genomic analysis in clinical and research settings. She is a consultant on national and international projects to promote nurses' research, education, and practice regarding genetics.

DIANE SEIBERT, PhD, APRN, FAANP

Dr. Seibert has spent two decades working on improving the genomic competencies of advanced practice nurses, particularly the nurse practitioner community. She has developed novel genetics curricula that are shared with faculty across the country, and has served as a consultant for the NINR genomic research advisory group. She was a member of the team that developed the G2C2 and the G3C. She was co-editor for the *Essential Genetic and Genomic Competencies for Nurses with Graduate Degrees*, which provided a framework for a curriculum structure for graduate nurses. Her work has contributed significantly to genomic education, impacting current/future generations of nurse educators/students and creating critical resources to expand genomics education, practice, and research.

Nursing Leadership in Quality, Safety, and Public Health

According to the World Health Organization (WHO), "Quality of care is the degree to which health services for individuals and populations increase the likelihood of desired health outcomes. It is based on evidence-based professional knowledge and is critical for achieving universal health coverage. As countries commit to achieving Health for All, it is imperative to consider the quality of care and health services carefully." Here are some of the nurses making momentous strides in *quality*, *safety*, and *public health*. Several nurse leaders have made an enormous impact in this area.

SUSAN HASSMILLER, PhD, RN, FAAN

Dr. Hassmiller is the Senior Adviser for Nursing, Robert Wood Johnson Foundation (RWJF), and the Senior Scholar-in-Residence and Senior Adviser, National Academy of Medicine, where she was director of both Future of Nursing Reports (see Chapter 1). Dr. Hassmiller has spent a quarter of a century creating, delivering, and evaluating the higher quality of care for the American people, families, and communities. Dr. Hassmiller works with the American Association of Retired Persons (AARP) Future of Nursing: Campaign for Action, creating healthcare systems where nurses are seen as essential partners in providing care and promoting health as charged by the IOM Future of Nursing. Serving as the executive director of the US Public Health Service (USPHS) Primary Care Policy Fellowship, Dr. Hasmiller was a member of the National Board of Governors for the American Red Cross and served as chair of the Disaster and Chapter Services Committee and as national chair of the 9/11 recovery program.

PETER BUERHAUS, PhD, RN, FAAN

Dr. Buerhaus is the director of the Center for Interdisciplinary Health Workforce Studies at Montana State University College of Nursing and a healthcare economist renowned for his studies on the nursing and physician workforces in the United States. While chairing the National Health Care Workforce Commission, he advised Congress and the Administration on health workforce policy for the Healthcare Care Workforce Commission. He serves on the Board of Directors for the Bozeman Deaconess Health System and is a member of the National Academies of Medicine Committee on the Future of Nursing, 2020–2030.

LORETTA FORD, PhD, FAANP, FAAN

Dr. Loretta Ford created the role of the nurse practitioner. This initiative was born out of her experiences as a nurse in World War II and solidified in the early 1960s, when, as a public health nurse, she realized that rural children and families were not receiving timely care due to a shortage of physicians. She believed nurses could fill that gap, so in 1967 she partnered with Dr. Henry Silver, a pediatrician at the University of Colorado Medical Center, to create and implement the country's first nurse practitioner program. In the early 1970s, she was recruited to New York, where she served as Founding Dean of the University of Rochester School of Nursing and continued to advocate for the role of the nurse practitioner.

Nursing Leaders in Public Policy

Well-crafted and forward-thinking policy shapes healthcare in massive and subtle ways. Policy molds how healthcare is delivered and accessed at the national or state level and influences how healthcare is delivered at the bedside or an outpatient clinic. Thoughtful and comprehensive policies articulate the healthcare goal while identifying intermediate (or reference) points for short- and medium-term outcomes. Health policy clarifies priorities, establishes roles and expectations for different groups of providers, and builds consensus among the various stakeholders (recipients and providers of care) within a community, population, or health system. Some key nursing leaders in the policy arena follow.

MARY WAKEFIELD, PhD, RN, FAAN

Dr. Wakefield is the Visiting Distinguished Professor in the Practice of Health Care at Georgetown University and a Visiting Professor and Distinguished Fellow at The University of Texas at Austin. Over her career, she has served as the Acting Deputy Secretary of the HHS, where she oversaw management and operations to include a $1 trillion budget and 80,000 employees while leading department-wide initiatives in key health policy areas, mainly focusing on programs for vulnerable populations. Prior to that, she served for 8 years as a legislative assistant and chief of staff to two North Dakota senators and as a consultant to the WHO's Global Program on Acquired Immunodeficiency Syndrome (AIDS) in Geneva, Switzerland. As a member of the National Academy of Medicine, she served on the IOM committee that produced two landmark reports, *To Err Is Human* and *Crossing the Quality Chasm*, and co-chaired IOM committees that produced two others: *Health Professions Education a Bridge to Quality* and *Quality Through Collaboration: Health Care in Rural America*. She either chaired or served as a member of the Medicare Payment Advisory Commission, the National Advisory Council for the Agency for Healthcare Research and Quality, the Advisory Commission on Consumer Protection and Quality in the Health Care Industry, the National Advisory Committee to the Health Resources and Services Administration (HRSA)'s Office of Rural Health Policy, and the Commonwealth Fund's Commission to Create a High Performing Health System.

LINDA H. AIKEN, PhD, RN, FAAN, FRCN

Dr. Aiken is the Center for Health Outcomes and Policy Research Director and Senior Fellow of the Leonard Davis Institute for Health Economics. She has made contributions to nursing by demonstrating that baccalaureate-prepared nurses have better outcomes, and that unhealthy work environments, including the number of hours worked or patient responsibilities a nurse has, worsened the outcomes for inpatients. Her research showed that as the number of nurses with BSN degrees increased, there was a statistically significant drop in risk-adjusted mortality, and demonstrated that patient outcomes are better in organizations that involve nurses in decision-making.

Nursing Leadership in Military and Public Health

Modern healthcare evolved from war and involved the nurses serving alongside the service members. American nurses have been present on the battlefield since the Revolutionary War and before Florence Nightingale and the Crimean War. Although they are not officially recognized or rewarded for their service, Congress approved General Washington's request to add a nurse for every 10 patients in military hospitals during the Revolutionary War.

REAR ADMIRAL (RET) CAROL ROMANO, PhD, RN, FAAN

Dr. Romano is currently the Dean at the Uniformed Services University of the Health Sciences, but prior to that had a long career in the Public Health Services, culminating in her being selected as the Chief Nurse of the Public Health Services. The chief nurse role is not a full-time job for any of the Nursing Service Chiefs, so while she was serving as chief nurse, her major responsibility was the Deputy Chief Information Officer (CIO) for Clinical Research Informatics at the Clinical Center of the NIH, and Acting Chief of Staff for the Office of the Surgeon General. Many of the features of today's healthcare technology can be traced back to Dr. Romano's work with information systems in the late 1970s, when she designed a model for a computerized database, defined the quality improvement role for clinical information systems, and represented nursing informatics on interdisciplinary federal committees, including the government representative to the Informatics Committee of Clinical Translational Science. Dr. Romano co-created the first graduate curriculum in nursing informatics at the University of Maryland, a program that continues to graduate hundreds of nurse informaticians every year.

REAR ADMIRAL SUSAN ORSEGA, RN, FNP-BC, DNP (HON), FAANP

Rear Admiral (RADM) Orsega is the principal advisor to both the Assistant Secretary for Health and the US Surgeon General on a full range of United States Public Health Service (USPHS) Commissioned Corps programs, policies, and activities. During the transition from President Trump to President Biden, she served as Acting Surgeon General (SG) of the United States, pending the Senate confirmation of Dr. Vivek H. Murthy. Prior to that, RADM Orsega was the Director of Commissioned Corps Headquarters (CCHQ), managing the activation of the largest deployment of the USPHS Commissioned Corps in support of international and national COVID-19 efforts and, as mentioned above in Dr. Romano's biography, she also served as the Corps Chief Nurse Officer, advising the SG and providing leadership to 4500 USPHS nurses and HHS nurse civilians.

Nursing Leadership in Global Health

Like military nurses, other nurses have worked to improve global health but have chosen to do so differently. Here are some of the nurses who have shaped care around the world.

LINDA MACINTYRE, PhD, RN, PHN, FAAN

Dr. MacIntyre is the Chief Nurse of the American Red Cross, where she provides leadership, vision, direction, and support in meeting the Red Cross mission. She is responsible for overseeing the recruitment process for health professionals wanting to serve the Red Cross and provides oversight for Academic Service-Learning as a volunteer engagement strategy.

AFAF I. MELEIS, PhD, RN, DrPH (HON)

Dr. Meleis is an expert in global health and immigrant and women's health, ensuring that vulnerable populations (mainly women) are given a voice. She was Dean of the University of the Pennsylvania School of Nursing for a decade and was faculty at University of California San Francisco for decades prior to that. Her work has redefined women's work, health, and contributions internationally with her renowned quote, "Give nurses, as we give women more power, give them better compensation, give them more autonomy, and some of that translates to their ability to do even better work in supporting the patients and in making a difference in society, making a difference in the health care system." Dr. Meleis developed a Transitions Theory, used globally in education, policy, research, and evidence-based practice for which she received the 2020 Carnegie Great Immigrants Award.

BARBARA STILWELL, PhD, RN, FRCN

Early in her career, Barbara Stilwell worked in the inner city of Birmingham, United Kingdom, and recognized that many of her patients (mostly immigrants) lacked preventive care services. She earned a nurse practitioner degree in the United States and an honorary doctorate from the RCN at London South Bank University

(LSBU) in 2000. Dr. Stilwell established England's first nurse practitioner training program. Dr. Stilwell worked with the WHO to change the organization's approaches to performance improvement, particularly in health worker migration. Dr. Stilwell guides countries in Eastern Europe and Africa to develop their healthcare workforces. As a nurse consultant, Dr. Stilwell guides teams to navigate complex nursing issues, improve health systems, address the global health workforce shortage, and optimize workforce design to support nonphysician clinicians in sub-Saharan Africa. She currently serves as the senior director of health workforce solutions at IntraHealth International.

Summary

Now that you have caught a glimpse of the wide-open horizons and possibilities, consider how and where your nursing career might take you. The growth of the DNP degree promises to amplify further the reach and innovation of doctoral-prepared nurse leaders, educators, clinicians, and scientists serving around the world. To learn more (or find a mentor), review the bios of nurses inducted as fellows in different nursing organizations (Table 2.4). Reach out to clinicians, administrators, educators, and researchers who inspire you, explore the many thought-provoking and inspirational narratives of doctoral-prepared nurses in our text, and learn how to make your mark on the nursing profession and people's health around the world. You are the future of our profession, and we are proud you are joining us to continue to work toward a world in which more people enjoy longer, healthier, happier lives.

TABLE 2.4 ■ **Professional Organizations and Nomenclature**

FAAN	Fellow in the Academy of Nursing	American Academy of Nursing www.aan.org
FAANP	Fellow in the Academy of Nurse Practitioner	American Association of Nursing Practitioners www.aanp.org
FNAP	Forum of Nurses in Advanced Practice	https://fnap.enpnetwork.com/

Bibliography

Alligood MR. *Nursing Theorists and Their Work–e-Book*. Elsevier Health Sciences; 2017. https://brand.amia. org/m/5c77f33de1cbef8b/original/Carol-Romano-NIWG-pdf.pdf.

American Association of Colleges of Nursing. *Doctor of Nursing Practice (DNP) Tool Kit*. 2021a. Available at: https://www.aacnnursing.org/DNP/Tool-Kit.

American Association of Colleges of Nursing. *The Essentials: Core Competencies for Professional Nursing Education*. 2021b. Available at: https://www.aacnnursing.org/Portals/42/AcademicNursing/pdf/Essentials-2021.pdf.

American Medical Informatics Association Nursing Informatics History project. Available at: https://brand.amia. org/m/5c77f33de1cbef8b/original/Carol-Romano-NIWG-pdf.pdf.

Ervin SM. History of nursing education in the United States. *Curriculum Development and Evaluation in Nursing*, (2015). 3-32.

Harker M. History of nursing education evolution Mildred Montag. Teach Learn Nurs. 2017;12(4):295-297.

International Academy of Nursing Editors (INANE). Available at: https://nursingeditors.com/2018/06/08/how-many-nursing-journals-are-there/. Retrieved April 16, 2022.

Langevin K. Doctoral education for the nurse educator. *Nurs Made Incredibly Easy*. 2021;19(6):18-21. doi:10.1097/01.NME.0000753068.50489.dc.

Montag ML, Gotkin LG. *Community College Education for Nursing*. New York: McGraw Hill Book Company, Inc; 1959.

Nightingale F. *Notes on Nursing. What It Is and What It Is Not, 1860*. 1947.

Olubadewo J. The Pharm. D. Degree and the Title by Which Pharmacists are Addressed. *Int J Appl Sci Technol*. 2012;2(1):226.

Stanhope M, Lancaster J. *Foundations for Population Health in Community/Public Health Nursing*. 6th ed. St Louis, MO: Elsevier; 2022.

CHAPTER 3

Building Nursing for the Future

Marisa L. Wilson, DNSc, MHSc, RN-BC, CPHIMS, FAMIA, FIAHSI, FAAN ◼ Mary F. Terhaar, RN, PhD, ANEF, FAAN ◼ Laura A. Taylor, PhD, RN, ANEF, FAAN

We cannot become what we need by remaining what we are.
—John C. Maxwell

There are so many ways to enter into a discussion of the future, and such discussions are important for nursing and for society, because one needs to have a clear and detailed vision of the future in order to create it. The more vibrant and positive the vision, the greater our potential to achieve it. That is the purpose of this chapter. We will describe significant trends in healthcare and society and forecast their implications for the future. Some of the future trends, in fact, will take us back to the roots of nursing.

Moving nurses out of the four walls of acute care settings is imperative (Sawin and O'Connor, 2019). Nurse leaders need to look to our history and to the important roles nursing is being called to work in the home, in the community, and among populations to meet the challenge of accomplishing this move. Doctorally prepared nurse leaders will be relied upon to creatively, innovatively, and with disruptive intent advance nurses and nursing into areas where we have not been for decades or have never been before. One notable difference between the past and the present is the vast array of technologies and strategies available to those emboldened to embrace them. Maxwell challenges us to envision a positive future and then enact strategies to achieve that future. This is design thinking and it guides the text in this chapter and this book (Liedtka, 2018). Earning a doctorate, developing a bold outlook, creating a future vision, and taking the steps to create it are the ways to rise to the challenges facing nursing and society. This is the path to an exciting and impactful career.

As you move through this chapter, you will be able to anticipate the challenges and opportunities doctoral-prepared nurses will face, as well as:

1. appreciate the social contract of nursing as a foundation for its future,
2. discuss key societal trends that have significance for nursing,
3. recognize the incredible opportunities open to nursing, and
4. explore opportunities for nurses in nontraditional roles.

Nursing's Social Contract as a Foundation for Its Future

Nursing has always been grounded in service and, even though the places and the forms that service has taken have evolved over time, the mission has held steady. Like many professions, we have an implicit agreement with a society that allows us privileges and assigns us responsibilities to benefit members of that society. Extending back in history, we have enjoyed the highest level of trust and, as evident in times of COVID-19, great respect.

From as far back as the crusades in the 12th century, those who tended the sick and wounded were presented badges and became knights of the Order of the Hospital of St. John the Baptist (Barber, 1937). Each knight took the monastic vow to become "*serf and slave*" of their lords and were presented a Maltese cross that was worn on their black habit and draped over their armor. This commitment is the foundation for the pinning ceremonies still conducted in nursing schools today.

In ancient times nursing was aligned with more commonsense actions conducted by caring individuals to benefit and comfort other vulnerable individuals.

Nursing is one of the oldest arts. There has always been helplessness of one sort or another and to a greater or lesser degree: wounds have demanded attention: babies and old people have needed care, and disease in some form — due to willful or ignorant disregard of natural laws—has always been present in the world. The great universal mother-instinct has met these emergencies by what we call "nursing."

—GOODNOW (2020)

At this time, interventions included cleansing wounds, releasing content of abscesses, bleeding, leeching, cooling fevers, and providing comfort. These helping individuals often followed directions of another individual who was recognized in society as a healer. A great range of human needs and vulnerabilities claimed the attention of those who worked as nurses. Christian women and men dedicated their lives to service and provided care for the ill for centuries. Hospitals formed and formal home visiting began. Apprenticeships continued, and philanthropic support became available in the form of donations and almsgiving (Goodnow, 2020). Importantly, in the earliest times, nursing practice would have lacked any scientific, evidentiary, or technologic foundation and would have relied on observation, trial and error, and apprenticeship training (Goodnow, 2020).

In the 1800s, nursing care was still provided by women of the lower class, such as Charles Dickens's character Sairey Gamp (Dickens, 2009). Women arrested for drunkenness and disorderly conduct would spend 10 days in jail, sober up, and work it off as nurses in the wards. No training. No intent to serve. No choice (Dickens, 2009).

Florence Nightingale (1820–1910) was the ultimate image consultant who had a task before her to improve the image of nurses from that of drunken indolent care providers. When Florence Nightingale established her school to "train" nurses, not only was she applying data and analytics to identify risks and conditions in the community that disposed its members to illness, but she also began to identify practices that effectively improved outcomes like handwashing and rest. During this time, our profession made its first steps toward evidence-based practice and epidemiology (Goodnow, 2020).

Because of this forward-thinking of nursing leaders in the 19th and early 20th centuries, nurses have earned the highest level of trust and respect as society has experienced global pandemics of exceptional magnitude: the Spanish Flu of 1918, the polio epidemic of the 1940s and 1950s, the human immunodeficiency virus (HIV), aka HIV/AIDS, in the 1980s and 1990s, and, most recently, the COVID-19 pandemic of 2020–2023.

The vulnerability in society today is more fully understood as extending beyond physical maladies to include psychological, developmental, immunological, and sociocultural conditions such as poverty, policy, and politics. These challenges demand the attention of the nurse and all members of a well differentiated and highly specialized healthcare team. The natural and human-made environments, technologies, genetics and genomics, and social policy have impacts far beyond the conditions identified by Nightingale. Our social contract in the future depends on the ways our profession responds to these needs and seizes opportunities in each. Our social contract will extend our services back into homes, communities, and populations. However, the platforms will continue to evolve as they have since the origin of our profession.

Key Social Trends That Have Significance for Nursing

Across disciplines, thought leaders forecast priorities in healthcare that paint the landscape for the future of nursing practice and scholarship. A high-level summary of select position papers and scholarship is presented in Table 3.1.

The most encompassing and specific assertions about the demands and opportunities for nurses are presented in *The Future of Nursing 2020–2030 Report* (National Academy of Medicine, 2021). The report makes the case for an aggressive response to increase the quantity and quality of the nursing workforce. It asserts that this workforce needs to be prepared to help mitigate the impact of the social determinants of health and promote equity, which requires the support of data and leadership. Nurses need to be effective, efficient, and highly collaborative, and we need to achieve meaningful diversity in gender, race, and ethnicity. We must be prepared to move beyond the acute care setting and out into communities in order to ensure connected systems that can deliver care that is responsive and focused on promoting a culture of health while still responding to episodic need.

TABLE 3.1 ■ **Priorities for Nursing Identified in Select Papers and Scholarship**

Sector	Forecasted Priorities	Author
Future of Nursing	Social determinants of health	National Academy of Sciences (2021)
	Effectiveness	
	Efficiency	
	Equity	
	Access	
	Collaborative practice	
	Culture of health	
	Workforce diversity (gender, race, and ethnicity)	
	Community voice in design and operations	
	Developing competency of educators	
	Prepare nurses to work outside acute care	
	Prepare nurses to lead	
	Nursing shortage—globally	
Nursing	Home care	Morris (2021)
	Tele health	
	Increasingly agile care models	
	Simulation and technology in education	
	Well-being and self-care	
	Resilience	
	Negative consequences of the shortage	
	Demand for higher education	
Nursing Education	Four spheres of care	AACN (2020)
	Enhanced focus on primary care	
	Diversity, equity, and inclusion	
	Systems-based practice	
	Informatics and technology	
	Population health	
	Academic-practice partnerships	
	Career-long learning	

Continued

TABLE 3.1 ■ **Priorities for Nursing Identified in Select Papers and Scholarship—cont'd**

Sector	Forecasted Priorities	Author
Geriatricians	Personalized healthcare	Gandarillas and Goswami (2018)
	Predictive care	
	Information and communication technologies	
	Home-based care	
	Prevention and promotion through patient empowerment	
	Care coordination	
	Community health networks	
	Community governance	
Health Policy	Made in America	Devore (2021)
	Value-based care	
	Strengthening the public health infrastructure	
	Tele-health	
	Maternal health	
Scholars & Advocates	Reliable information to support decisions	Nuti et al. (2014)
	Open access to information	
Hospitals	Cooperative competition	Martin (2021)
	Agile supply chains	
	Patient consumerization	
	Personalized care	
	Workforce safety and diversity	
	Virtual care	
	Automation and artificial intelligence	
	Revenue diversification	
	Mergers and integration	
	Payer shifts	
Patient Advocates	Access to care	Kavanaugh et al. (2017) Apeter et al. (2017)
	Fewer deaths due to medical errors	
	Symptom control	
Pharma	Risk reduction	Vogenberg and Santilli (2019)
	Cost containment	

TABLE 3.1 ■ **Priorities for Nursing Identified in Select Papers and Scholarship—cont'd**

Sector	Forecasted Priorities	Author
Reducing Racial Disparities	Neighborhood and physical environment	Harrison (2021)
	Access to quality healthcare	
	Occupational and job conditions	
	Income and wealth	
Healthcare Technology Trends	Remote healthcare and telemedicine	Marr (2022)
	Extended reality for clinical training and treatment	
	Artificial intelligence and machine learning	
	Personalized medicine and genomics	
	Digital twins and simulations	

This will require more doctorally prepared nurses in all roles who practice at the top of their license as well as more faculty to educate this workforce with all the competencies they will need. This will require faculty who are competent, confident, and capable to teach future nurses and nurse leaders to think beyond skills and become bold disruptors of current practice using the tools and techniques available.

Policy makers and industry leaders identify implementing value-based care, producing needed materials domestically, building and strengthening the systems and infrastructure required to effectively promote public and population health, offering technology mediated services such as telehealth to improve access to healthcare and mitigate the impact of health disparities, and correcting abysmal maternal health outcomes. All are seen as priorities that require attention in the United States (Devore, 2021).

Patients, caregivers, and communities require support and education in order to improve the health outcomes of the nation. Scholars and advocates emphasize the importance of open access to reliable health information and literature (Nuti et al., 2014). The U.S. Department of Health and Human Services Office of Disease Prevention and Health Promotion (2021) has offered to the nation the Health Literate Care Model to assist in increasing engagement in prevention, decision making, and self-management. Doctorally prepared nurse leaders need to create a path to achieve health literacy not just with individual patients but with entire communities and populations beyond the acute care four walls.

Patient advocates prioritize eliminating deaths due to medical error, symptom management while increasing access (Kavanagh et al., 2017; Apter et al., 2017). This requires careful consideration of the appropriate data and information that can make this happen. PhD-prepared nurse leaders must be at the forefront of building the evidence for the information systems to be used in the correct cognitive and workflow processes that can reduce risk and harm while not adding to documentation burden. Doctor of Nursing Practice (DNP)-prepared nurse leaders will need to use translation, implementation, and evaluation competencies to make this happen at various points of care.

Nursing's allied partners understand the vital contributions of innovative, disruptive, and highly educated leaders who can work effectively and efficiently as interdisciplinary team members. The pharmaceutical industry prioritizes risk reduction and cost containment (Vogenberg and Santilli, 2019). The pharmaceutical industry has had structures and operations in place led by PhD- and PharmD-prepared providers to educate potential prescribers by going out into the communities and offices to conduct evidence-based educational approaches that will result in sustainable practice changes and improved decision making to increase benefit and decrease harm (McKeirnan, 2019).

Opportunities Open to Nurses

The future forecasted by a broad coalition of stakeholders points to the need for nurses with highly specialized and well-developed knowledge and expertise. There is agreement that society needs nurses prepared to lead efforts in the areas of informatics, population health, genomics, system reform, health of the environment, social policy, diversity and inclusion, quality, cost containment, improving outcomes, and achieving innovation. This will require the teaming of nurses prepared to generate new knowledge through PhD preparation and the DNP-prepared nurses with deep yet broad systems understanding, translation, implementation, and evaluation to activate the future opportunities in and across all of the American Association Colleges in Nursing (AACN, 2021) four spheres of care which are:

1. Wellness and Disease Prevention,
2. Chronic Disease Management,
3. Regenerative/Restorative Care, and
4. Hospice and Palliative Care.

INFORMATICS AND HEALTHCARE INFORMATION TECHNOLOGY

Informatics simply stated is a process that takes data and turns it into information and knowledge. The Data to Information to Knowledge to Wisdom (DIKW) model provides a theoretical framework for practice for not only nurses with advanced informatics competency but for all nurses and nurse leaders who make data-driven decisions (Nelson, 2021). The key word is "process." The DIKW process does not require technology. In fact, for 200 years visionary nurses have done this using paper and pencil. Not so long ago records of patients were kept in large ledger books and outcome data were extract from paper medical records. Today, electronic health records and other healthcare technologies are the tools used in that same pursuit. The difference is that the volume and velocity of that data are growing exponentially.

The health information technologies (HIT) in use today are substantially different from the HIT of only 15 years ago, and promise to be substantially different from those used in the future. Remaining vigilant to the ever-present adaptions and rapid growth of technology will be instrumental in successfully navigating the complexities of current HIT: electronic health records, personal health records, mobile devices, wearable devices, monitors, social media, robotics, nanotechnology, and genomics. Each is made available due to the rapid advancements in hardware, software, and technology, all enabling infrastructure underpinned by best evidence for use in a variety of settings across the AACN (2021) Four Spheres of Care. Doctorally prepared nurses are well positioned to ensure that these technologies, as well as ones on the horizon, are implemented based on evidence. Goals for optimal HIT are established to drive/support targeted outcomes, quality, safety, and efficiency not just for patients and caregivers but also for clinicians, communities, and populations (Table 3.2).

Each of these technologies collects data through a variety of methods such as direct data entry by an individual or by interfaces that collect the data ubiquitously without the individual being specifically aware of the collection. This data collection requires nurse leaders at the helm considering which data is being collected, its accuracy, and the decision making surrounding the information garnered as well as how that information be accessed and used to form knowledge.

The volume of the data generated by our HIT has only highlighted the need for more innovative and future-focused nurses to consider the implications of collecting and storing vast amounts of data. These pools, lakes, and warehouses of data have been termed Big Data. Big Data is not just the data contained in one Electronic Health Record, but it transcends that one application in one organization. Big Data is a combination of structured, semistructured, and unstructured data collected by organizations that can be mined for information and used in machine learning and predictive analytics. Big data is characterized by large volumes coming from many environments, a wide variety of data types, and arriving at a greater velocity for storage and processing. The challenge to the future-oriented, doctorally prepared nurse is to find ways to use the tools available to us to drive outcomes, improve quality and safety, and maximize efficiencies. Future nurse leaders must be willing and able to actively collect and analyze data to answer questions that lead to improvements in business processes, finance, care delivery, safety, and outcomes as well as methods to support seamless care coordination across the care continuum. The critical role of nursing informatics requires strength in learning with, from, and about our healthcare team colleagues and exploring inter-/intraprofessional feasibility assessments to identify potential areas of system improvement (American Nursing Informatics Association [ANIA], 2015).

TABLE 3.2 ■ **Some Key Health Information Technologies Currently Available and in Use**

Technology	Description	Resource
Electronic Health Record	An electronic version of a patient's medical history that is maintained by the provider over time.	https://www.cms.gov/Medicare/E-Health/EHealth Records
Personal Health Record	A personal health record (PHR) is an electronic application through which a patient can maintain and manage their health information, communicate with providers, schedule appointments, receive health information, and other functions to improve their engagement.	CMS.gov (2021). Personal Health Records. https://www.cms.gov/Medicare/E-Health/PerHealthRecords
Social Media in Healthcare	Social media provides an opportunity for healthcare organizations to increase education and awareness about the most pressing healthcare problems of the time. Social media can strengthen counseling and empower patients to learn about their conditions. It is a driving force in the industry for disseminating information.	Kirstel (2022). Healthcare social media trends to watch in 2022. https://www.forbes.com/sites/forbesbusinesscouncil/2022/01/24/healthcare-social-media-trends-to-watch-in-2022/?sh=192cad18434d
Mobile health (mHealth) information devices	mHealth devices are a subset of electronic devices that are portable and wireless and are capable of transmitting, storing, processing, and communicating with other devices. mHealth solutions can improve collaboration between patients and providers. An mHealth device can be carried in the hand or worn on the body.	mHealth: A Journal for Research, Validation, and Discussion of Mobile Technology, Digital Health, and Medicine
Robotics	Robots are programmed to perform a variety of critical functions and may help to relieve clinicians for routine tasks.	Advent Health University (2022). Robotics in Healthcare: Past, Present, and Future. https://online.ahu.edu/blog/infographic/robotics-in-healthcare/
Nanotechnology	Nanotechnology is basically the science of the use of extremely small nanoparticles that can be used in diagnosis and treatment. Nanotechnology is already in use to target tumors, in drug delivery, and to improve medical imaging.	Anjum, Ishaque, Fatima, Farooq, Hano, Abbasi, & Anjum (2021). Emerging applications of nanotechnology in healthcare systems: grand challenges and perspectives. https://doi.org/10.3390%2Fph14080707

Population Health

Population health is defined as the health of outcomes of a group of individuals, including the distribution of such outcomes within the group, which includes the study of those outcomes along with patterns of health determinants, policies, and interventions (Kindig and Stoddard, 2003). Today population health is transforming and diversifying depending on the agency in which the program lies. However, the hallmark of population health is the significant attention focused on the multiple determinants of health outcomes. Population health program leadership seeks to ameliorate the impact of factors such as access to care, the social environment, and the physical environment on outcomes, not by assessing and treating patients one by one but by devising solutions for the problems common to groups of individuals.

The innovative and future-oriented nurse leader will actively team build and seek opportunities across the broad array of healthcare sectors to create programs that address population needs. Teammates on this population needs-based, opportunity-spanning adventure include insurance companies, nonprofit organizations, advocates, academics, and providers working in collaboration with the many different disciplines comprising the full healthcare team and span all points of care. Doctorally prepared nurses will be needed to lead population-based programs that are based on evidence. They will need to promote these programs at state and federal levels while advocating using data as a leverage.

Population health nursing leadership is needed across all healthcare systems, striving to reduce hospitalizations and emergency room visits in order to turn a sick care system into a true healthcare system. In thinking back to nursing's past, this is where the root of nursing started: knowing the community, knowing its needs, and determining solutions that go beyond medication and treatment to promote health and wellness.

Genomics

The Office of Disease Prevention and Health Promotion in Healthy People 2030 (ODPHP, 2022) reminds leaders that the overall determinants of health consist of several broad categories:

1. Policy Making
2. Social Factors
3. Health Services
4. Individual Behavior
5. Biology and Genetics

Our genetics contribute approximately 30% to our overall health status (Hayes & Delk, 2018). Some of this genetic input is based on what we inherit from our parents. Many are familiar with this germline testing that seeks to gain information for an individual on birth defects, cancer, cystic fibrosis, Huntington disease, and other conditions that are inherited. But there also exists genomics that describes the study of all of the person's genes (or genome) to include interactions of those genes with each other and with the person's internal and external environments. This is the basis for precision medicine, which uses this information about a person's unique genetics, environment, and lifestyle to offer each person more accurate and effective disease treatment and prevention. Doctorally prepared nurses are being called to lead innovative responses to this unique opportunity to provide patients what they need to treat disease, maintain health, and increase productive years of life by learning the specifics of how genomics drives many conditions. Probably the best-known use of genomics is in cancer treatment, in which patients are receiving targeted treatments based on their genomics and specific biomarkers. This process potentially gives patients a better chance at life while providing a fiscal benefit for the healthcare system by avoiding the use of treatments that will not make a difference for the patient but may also increase risk of harm. The AACN (2021) Essential Core Competencies for Professional Nursing Education does, under Domain 2, call for the advanced nurse to apply individualized information such as genetic/genomic, pharmacogenetics, and environmental exposure in the delivery of care. It will be for the doctorally prepared nurse to forge that path for all nurses so that they can assist patients whether they are seeking care for cancer, mental health disorders, neurodegenerative diseases, respiratory ailments, pain, or post-traumatic stress disorder (PTSD). A foundation for this work can be found through the Office of Research and Development of the U.S. Department of Veterans Affairs Million Veterans Program (U.S. Department of Veteran's Affairs, 2022)

HEALTH OF THE ENVIRONMENT

Florence Nightingale was ahead of her time when she identified an association between certain environmental conditions and patterns of illness. She taught that nursing practice *"ought to signify the proper use of fresh air, light, warmth, cleanliness, quiet, and the proper selection and administration of diet—all at the least expense of vital power to the patient"* (1860, p. 8). These concerns focused on homes and communities where sewage handling and air quality were problematic. When healthcare moved to hospitals, the environment of concern to nurses became constrained to the bedside and the operating room (OR), and our focus on the larger environment was lost (Kalisch and Kalisch, 1986).

More recently, nursing leaders have emphasized that healthcare is one of the largest sectors of industry that impacts the environment, and they advocated action. A panel of educators set three priorities for the discipline with regard to the environment (Pope et al., 1995). These priorities included: raising awareness of the environment as a primary determinant of health with hazards found in it as detrimental to all; emphasizing that nurses can make important contributions to alleviating health concerns of those negatively impacted by their environment; and raising awareness of the importance and impact of environmental threats. This team and the panel they represent identified a list of environmental hazards for society and nursing to address across all living environments, including the

TABLE 3.3 ■ **Environmental Hazards of Importance to Public Health and Nursing**

Area	Hazard
Living problems	Environmental tobacco smoke
	Noise exposure
	Urban crowding
	Residential lead-based paint
Work hazards	Toxic substances
	Machine operation hazards
	Repetitive motion injuries
	Carcinogenic work exposures
Atmospheric quality	Greenhouse gasses and global warming
	Depletion of the ozone layer
	Arial spraying of herbicides and pesticides
	Acid rain
Housing conditions	Rodent infestation
	Particulates from wood-burning stoves
	Houses and buildings with poor ventilation (sick building syndrome)
	Off gasses from plastics and carpets used in construction

Source: Pope AM, Snyder MA, Mood LH. *Nursing, Health, and the Environment.* Committee on Enhancing Environmental Health Content in Nursing Practice, Institute of Medicine. The National Academies Press; 1995. http://www.nap.edu/catalog/4986.html http://www.nap.edu/catalog/4986.html.

home, place of work, atmosphere, climate, and buildings. More detail is presented in Table 3.3.

Subsequently, a thorough review of policy statements and white papers from government agencies and health professions established strong agreement on areas in which healthcare professionals have opportunities to protect the environment and promote health (Kangasniemi et al., 2014) (Table 3.4).

Based on this review, Kallo (2020) recommends nurses expand their scope of responsibility and influence beyond traditional expectations to encompass responsibility for the environment that influences the health of those in our care and in which we practice (2020). This model for nursing practice in relation to the environment is presented in Fig. 3.1.

The scope and standards of practice from the American Nurses' Association explicitly state that *"The registered nurse practices in an environmentally safe and healthy manner"* (ANA, 2022a). This is seen as completely consistent with our social contract and with the Hippocratic Oath which emphasizes *"Above all else, do no harm"* (Hippocratic Oath, https://www.nlm.nih.gov/hmd/greek/greek_oath.html).

TABLE 3.4 ■ **Position Papers From Health Professions Addressing Environmental Protection**

Theme	NHS	HCHW	EPA	PGh	UNEP
Energy efficiency in water use	*	*	*	*	
Purchasing environmentally friendly products		*	*	*	
Sustainable waste management	*	*	*	*	*
Food	*	*		*	
Chemicals		*		*	
Pharmaceuticals		*			
Travel and transport	*	*			
Design of the built environment	*	*		*	

EPA, Environmental Protection Agency; *NHS*, National Health Services; *PGh*, Practice Greenhealth; *UNEP*, United Nations Environment Programme.
Source: Kangasniemi M, Kallio H, Pietilä AM. Towards environmentally responsible nursing: a critical interpretive synthesis. *J Adv Nurs.* 2014;70(7):1465–1478. doi:10.1111/jan.12347.

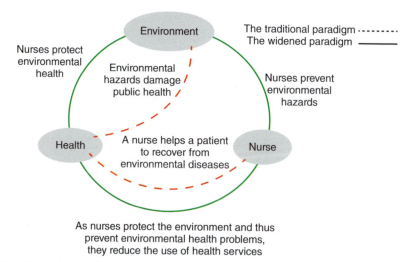

As nurses protect the environment and thus prevent environmental health problems, they reduce the use of health services

Fig. 3.1   Expanding the nurse's role in relation to the environment. (Source: Kallo H. Environmental Responsibilities of Nurses in Hospitals. *Dissertations in Health Sciences.* University of Eastern Finland; 2020. https://www.researchgate.net/publication/341398201.)

SOCIAL POLICY

Nurses in the United States and across the globe lament that their concerns and contributions are underrepresented in policies related to healthcare, even though those same policies have significant impact on practice and outcomes (Tønnessen et al., 2020). The American Nurses Association https://www.nursingworld.org/

practice-policy/health-policy/, American Academy of Nursing https://www.aannet. org/about/about-the-academy, American Association of Colleges of Nursing https://www.aacnnursing.org/Policy-Advocacy/Federal-Policy-Agenda, and National Academy of Sciences https://www.nationalacademies.org/home all advocate for greater engagement and highlight the impact of nurses in advocacy, crafting of legislation, implementation of policies that support accessible, equitable, safe, and effective healthcare, and monitoring the implementation and innovation that advance the health of society.

Nurses may be hesitant to engage in the work of creating policy. Still their perspective is valuable and their ability to advocate for members of society who are in need is valued because it increases the relevance of the policy created. Once nurses catch the bug, they tend to remain engaged and their voice becomes indispensable (Gebbie et al., 2004).

NURSES SERVING ON BOARDS

Nurses have much to contribute to the design, operations, foci, and impact of healthcare systems in part because of their proximity to the problems faced by members of the public and in part because they are embedded in and across these systems, making them fully aware of the strengths and weaknesses of those systems. Doctorally prepared nurses become experts in their areas of practice and carry knowledge of the science as well as the responsibilities of providing care and advocating for those in need. It is this intimacy, knowledge, and expertise that positions nurses to be strong contributors to the work of any board. It is the deep trust of society in the ethics and integrity of the nursing profession that makes boards welcome nurses to membership (Sundean et al., 2017).

Nurses serving on boards can bring evidence into the conversation in particularly effective ways. Over time their roles have evolved from passive ones characterized by observation and representation to more active roles that bring curiosity and inquiry to the table and invite application of scientific evidence to complement financial, market, and operational data to the work of the board (Murt et al., 2019). As society demands accountability for quality and value, nurses can provide perspective and experience with using data to improve outcomes and to promote responsiveness to the needs of the population served (Fox, 2021). For all these reasons, nurse participation on boards is on the rise, the trend promises to continue, and doctoral education positions nurses to achieve full impact that serves the board, the institution, the profession, and those in our care.

ACHIEVING DIVERSITY AND INCLUSION

In preparing for optimal healthcare delivery in the 21st century, more than ever nursing will need to build structures to increase diversity in our workforce that more adequately reflect the growing diversity of our national and global populations (Phillips and Malone, 2014).

This need to enhance diversity is not new to nursing and healthcare; however, the COVID-19 pandemic placed a spotlight on health disparities and their impact on care delivery. Now, more than ever, leadership is needed to effectively address this issue. Dr. Sullivan-Marx, President of the American Academy of Nursing noted in 2020, "*We must commit now to change, with fierce conviction, so that our profession can ease suffering and elevate health equity in our recovery*" (https://www.aannet.org/about/2020annualreport).

Growth in Minority Nursing

Ways to invite and bring more minority and ethnically diverse nurses into the workforce include factors such as pre-admission academic mentoring, financial support, and partnerships with community stakeholders. These are all deemed important to the successful recruitment and retention of underrepresented minority groups in nursing (Phillips and Malone, 2014). Structured programs such as the Guiding Initiatives for Doctoral Education (GuIDE program, www.guidetodegree.com) and Johnson & Johnson's Foundation of National Student Nurses Association Diversity Scholarships (https://nursing.jnj.com/our-commitment/diversify-and-strengthen-the-workforce), and resources designed to mentor men, ethnically, racially and culturally diverse nurses, have increased confidence among those considering doctoral education and led to impressive completion rates among participants (Taylor and Terhaar, 2018).

Best practices are guiding schools of nursing and places of employment to have institutional strategic plans that address recruitment and retention of nurses from underrepresented groups and build diversity in their organization. These efforts seek to create cultures in which diversity is embraced as value added. A clear focus on inclusion and belonging demands clear metrics that are tracked and evaluated to determine if performance is approaching and achieving targets for diversity (Kedge and Appleby, 2010). Numerous resources from our professional organizations are available to help your school/program/work institution build their diversity (Table 3.5).

Support for the development of cultural awareness, with specific attention to uncovering implicit biases, is a critical component of intrapersonal cultural humility. Implicit biases are deeply engrained learned stereotypes about people from diverse cultural and ethnic backgrounds that are often subconsciously developed (Fitzgerald and Hurst, 2017). Although they often occur outside of our conscious awareness, they can manifest in different ways, can go unnoticed, and can result in destructive conceptualizations of cultural difference. Nurturing a culture that fosters respect for cultural difference, appreciation of differing roles, and understanding of diverse backgrounds is critical for effective intercultural working (Markey et al., 2021). Nurse leaders need to empower staff to share and question differing perspectives in nonjudgmental manners as a means of supporting openness and respect for differences of all kinds. This requires the development of trusting working relationships, where shared understanding of social cohesion and respect for differences are flourished (Foronda et al., 2016).

TABLE 3.5 ■ Select Resources to Achieve Diversity in Nursing

Resource	Source
New Careers in Nursing scholarship program is supported by the Robert Wood Johnson Foundation and the American Association of Colleges of Nursing.	http://www.newcareersinnursing.org/
A range of webinars, programs, and publications are available through Minority Nurse.	www.minority.com
Statements condemning violence against Blacks, men, Asian Americans, and Pacific Islanders as well as other anti-racism resources are available from the National Coalition of Ethnic Minority Nurse Associations.	http://www.ncemna.org
Numerous resources and update on federal programs to promote diversity and combat racism, discrimination, and disparities are available through the U.S. Department of Health and Human Services, Health Resources and Services Administration, Bureau of Health Professions.	http://bhpr.hrsa.gov/grants/diversity
Information about the Minority Nurse Faculty Scholars Program sponsored by Johnson & Johnson Campaign for Nursing's Future in partnership with the American Association of Colleges of Nursing	http://www.aacn.nche.edu/students/scholarships/minority
Together We Advance an Inclusive Nursing Profession: A Model for Mitigating and Responding to Racism, Discrimination and Microaggressions is available from the American Academy of Nursing (AAN) Diversity and Inclusivity Committee.	https://www.aannet.org/about/about-the-academy/edu https://www.youtube.com/watch?v=zVDbFa5FPTI
Nurses Taking a Stand: A Tool Kit for Addressing Racism in Nursing and Healthcare Presented by ONL's Diversity, Equity, Inclusivity, and Belonging Task Force is available through the American Organization of Nurse Leaders. May 2022.	https://onl.memberclicks.net/assets/docs/DEIB/ONL-Tool-Kit-for-Addressing-Racism-in-Nursing-andHealthcare.pdf
A statement about accountability, racism, and reconciliation in nursing is available through the American Nurses Association.	https://www.nursingworld.org/practice-policy/workforce/racism-in-nursing/

The ability to navigate and construct multicultural environments that reflect our understanding and sensitivity to a population's experience and offer unbiased care has taken on a newer term: *Cultural Intelligence*. Richard-Eaglin (2021) offers the following:

Cultural intelligence (CQ—cultural quotient), which is the ability to efficiently traverse multicultural environments and interactions, can have a profound impact on cultural literacy and fluency. It is foundational in the embodiment of cultural awareness, sensitivity, humility, and competence, and in decreasing biased decision-making.

Improving Quality

Recognizing Quality Care

Although many nurses might not be able to provide a scholarly definition of quality care, we all know it when we see it. As a nursing student or practitioner, you have been exposed to literature or lectures that emphasize the critical importance of quality care. In your current position or once you graduate, you will choose to work for healthcare facilities that offer quality care and prioritize quality outcomes.

The doctorally prepared nurse takes responsibility for promoting quality in provision of 1:1 patient care and in the systems that support care. The future workforce will consistently use data and evidence to improve quality and the many parameters associated with it. As providers, we seek to achieve the best possible outcomes, reduce sequelae and complications, deliver a positive patient experience, coordinate care activities across all members of the team, and involve the patient and family in decisions. Tomorrow's nurse leaders will be leading teams that maintain focus on the goals of the patient and evaluate and address the care delivery regardless of setting, race, culture, age, beliefs, or other individual differences or sources of health disparities.

Effective care and services should be based on scientific knowledge and best available evidence. Using the resources from Agency for Healthcare Research and Quality (AHRQ, 2019) quality care will be:

- Safe: Risk of harm to users is to be minimized or removed. Injuries are to be prevented and medical errors eliminated.
- Timely: Delays in providing and receiving healthcare are to be kept to a minimum.
- Equal opportunity: Quality and access of care should not differ depending on gender, ethnicity, race, beliefs, geographical location, or socioeconomic status.
- Efficient: Waste is to be minimized and avoided, and resources are to be maximized.
- Effective: Achieving, restoring, or promoting the highest state of wellness, comfort, and function is always the goal.
- People and culture centered: Cultural preferences and personal preferences and aspirations of the individual and the community being served are always used to inform care.
- Ethical: The rights of the individual to privacy, autonomy, and respect are universal and unimpeachable.

Around the world, nurses and healthcare delivery systems are actively engaged in exploring what defines quality. A study of six European hospitals revealed that there is a positive correlation between the proportion of professional nurses at the bedside who had earned a baccalaureate degree or higher and the quality of the outcomes for patients and for nurses (Aiken et al., 2017). The AACN and numerous organizations are aligned in the conviction that education has a substantial impact on a nurse's ability to practice and that patients deserve the best-educated nursing workforce possible. The 2019 position statement, Academic Progression in Nursing: Moving Together Toward a Highly Educated Nursing

Workforce, highlights the need for collaborative solutions encouraging nurses to take the next step in their educational development to serve the nation's health needs (https://www.aacnnursing.org/News-Information/Fact-Sheets/Nursing-Workforce).

O'Connor et al. (2021) devised quality care process metrics (QCP-Ms) and indicators for practice areas: searching the evidence, selecting relevant documents, data extraction, validating findings, synthesizing, and refining nursing educational program theory. It is essential that nurses take advantage of the fast-developing technology and fully incorporate information technology across nursing education so that our profession will be better prepared to measure, evaluate, and track outcomes in order to drive improvement and achieve a higher quality of healthcare (Darvish et al., 2014). To prepare the future nurse workforce to identify, define, and evaluate quality care, nursing curricula will need to establish short-term and long-term specialized data driven informatics courses focusing on the primary target groups (Box 3.1) across curriculum: senior undergraduate (pre-licensure), working nurses, graduate, and doctorally educated nursing curriculum (Darvish, 2014).

The Primary Care Medical Home (PCMH) demonstrates a commitment to quality and quality improvement by ongoing engagement in activities such as using evidence-based medicine and clinical decision-support tools to guide shared decision-making with patients and families (AHRQ: https://www.ahrq.gov/ncepcr/tools/pcmh/defining/index.html). Yet, the U.S. healthcare system is facing a growing healthcare provider shortage in primary and specialty care settings as well as a burgeoning data management shortfall (AHRQ, 2015). Together with our healthcare partners, nursing is seeking to maximize quality in the future critical areas that we described in Box 3.2.

Sharing robust quality and safety data and improvement activities are important markers of a system-level commitment to quality. The ANIA recognizes that the

---

BOX 3.1 ■ Information Technology Is Critical to Ensuring Quality Care

Quality care involves using data and feedback:
1. to track and assess performance over time, and
2. to make necessary changes in processes to improve performance (Taylor et al., 2013b). Examples of activities to support continuous quality improvement (QI) include:
   - having a standing QI committee within the practice that meets regularly and reports back to the entire staff on QI activities and progress,
   - implementing a system for providing and acting on provider and practice-level feedback on selected quality measures,
   - developing an approach for identifying preventive service needs and gaps in care by running daily reports on patients with scheduled visits,
   - using decision support tools to remind providers to address these needs at the point of care, and
   - monitoring progress toward meeting quality goals over time. Health IT can support QI in many ways through data extraction and analysis enabled by electronic health records (EHRs), registries, and health information exchange (HIE).

BOX 3.2 ■ Medicare Shared Savings Program Quality Measures Methodology and Resources

Quality Domains and Measures for Performance Year 2019.

CMS will measure quality of care using 23 nationally recognized quality measures that span four key domains:

1. Patient/Caregiver Experience (10 measures)
2. Care Coordination/Patient Safety (4 measures)
3. Preventive Health (6 measures)
4. At-Risk Population (3 measures)—
   Mental Health (1 measure) —
   Diabetes (1 measures) —
   Hypertension (1 measure)

Source: CMS. *Medicare shared savings program.* Quality Measurement and Methodology Resources. Specifications Program. 2020. https://www.cms.gov/files/document/2020-quality-measurement-methodology-and-resources.pdf.

---

future healthcare workforce must be able to build and lead knowledge development in the area of clinical practice, people alignment, processes, and technology to support evidence-based information systems that enable the delivery of efficient and effective nursing care across the organization. New models for influencing quality improvement are needed and require nurses educated at the highest level possible to lead the planning and implementation of improvement efforts. Doctorally prepared nurses will use evidence and data to examine the pervasive barriers of constant change. Addressing the culture of quality and characteristics of the healthcare team will further enhance and sustain improvement efforts related to quality care and management (Tavernier et al., 2018).

CONTROLLING COST

Accomplishing the best possible value, not simply containing cost, must become the top priority for all members of the healthcare team. All disciplines have embraced the Quadruple Aim that charges us to *improve the experience of care, increase the health of populations, reduce the associated per capita costs,* and *focus on the quality of the work experience of the professionals providing care* in order to retain talent and perpetuate quality (Berwick et al., 2008; Bodenheimer and Sinsky, 2014). This focus on the experience of the members of the healthcare team emphasizes each caregivers' ability to find meaning in their work (Sikka et al., 2015).

Value-based care is a new development that relies on the voice of the patient and the community to influence decisions about the care offered and the design of the systems that deliver that care. This approach ensures that choices focus on health outcomes that matter to patients and consider the cost of interventions required to achieve those outcomes (Porter and Teisberg, 2006; Teisberg, 2020). This work requires open and ongoing dialog between clinicians (nurses included) and those in their care, and these conversations take the form of qualitative research, focus groups, and assessments conducted in collaboration with advocacy groups. The potential for nurses and nurse researchers to lead and have impact here is tremendous, and the work is new and waiting for talented professionals to take it forward.

INNOVATION

Innovation is a portal to increased satisfaction and retention among nurses, the redesign of healthcare, and improved outcomes for patients (Garson and Levin, 2001; Barr and Nathenson, 2022). Prioritizing innovation and unlocking its potential represent a relatively recent point of emphasis in our discipline. Some propose that the pandemic will have served as a disruptive force that opened the portal and brought down intrinsic resistance to innovation in healthcare practice settings (ANA, 2022b). Maintaining an environment that is hospitable to curiosity and innovation will be the leadership challenge that must be met in order to support innovation.

Learning the mindset for innovation promises to help achieve improvements at a pace that sustains the energy required to do so and reinforces both the need and the potential for progress in order to remain relevant in any fast-paced industry (Gutsche, 2020; https://nursing.jnj.com/innovate-with-us/nurses-innovate-quickfire-challenge).

Nontraditional Roles for Nurses and the Opportunities They Present

Doctorally prepared nurses at either the PhD or DNP level will need to prepare themselves to step out of the usual and into the innovative. The nurse leaders will need to forge paths in informatics and technology development and population health program development both inside and outside of the traditional healthcare enterprises. These nurse leaders will need to take a deep look at the Hospital at Home programs springing up across the nation. These programs seek to offer and deliver acute level care to patients in their homes and not in hospitals (https://www.aha.org/hospitalathome). Much of the work to success with a Hospital at Home rests with nurses. Doctorally prepared nurses will need to be in the communities organizing, educating, and leading the development of networks of resources to address the population health needs of the targeted communities. These uniquely qualified nurse leaders will need to take an even bigger leap into entrepreneurship creating new forms of healthcare provision using "out of the box" and innovative thinking, disruption, data, evidence, and vision.

Summary and Conclusions

Tremendous agreement exists among policymakers, scholars, various health professions, and nursing leadership regarding the vision for the future of nursing. This vision calls for nurses to be prepared for and fully engaged in informatics, population health, genomics, system reform, the health of the environment, social policy, achieving diversity and inclusion, improving quality, controlling cost, improving outcomes, and advancing innovation. Every aspect of the forecasted future invites nurses to develop deep knowledge and expertise and to create great impact. Pursuing your doctorate is an important step toward a future where you can contribute to fulfilling the social contract of our discipline and having a substantial impact.

Having earned your doctorate, you will be called upon to help visualize the future as we have done here in relation to those in your care, those in your community, and in your profession. Opportunity comes dressed as work. Your education will prepare you for both.

Bibliography

Agency for Healthcare Research and Quality. *Using Healthcare Information Technology to Support Quality Improvement in Primary Care.* 2019. Available at: https://www.ahrq.gov/sites/default/files/wysiwyg/ncepcr/tools/PCMH/using-health-it-to-support-qi.pdf.

Aiken LH, Sloan D, Griffiths P, et al. Nursing skill mix in European hospitals: association with mortality, patient ratings, and quality of care. *BMJ Qual Saf.* 2017;26(7):559-568. doi:10.1136/bmjqs-2016-005567.

American Association Colleges in Nursing. *Academic Progression in Nursing: Moving Together Toward a Highly Educated Nursing Workforce.* 2019. Available at: https://www.aacnnursing.org/News-Information/Position-Statements-White-Papers/Academic-Progression-in-Nursing.

American Nurses Association. Social contract theory this profession called "nursing," and its rights, privileges, and obligations. In: *Nursing's Social Policy Statement.* Sewell, NJ: American Nursing Informatics Association; 2015:1-28.

American Nurses Association. Standards of professional nursing practice found. In: *Nursing: Scope and Standards of Practice.* 3rd ed. Washington, DC: ANA; 2022a.

American Nurses Association. *ANA Innovation.* 2022b. Available at: https://www.nursingworld.org/practice-policy/innovation/education/.

American Nursing Informatics Association. *HIT Safety Position Statement. Addressing the Safety of Electronic Health Records.* 2015. Available at: https://www.ania.org/sites/default/files/assets/documents/aniaOverview.pdf.

Apter AJ, Morales KH, Han X, et al. A Patient Advocate to facilitate access and improve communication, care, and outcomes in adults with moderate or severe asthma: rationale, design, and methods of a randomized controlled trial. *Contemp Clin Trials.* 2017;56:34-45. doi:10.1016/j.cct.2017.03.004.

Barber H. The symbol of the cross as used in nursing. *Am J Nurs.* 1937;37(7):n788-n792.

Barr T, Nathenson SL. A holistic transcendental leadership model for enhancing innovation, creativity, and well-being in health care. *J Holist Nurs.* 2022. Available at: https://doi.org/10.1177/08980101211024799.

Berwick DM, Nolan TW, Whittington J. The triple aim: care, quality and cost. *Health Aff.* 2008;27(3):759-769. doi:10.1377/hlthaff.27.3.759.

Bodenheimer T, Sinsky C. From triple to quadruple aim: care of the patient requires care of the provider. *Ann Fam Med.* 2014;12(6):573-576. doi:10.1370/afm.1713.

CMS. *Medicare Shared Savings Program. Quality Measurement and Methodology Resources. Specifications Program.* 2020. Available at: https://www.cms.gov/files/document/2020-quality-measurement-methodology-and-resources.pdf.

Darvish A, Bahramnezhad F, Keyhanian S, Navidhamidi M. The role of nursing informatics on promoting quality of health care and the need for appropriate education. *Glob J Health Sci.* 2014;6(6):11-18. Available at: https://doi.org/10.5539/gjhs.v6n6p11.

Devore S. *Health Care in 2021: Five Trends to Watch.* Health Affairs; 2021. Available at: https://www.healthaffairs.org/do/10.1377/forefront.20210119.724670/full/.

Dickens C. *The Life and Adventures of Martin Chuzzelwit.* Oxford, England: Oxford University Press; 2009.

FitzGerald C, Hurst S. Implicit bias in healthcare professionals: a systematic review. *BMC Med Ethics.* 2017;18:19.

Foronda C, Baptiste DL, Reinholdt MM, Oursman K. Cultural humility: a concept analysis. *J Transcult Nurs.* 2016;27(3):210-217. Available at: https://doi.org/10.1177/1043659615592677.

Foxx M, Garner C. Qualifications of executive nurses for service on hospital boards. *J Nurs Admin.* 2021;51(12):626-629. doi:10.1097/NNA.0000000000001085.

Gandarillas MA, Goswam N. Merging current health care trends: innovative perspective in aging care. *Clin Interv Aging.* 2018;13:2083-2095.

Garson Jr A, Levin SA. Ten 10-year trends for the future of healthcare: implications for academic health centers. *Ochsner J.* 2001;3(1):10-15.

Gebbie KM, Wakefield M, Kerfoot K. *Nursing and Health Policy.* 2004. Available at: https://doi.org/10.1111/j.1547-5069.2000.00307.x.

Goodnow M. *Outlines of Nursing History.* 3rd ed. Westphalia Press. 2020. https://westphaliapress.org/editorial-advisory-board/ Re-release from 1926 publication.

Gutsche J. *Create the Future & Innovation Handbook: Tactics for Disruptive Thinking.* New York: Fast Company Press; 2020.

Harrison M. *5 Critical Priorities for the U.S. Health Care System.* Harvard Business Rev; 2021. Available at: https://hbr.org/2021/12/5-critical-priorities-for-the-u-s-health-care-system.

Hayes, T. & Delk, R. (2018). Understanding the social determinants of health. American Action Forum. https://www.americanactionforum.org/research/understanding-the-social-determinants-of-health/#_edn8.

Hippocrates. *Hippocratic Oath.* Available at: https://www.nlm.nih.gov/hmd/greek/greek_oath.html.

Johnson & Johnson Nursing. Available at: https://nursing.jnj.com/innovate-with-us/nurses-innovate-quickfire-challenge.

Kalisch PA, Kalisch BJ. A comparative analysis of nurse and physician characters in the entertainment media. *J Adv Nurs.* 1986;11:179-195.

Kallo H. *Environmental Responsibilities of Nurses in Hospitals. Dissertations in Health Sciences.* University of Eastern Finland; 2020. Available at: https://www.researchgate.net/publication/341398201.

Kangasniemi M, Kallio H, Pietilä AM. Towards environmentally responsible nursing: a critical interpretive synthesis. *J Adv Nurs.* 2014;70(7):1465-1478. doi:10.1111/jan.12347.

Kedge S, Appleby B. Promoting curiosity through the enhancement of competence. *Br J Nurs.* 2010;18(10):584-587. doi:10.12968/bjon.2010.19.9.48058.

Kavanagh KT, Saman DM, Bartel R, Westerman K. Estimating hospital-related deaths due to medical error: a perspective from patient advocates. *J Patient Saf.* 2017;13(1):1-5. doi:10.1097/PTS.0000000000000364.

Kindig D, Stoddard G. What is population health. *Am J Public Health.* 2003;93(3):380-383. doi:10.2105/ajph.93.3.380.

Liedtka J. *Why Design Thinking Works.* Harvard Business Review; 2018. Available at: https://hbr.org/2018/09/why-design-thinking-works. Accessed September 28, 2022.

Markey K, Prosen M, Jamal EM. Fostering an ethos of cultural humility development in nursing inclusiveness and effective intercultural team working. *J Nurs Manag.* 2021. Available at: https://doi.org/10.1111/jonm.13429.

Marr B. *The Five Biggest Healthcare Tech Trends in 2022.* Forbes. Enterprise Technology; 2022. Available at: https://www.forbes.com/sites/bernardmarr/2022/01/10/the-five-biggest-healthcare-tech-trends-in-2022/?sh=3d2ccab754d0.

Martin G. *Top 10 Emerging Trends in Health Care for 2021: The New Normal.* 2021. Available at: https://trustees.aha.org/system/files/media/file/2021/01/Martin_Top%2010%20Emerging%20Trends.pdf.

McKeirnan K. Examining the role of academic detailing in improving immunization practices. *Pharmacy Times.* 2019;1(2). Available at: https://www.pharmacytimes.com/view/examining-the-role-of-academic-detailing-in-improving-immunization-practices.

Medicare Shared Savings Program. *Quality Measurement and Methodology Resources CMS Specifications.* 2019. https://www.cms.gov/Medicare/Medicare-Fee-for-Service-Payment/sharedsavingsprogram

Morris G. Nursing and healthcare trend we can expect to see in 2022. *Nurs Healthc J.* 2021. Available at: https://nursejournal.org/articles/2022-nursing-healthcare-trends/.

Murt MF, Krouse AM, Baumberger-Henry ML, Drayton-Brooks SM. Nurses at the table: a naturalistic inquiry of nurses on governing boards. *Nurs Forum.* 2019;54(4):575-581. doi:10.1111/nuf.12372.

National Academy of Medicine. *Future of Nursing Report: 2020–2030.* 2021. Available at: https://nam.edu/publications/the-future-of-nursing-2020-2030/.

Nelson R. Informatics: evolution of the Nelson data, information, knowledge, and wisdom model: part 2. *Online J Issues Nurs.* 2021;25(3). Available at: https://doi.org/10.3912/OJIN.Vol25No03InfoCol01.

Nightingale F. *Notes on Nursing: What It Is and What It Is Not.* First American Edition. D. Appleton Company; 1860. Available at: https://digital.library.upenn.edu/women/nightingale/nursing/nursing.html.

Nuti, S. V., Wayda, B., Ranasinghe, I., Wang, S., Dreyer, R. P., Chen, S. I., & Murugiah, K. The use of google trends in health care research: a systematic review. *PloS one.* 2014;9(10):e109583. https://doi.org/10.1371/journal.pone.0109583.

O'Connor L, Coffey A, Lambert V, et al. Quality care process metrics (QCP-Ms) in nursing and midwifery care processes: a rapid realist review (RRR) protocol. *HRB Open Res.* 2021;3:85. Available at: https://doi.org/10.12688/hrbopenres.13120.2.

Office of Disease Prevention and Health Promotion [ODPHP]. Determinants of health. 2022. Available at: https://www.healthypeople.gov/2020/about/foundation-health-measures/Determinants-of-Health#biology%20and%20genetics.

Office of Veterans Affairs. *Genomics.* 2022. Available at: https://www.research.va.gov/topics/genomics.cfm#research2.

Phillips JM, Malone B. Increasing racial/ethnic diversity in nursing to reduce health disparities and achieve health equity. *Public Health Rep.* 2014;129(suppl 2):45-50. doi:10.1177/00333549141291S209.

Pope AM, Snyder MA, Mood LH. *Nursing, Health, and the Environment.* Committee on Enhancing Environmental Health Content in Nursing Practice, Institute of Medicine. The National Academies Press; 1995. Available at: http://www.nap.edu/catalog/4986.html.

Porter ME, Teisberg EO. *Redefining Healthcare: Creating Value-Based Competition on Results.* Boston: Harvard Business School Press; 2006.

Richard-Eaglin A. The significance of cultural intelligence in nurse leadership. Nurse Leader; 2021. Available at: https://doi.org/10.1016/j.mnl.2020.07.009.

Sikka R, Morath JM, Leape L. The quadruple aim: care, health, cost and meaning. *Br Med J Qual Saf.* 2015;24:608-610. doi:10.1136?bmjqs-2015-004160.

Sawin G, O'Connor N. Primary care transformation. *Prim Care.* 2019;46(4):549-560. doi:10.1016/j.pop.2019.07.006.

Sundean LJ, Polifroni EC, Libal K, McGrath JM. Nurses on health care governing boards: an integrative review. *Nurs Outlook.* 2017;65(4):361-371. Available at: https://doi.org/10.1016/j.outlook.2017.01.009.

Tavernier S, Guo J, Eaton J, Brant J, Berry P, Beck S. Context matters for nurses leading pain improvement in U.S. hospitals. *Pain Manag Nurs.* 2018;19(5):474-486.

Taylor LA, Terhaar MF. Mitigating barriers to doctoral education for nurses. *Nurs Educ Perspect.* 2018;39(5):285-290. doi:10.1097/01.NEP.0000000000000386.

Teisberg E, Wallace S, O'Hara S. Defining and implementing value-based health care: a strategic framework. *Acad Med.* 2020;95(5):682-685.

Tønnessen S, Christiansen K, Hjaltadóttir I, et al. Visibility of nursing in policy documents related to health care priorities. *J Nurs Manag.* 2020;28:2081-2090.

U.S. Department of Health and Human Services, Office of Disease Prevention and Health Promotion. *Health Literate Care Model.* 2021. Available at: https://health.gov/our-work/national-health-initiatives/health-literacy/health-literate-care-model.

Van Dover TJ, Kim DD. Do centers for Medicare and Medicaid services quality measures reflect cost-effectiveness evidence? *Value Health.* 2021;24(11):1586-1591. Available at: https://doi.org/10.1016/j.jval.2021.03.017.

Vogenberg FR, Santilli J. Key trends in healthcare for 2020 and beyond. *Am Health Drug Benefits.* 2019; 12(7):348-350. Available at: https://www.britannica.com/topic/Sairey-Gamp.

CHAPTER 4

Reflection on Challenges: The Nursing Workforce Shortage

Mary F. Terhaar, RN, PhD, ANEF, FAAN

Ah, the nursing shortage. It is a problem that ebbs and flows over time and will continue to do so across the span of your career. As this book goes to print, the American Nurses Association (ANA) reports that there are 4.3 million nurses in the United States (U.S.). We are the largest segment of the healthcare workforce. That number may seem like a lot, but the ANA forecasts that every year for the next decade there will be close to 200,000 openings for nurses (ANA, 2022).

Competition for bright and talented young people and aspirations for better working conditions, better pay, and more respect commonly call people who want careers in service away from nursing. Each of these facts alone is concerning. Together they paint a picture of a crisis in need of action. These are conditions that nurses who earn doctorates are prepared to overcome. You are needed to do the important work to mitigate these conditions and help our profession thrive and contribute to its fullest potential.

In this chapter, we provide a detailed picture of the nursing shortage and the kinds of solutions being implemented to address it. By the time you turn the last page of this chapter you will be able to:

1. critically consider the data that assert there is a shortage of nurses;
2. discuss the conditions that contribute to and perpetuate the shortage;
3. understand the importance of achieving diversity, inclusion, and belonging among nurses as we respond to the shortage;
4. discuss some of the strategies being implemented to address the shortage; and
5. identify the ways that your joining the workforce of doctorally prepared nurses contributes to overcoming the shortage now and in the future.

Data-Based Picture of the Nursing Shortage

Many entities are observing and analyzing the state of the nursing workforce and projecting a growing shortage. Data from multiple sources tell a compelling story.

- Nurses comprise the largest single segment of the healthcare workforce. In the United States there are some 4.3 million nurses (ANA, 2022), and globally there are 29 million nurses and midwives (World Health Organization, 2020).

- More than 275,000 additional nurses will be needed in the United States between 2020 and 2030 (U.S. Bureau of Labor Statistics, 2020).
- One million additional nurses will be needed globally by 2020 (World Health Organization, 2020).
- The need for nurses far exceeds the need for any other health professionals (American Nurses Association, 2020).
- Projections call for nurse employment opportunities to grow at a rate of 9% from 2016 through 2026, far faster than all other occupations (U.S. Bureau of Labor Statistics, 2020).
- The United States alone is expected to face a shortfall of 200,000 to 450,000 nurses for direct patient care roles by 2025 (Hagland, 2022).
- This 10% to 20% gap will require schools of nursing to double the number of nurses they *prepare and graduate* now for 3 years running (Hagland, 2022).
- More importantly, all those new nurses would need to continue to provide direct care in order for the gap to be resolved (Hagland, 2022).
- The shortage of nurses cuts across the entire profession impacting all specialties, roles, and practice settings.
- Nursing and society need more men, more women, and more people who identify as LGBTQ. We need more black, brown, yellow, and white individuals to provide the very best care in order to effectively meet society's needs in the near and long term.

The good news is that the number of millennials joining the nursing profession is on the rise just as pre-boomers, boomers, and Gen Xers are leaving the profession. These data are presented in Fig. 4.1.

Conditions That Perpetuate the Shortage

Many factors drive the nursing shortage, including population demographics, geographic distribution, and work conditions (Haddad et al., 2022). Let's consider those factors impacting practice now and those that will have impact in the future.

IN THE NOW

Three factors contribute to the shortage in the near term. They are the aging of the population, the pandemic, and the shortage of educators, placements, and preceptors. The impact of these factors in the near future will have downstream consequences that persist well into the future.

First, aging reduces the number of nurses in practice. Sadly, retirements far outpace graduations. Today, 1 million nurses are over the age of 50 that is, fully 25% of the nursing workforce (ANA, 2020). No professional football or soccer

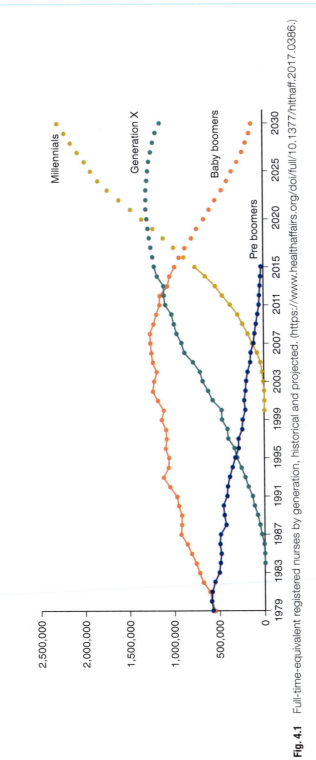

Fig. 4.1 Full-time-equivalent registered nurses by generation, historical and projected. (https://www.healthaffairs.org/doi/full/10.1377/hlthaff.2017.0386.)

enterprise would want to field a team with predominantly older players. These sports teams all have expansive farm teams and junior leagues in which they develop and groom new, younger players in preparation for the time when the experienced, seasoned players retire or are recruited away. Nursing needs a "farm league" too. We need a model and processes to develop our younger talent, to groom younger nurses for leadership and for growth in our profession (Poindexter, 2022).

Second, the pandemic has caused many premature departures from our profession. For those providing direct care, it has been especially difficult to see that society had access to, but did not effectively use, the tools needed to stop the spread of disease, avoid suffering, and prevent deaths. This crisis made clear to many who had not been paying attention that health disparities adversely impact people of color. We need to tackle this inequity and ensure that the benefits of science reach all. Doctorally prepared nurses will be on the front line of those efforts. As a result of the tremendous burden introduced by COVID-19, many in healthcare burned out and made career choices that took them away from the bedside and from nursing altogether (Haddad et al., 2022). The pandemic also resulted in an abrupt educational paradigm shift. The need for social distancing and prevention of the spread of disease demanded new curriculum delivery and new andragogy to prepare knowledgeable, competent, inclusive graduate nurses to serve a more diverse population. This needed to be accomplished at the same time clinical placements were difficult to provide and clinical instructors felt compelled to put in extra hours to help their teams cover staffing rather than serving as clinical faculty. Data support the conclusion that distance learning and other innovative pathways are critical to the preparation of new nurses and they support that baccalaureate preparation is a must (Porat-Dahlerbruch et al., 2022; Sokolowich et al., 2022).

Third, the shortage of nurse educators is significant and widespread. Noncompetitive salaries, lack of understanding of the role, and lack of respect for faculty all contribute to this shortage. Despite federal and philanthropic funding, the shortage of faculty persists (National Advisory Council on Nurse Education and Practice, 2022). As a result, nursing programs are declining interested and qualified applicants because they do not have enough teachers, which translates to an insufficient number of nurses graduating to meet the market's needs (Feldman et al., 2015). The problem is exacerbated by a coincidental lack of preceptors, competition for clinical sites, and pressured staff on units. All compound the challenge of educating the next generation of nurses and mitigating the shortage.

IN THE FUTURE

In addition to the factors that contribute to the shortage in the near term there is a group of factors that will impact our workforce and the health of society in the longer term. This group includes approaching retirement, geographic maldistribution, and lack of diversity.

Fully one-third of the nursing workforce is expected to retire within the next decade. The foreseeable lack of nurses will lead to high workloads, further stress at work, burnout, and even more departures from the direct care arena. These conditions beg for doctorally prepared nurses who will seek new solutions, discover new strategies, and translate evidence into practice. Opportunity usually comes dressed as work, and that is where you come in. The profession needs fresh eyes, new thoughts, and new collaborations that will result in finding new solutions and breaking free from patterns that have become ineffective.

Uneven distribution of nurses geographically leads to areas where the shortage is keenly felt. Data from the National Center for Health Workforce Analysis, which creates statistical models predicated on the assumption that healthcare utilization and consumption patterns hold, identifies seven states whose shortage will be most acute by 2030. These include California, which will need 44,500 nurses; Texas, which will need 15,900; New Jersey, which will need 11,400; South Carolina, which will need 10,400; Alaska, which will need 5400; Georgia, which will need 2200; and South Dakota, which will need 1900 (Health Resource Services Administration [HRSA], 2017). Based on these same assumptions regarding utilization, several states are predicted to experience a surplus of nurses. This group includes Florida, which will experience a surplus of 53,700; Ohio will experience a surplus of 49,100; Virginia will experience a surplus of 22,700; and New York will experience a surplus of 18,200 (HRSA, 2017).

There is a joke that goes like this. A statistician is one who stands with his head in the oven and his feet in the freezer and then says "on average I feel fine." If you are in an area of acute shortage, the impact is real and palpable even if the numbers on a macro level do not paint that picture. The innovations and strategies we develop and deploy will need to address the nuances and full scope of the problem. Doctorally prepared nurses will contribute to development of such solutions to all dimensions of the challenge.

Achieving Diversity, Inclusion, and Belonging in Nursing

Every day our society becomes more diverse. Between 2010 and 2019, the growth of diversity in associates and baccalaureate students grew as well. According to the National Center for Education Statistics 2020 report, we are making progress. RNs self-reported the following:

- 9.4% identified as male (0.3% higher than in 2017).
- 0.1% selected a third gender response option of "other" newly added to the survey.
- Nearly 81% reported being White/Caucasian.

- 7.2% reported being Asian, which represents the largest non-Caucasian racial group in the RN workforce.
- 6.7% identified as Black/African American.
- 5.6% reported being Hispanic/Latinx.

The number who identify as white is 12% lower, the number who identify as black is 14% higher, and the number who identify as Hispanic is 16% higher than the last survey, which was conducted in 2013 (National Center for Education Statistics, 2020). This is not a blip in the data, not a flaw in the fabric of our world and our communities today: Diversity is a defining feature. It is a strength upon which we can call to increase the quality and effectiveness of our problem solving, creativity, and innovation. That is true in the arts, in sports, and in science. Think of the rainforests. They are a microcosm defined by diversity. Each species living in the rainforest contributes to the environment and the community as a whole to the benefit of every species in it. The same applies to healthcare and its workforce.

The challenge we face is finding ways to achieve meaningful diversity and inclusion in the healthcare workforce so that those we serve in the clinical setting and in our classrooms see themselves in the faces, voices, and narratives of the professionals who serve them (Sokolowich et al., 2022).

We all want something to offer. This is how we belong. It's how we feel included. So, if we want to include everyone, we have to help everyone develop their talents and use their gifts for the good of the community. That's what inclusion means— everyone contributes.

—MELINDA GATES

Achieving diversity in the nursing workforce is the right thing to do, and your decision to pursue a doctoral degree promises to add to the diversity regardless of your gender identity, race, age, the language you speak, or the place you call home. To meet this challenge, we must create safe and inclusive spaces where everyone can learn, collaborate, solve problems, and thrive together. This will require new skills, norms, patterns, tenacity, and intent. Today's nurses are charged with identifying how tomorrow's workforce of doctorally prepared nurses will be made to feel included. As Melinda Gates shares, inclusion means everyone contributes and must contribute if we are to combat and overcome the shortage now and in the future (Fig. 4.2).

Strategies Being Implemented to Address the Shortage

A broad range of strategies are being embraced in efforts to mitigate the nursing shortage. They fall into three clusters: those related to academe and education, those related to the practice environment, and those related to professional organizations.

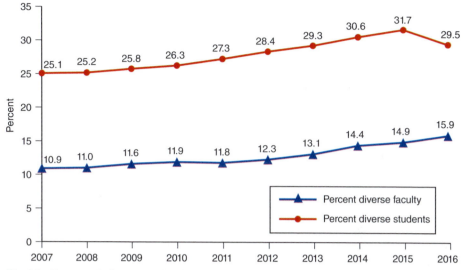

Fig. 4.2 Percent of diverse nursing faculty vs. percent diverse students, 2007–2016.[1,2] (From Nursing Faculty: A Spotlight on Diversity. American Association of Colleges of Nursing Policy Brief. Washington, DC: American Association of Colleges of Nursing; March 2017. Retrieved from https://www.aacnnursing.org/Portals/42/Policy/PDF/Diversity-Spotlight.pdf.)

STRATEGIES FOR ACADEME

Online and Blended Learning

Even before the COVID-19 pandemic, the number of students participating in distance learning was reported to be reaching nearly 20% (National Center for Education Statistics, 2019). Experts tell us that the prevalence of distance learning delivery has been accompanied by an increase in diversity. This is attributed to "convenience and accessibility for previously unreached groups, such as those who come from a rural setting or are underrepresented" (Sokolowich et al., 2022, p. 153). The pandemic itself catapulted nursing faculty into the 21st-century educational environment, creating the need for distance learning, online approaches, and blended pedagogies. Adopting evidence-based practices for distance learning fostered student engagement, a sense of community, effective collaboration, and

[1]American Association of Colleges of Nursing. (2017). 2016-2017 *Salaries of Instructional and Administrative Nursing Faculty*. Washington, DC. Percent Diverse is calculated using the percent of faculty that are American Indian or Alaskan Native, Asian, Native Hawaiian or Pacific Islander, Black or African American, Hispanic or Latino, and two or more races.

[2]American Association of Colleges of Nursing. (2017). 2016-2017 *Enrollment and Graduations in Baccalaureate and Graduate Programs in Nursing*. Washington, DC. Percentages will not add up to 100% due to the exclusion of students that had unknown race/ethnicity. Percent diverse is calculated using the percent of students that are American Indian or Alaskan Native, Asian, Native Hawaiian or Pacific Islander, Black or African American, Hispanic or Latino, and/or two or more races. Totals are derived from generic baccalaureate, MSN, PhD, and DNP.

meaningful inclusivity. Creating a community of scholars has been demonstrated to retain students and reduce attrition. The impact is particularly powerful among students from diverse backgrounds and those with lesser economic means. Retaining more diverse baccalaureate and graduate nursing students will lead to greater racial, cultural, and thought diversity in the profession, which can be expected to serve our nation's health: Greater workforce diversity is considered a strength when the goal is to improve access and mitigate health disparities (American Association of Critical-Care Nurses [AACN], 2017; National Academies of Science, 2021).

Mentoring

Nurse leaders in education administration agree that mentors have a significant positive impact on all new nurses, especially the new generation of minority nurses (Van Dyke, 2016). Consider this quote from Alexander Den Hijer: *"When a flower doesn't bloom, you fix the environment in which it grows, not the flower."*

Now, consider that sentiment in the context of healthcare: "When a team member doesn't bloom, fix the context in which they are not growing, not the team member."

Mentors help us find ways to fix the system and adapt our responses to the features of those systems that are fixed. They provide a fresh view to challenges and offer experience-based, evidence-based ideas for consideration. In the end it is the protégé's decision which wisdom fits and how to take steps to embrace it.

Finding a mentor may feel like a tall order. It is not uncommon to feel like asking someone to serve as your mentor is placing a burden on that person. In fact, many accomplished professionals seek protégées. Many professionals view mentorship as a responsibility and often a very rewarding endeavor. Most see the opportunity to mentor others as a way of giving back for mentorship given to them.

Still, initiating a dialogue about mentorship can feel like a very big first step. So, we offer some proven ways to explore mentorship in your place of work and doctoral educational environment.

1. Reach out to alumni. Ask if your school has an alumni program, and explore ways to engage with members there.
2. Ask leadership in your organization if nurses working in your facility are available to serve as mentors.
3. Consider your faculty or other colleagues whose skills and expertise you admire and respect. Invite them to coffee and ask if they might serve as your mentor.
4. Consider using social media or an app to establish a connection that would help you find other nurses who might serve as mentors and share their expertise.

SUPPORT AND ASSISTANCE FROM CLINICAL PRACTICE

Leaders in clinical practice understand that inclusive mentoring yields more graduates, happier nurses who stay in nursing, and better outcomes (quality, safety, clinical, cost, and operational).

In practice, it is well understood that support for development and investment in lifelong learning makes a big difference in important ways. Healthcare enterprises invest in their nurses in many ways that have been well reported in the literature:

1. Onboarding programs are common.
2. Transition to practice programs is standard across many communities and markets.
3. Healthcare enterprises of all kinds invest significant resources in training, dedication to lifelong learning, and professional development that build commitment and community.
4. Stackable training is popular as a strategy to improve performance and retention. The intent is for nurses to stay and thrive at ever higher levels of training and performance (think clinical ladders and incentives for performance).
5. Many employers offer loan forgiveness programs to encourage learning and development.
6. Recruitment and retention strategies and data are routinely posted on web pages and internet sites. This can be a great source for information about available resources.
7. Altered shifts or "workshare" approaches may be available to help you as your pursue your education (e.g., 0900–1400 shifts or other flexible options).
8. Some hospitals have strong community relationships that can contribute to development and provide opportunities. For example, the Assuring Success with a Commitment to Enhance Nurse Diversity (ASCEND) Program and nurse residency program work closely with nurses throughout their senior year (https://careers.akronchildrens.org/ascend-nursing-program/). Though it may be too late to take advantage of one of these programs if the facility offers one, they are likely seeing and building a forward-thinking approach to addressing the nursing shortage in their facility.

Creating strategies to meet the needs of an aging workforce must become a bright focus of leadership. Challenges faced by this group of seasoned employees include things like weight problems, physical pain, personal healthcare needs, family responsibilities, visual and hearing impairments, and manual dexterity challenges. This group is concerned about shift work and long hours (Uthaman et al., 2016).

Nurses over the age of 50 who remain at the bedside continue to find meaning and satisfaction in the work. They value their experiences with patients and families and derive satisfaction from providing direct care. Having opportunities to be heard and respected by leadership plays an important role in their decisions to remain in practice (Witkoski-Stimpfel, 2020).

Retaining this group of nurses and promoting safe, high-quality care requires attention. These older nurses are at risk for musculoskeletal injuries from lifting, are exposed to workplace hazards like needle sticks and exposure to blood-borne pathogens, face verbal and physical abuse from patients and families, and carry the demands of long shifts and the need to work overtime (Witkoski-Stimpfel et al., 2020). Strategies to retain nurses over 50 in direct patient care include the privilege of choosing the best shift and schedule for them, promoting meaningful teamwork, offering opportunities to mentor younger nurses, and ensuring leadership is attentive and responsive to concerns (Witkoski-Stimpfel et al., 2020).

The American Association of Nursing Leadership offers guiding principles for retaining older nurses that can help stabilize the workforce as we prepare nurses and leaders to assume their places. The principles are as follows:

- Commitment for retaining the older nurse in the workforce occurs across all levels of the organization (Senior leadership, Nursing leadership, MD leadership, HR).
- Organizations know and understand internal demographics such as the ages of nurses, intent to retire, types of positions vacated, and succession plans.
- Human resource benefits are designed to entice the older nurse to stay in the organization (e.g., health benefits).
- Alternative roles for older workers are designed and evaluated.
- Flexible work schedules are developed.
- Programs involving both experienced and newer nurses promote knowledge transfer.
- Training for various alternative career options is available.
- Environmental modifications with an emphasis on injury prevention are provided.
- Phased retirement or rehiring post-retirement options for older nurses are available.

https://www.aonl.org/system/files/media/file/2020/12/for-the-aging-workforce.pdf.

PROFESSIONAL ORGANIZATIONS

Professional organizations are embracing the benefits of forming young professional special interest groups and providing mentoring programs. It is important to join your professional organization for so many reasons. First, you can keep abreast with current developments and collaborations. Second, you can help your organizations keep informed about your practice and career experiences. And third, you can take full advantage of the brain trust in your specialty. These organizations have networks that span the nation and the globe. Resourceful, Inclusive, Giant Think Tanks!! (https://www.webscribble.com/blog/4-reasons-associations-need-young-professionals-committee). These organizations and special interest groups have been shown to offer tremendous guidance for nurses on their professional journey. They have materials, leaders, programs, funding, scholarships, and an incredible array of resources that can be helpful as you refresh your "bag of tricks."

Young professional groups expand opportunities for more significant support and reinforcement for challenging times.

1. American Nurses Association- https://www.nursingworld.org/foundation/programs/
2. American Association of Nurse Practitioners (AANP)- https://www.aanp.org/search?addsearch=mentoring

3. National Black Nurses Association (NBNA): NBNA Collaborative Mentorship Program https://www.nbna.org/content.asp?contentid=212;
   - New nurses/student nurses *(beginners or fundamental)*
   - Nurses transitioning into new nursing roles *(intermediate)* and
   - Nurses advancing into leadership roles *(advanced)*
4. SIGMA—SIGMA mentoring cohort https://www.sigmanursing.org/advance-elevate/careers/sigma-mentoring-cohort
5. American Association of Critical Care Nursing https://www.aacn.org/
6. American College of Nurse Midwives: https://www.midwife.org/Student-Rep-role
7. Association of perioperative Room Nurses: AORN Member Mentor program https://www.aorn.org/article/2022-04-06-Periop-Nurse-Mentor
8. American Association of Colleges in Nursing: Graduate Nurse Student Academy https://www.aacnnursing.org/gnsa-conference

Your Earning a Doctorate Will Be Helpful as Our Discipline Responds to the Nursing Shortage

As you embark on your nursing journey, our message is honest: the journey can be difficult. There will be days of pure exhaustion where you will not remember how you got from the shower to the bed before the alarm went off and you are back up and at it again. There will be other days when you cannot believe what you have accomplished and how far you have come. Together these days comprise the journey. There will be plenty of both days. You will learn to enjoy the good and struggle through the bad. But with the correct strategies and colleagues and resources you will discover that there are far more good days than bad. We want you to know that at the start, and then work to earn the good days.

In nursing, nearly 50% of all new grads leave their first position before the end of their first year of practice (Labrague & McEnroe, 2018). There is a parallel loss in doctoral study. Among those who are not well prepared or do not have realistic expectations it is easy to become discouraged and impatient. Our purpose is to help you set realistic expectations, help you understand the commitment, help you line up your supports, eliminate nonessential commitments, and set yourself up for success. We encourage you to do all of the following:

1. Write your own ***personal vision statement*** and post it where you can revisit it and reflect on it often. Clear goals help sustain commitment.
2. Make a ***to-do list*** that clearly describes what you intend to do to reach your goals. Share it with family and friends. Post it prominently and read it often. Update as needed.
3. Make a ***don't do list.*** This is where you identify the nice to-do items that are not necessary to do and then manage your time and effort accordingly.
4. Write an ***inventory of your personal strengths*** and put them to use.
5. Make a ***list of people who love you and support you*** who you can call on if you need support, encouragement, and reminders of your progress.

6. Make a ***plan for how you will use your time***. Think of items for that list in three groups:

    i. Stones: These are the big and essential things in your life. Your partner, children, family, faith, exercise, nutrition, classes, workyou name it. Plan for those first.

    ii. Pebbles: These are the things that you value but you might need to edit a bit. Travels. Activities. Volunteering. Professional meetings. Committees. Service activities. Plan for some of those but be careful not to overcommit.

    iii. Sand: These are the nice to do but by no means necessary items. These are the things that can go on the back burner. That is where you need to put them. You may need to delegate some, reduce the frequency of some, or say goodbye to some. Perhaps you have the kids do the dishes. Perhaps you hire a housekeeper. Perhaps you tell your book club that you need a sabbatical. Select carefully what you keep from this group. Do not allow the small things to keep you from your goal. That is wisdom shared and lived by many.

The point here is to recognize the value you bring to our discipline, your unique perspective, your remarkable story, then find ways to ensure that your personal strengths marry to the knowledge, skill, and competency of a doctorally prepared nurse, and then show up to take our profession and the people we serve to higher levels of health and productivity. That is why we all are needed. That is why the journey is worth it.

Bibliography

AACN. *Employment of New Nurse Graduates and Employer*. December 13, 2017. Available at: https://www.aacnnursing.org/News-Information/News/View/ArticleId/20903/Employment-17. Accessed September 1, 2022.

American Nurses Association. *Nurses in the Workforce*. 2022. Available at: https://www.nursingworld.org/practice-policy/workforce/. Accessed September 1, 2022.

Auerbach DI, Buerhaus PI, Staiger DO. *Workforce*. 2017. Available at: https://www.nursingworld.org/practice-policy/workforce/. Accessed June 2, 2022.

Feldman HR, Greenberg MJ, Jaffe-Ruiz M, Revillard R. Hitting the nursing faculty shortage head on: strategies to recruit, retain, and develop nursing faculty. *J Prof Nurs*. 2015;31(3):170-178. Available at: https://doi.org/10.1016/j.profnurs.2015.01.007.

Haddad LM, Annamaraju P, Toney-Butler TJ. *Nursing Shortage*. StatsPearls; February 22, 2022. Available at: https://www.ncbi.nlm.nih.gov/books/NBK493175/. Accessed June 17, 2022.

Hagland M. *McKinsey Report: Nursing Shortage Will Become Dire by 2025*. Innovation in Healthcare; 2022. Available at: https://www.hcinnovationgroup.com/policy-value-based-care/staffing-professional-development/news/21268125/mckinsey-report-nursing-shortage-will-become-dire-by-2025.

Health Resource Services Administration. *National Advisory Council on Nurse Education and Practice*. 2017. Available at: https://www.hrsa.gov/advisory-committees/nursing.

Health Resource Services Administration. *National Center for Health Workforce Analysis*. 2017. Available at: https://bhw.hrsa.gov/sites/default/files/bureau-health-workforce/data-research/nchwa-hrsa-nursing-report.pdf.

Labrague LJ, McEnroe-Petitte DM. Job stress in new nurses during the transition period: an integrative review. *Int Nurs Rev*. 2018;65(4):491-504. doi:10.1111/inr.12425.

National Academies of Science and Medicine. *The Future of Nursing 2020–2030*. National Academy of Medicine: National Academies of Sciences, Engineering, and Medicine; 2021. https://doi.org/10.17226/25982.

National Advisory Council on Nurse Education and Practice. Preparing nurse faculty and addressing the shortage of nurse faulty and clinical preceptors. 17th Report to the Secretary of Health and Human Services and the U.S. Congress. December 2020. Available at: https://www.hrsa.gov/sites/default/files/hrsa/advisory-committees/nursing/reports/nacnep-17report-2021.pdf. Accessed June 17, 2022.

Poindexter K. Mentorship for new graduates: responding to the challenge of transition to practice in a tumultuous and demanding health care environment. *Nurs Educ Perspec.* 2022;43(3):143-144.

Porat-Dahlerbruch J, Aiken L, Lasater K, Sloane DM, McHugh MD. Variation in nursing baccalaureate education and 30-day inpatient surgical mortality. *Nurs Outlook.* 2022;70:300-308.

Smiley RA, Ruttinger C, Oliveira CM, et al. The 2020 National Nursing Workforce Survey. *J Nurs Regul.* 2021;12(suppl). Available at: https://www.journalofnursingregulation.com/article/S2155-8256(21)00027-2/pdf.

Sokolowich JR, Ferguson PE, Hendricks KR. Taking the temperature of distance learners: does university climate influence perceptions of belonging in a distance education environment? *Nurs Educ Perspec.* 2022;43(3):152-157.

Uthaman T, Chua TL, Ang SY. Older nurses: a literature review on challenges, factors in early retirement and workforce retention. *Proc Singap Healthc.* 2016;25(1):50-55.

Van Dyke M. Mentoring the next generation of minority nurses. *Minor Nurs.* 2016. Available at: https://minoritynurse.com/author/mvandyke/.

Witkoski Stimpfel A. *Work Ability Among Older Nurses.* NIOSH Science Blog; August 12, 2020. Available at: https://blogs.cdc.gov/niosh-science-blog/2020/08/12/older-nurses/.

Witkoski Stimpfel A, Arabadjian M, Liang A, Sheikkhzadeh A, Schecter Weiner S, Vaughan Dickson V. Organization work factors associated with work ability among aging nurses. *West J Nurs Res.* 2020;42(6):397-404.

World Health Organization. *World Health Organization and Partners Call for Urgent Investment in Nursing.* April 7, 2020. Available at: https://www.who.int/news/item/07-04-2020-who-and-partners-call-for-urgent-investment-in-nurses#:~:text=To%20avert%20the%20global%20shortage,capita%20(population)%20per%20year. Accessed June 5, 2022.

Choosing Your Path, Making Your Decision, and Developing Your Plan

CHAPTER 5

Clarifying Your Options

Kim D. Jones, RN, PhD, FNP, FAAN ■
Jonathan H. Aebischer, DNP, FNP, PhD (c)

…and above and beyond all is the personal and spiritual attitude, and realization that she is not only serving the individual, but promoting the interests of collective society.
—Lillian Wald, 1913

Introduction

The Doctor of Philosophy (PhD) and Doctor of Nursing Practice (DNP) are terminal degrees in nursing, and each is highly valued in myriad settings that influence heath and healthcare, yet fewer than 2% of nurses earn these credentials (Campaign for Action, 2020; Shapiro et al., 2019). Earning a doctoral education in nursing is an option for those holding a baccalaureate or higher degree in nursing or a related discipline. In fact, the National Academy of Science and the Robert Wood Johnson Foundation have called for schools to develop curricula and resources that will advance students toward attainment of their terminal degree at a pace that far exceeds the traditional 5- to 7-year program of study that has been common for decades. Advancing to a terminal degree earlier in nursing promises longer careers of greater impact, which will advance the health of the nation.

Nurses with either doctoral degree are eligible for academic positions relevant to their education, background, experience, and goals. The American Association of Colleges of Nursing (AACN) program finder helps identify schools that offer these programs by state, enabling applicants to explore the full range of schools and evaluate fit with individual goals and aspirations: https://www.aacnnursing.org/Students/Find-a-Nursing-Program.

Many nurses choose to pursue non-nursing doctorates such as the Education Doctorate (EdD), Doctor of Public Health (DrPH), or Juris Doctorate (JD). These three are also classified as practice rather than research doctorates. Each is a terminal degree, but none is a terminal degree in nursing. We will present these options as well to support your fully informed decision of which degree option best meets your needs.

Boyer (1990) provides a model to explain the various forms of scholarship demonstrated by nurses. This same framework can help organize our discussion of the various programs for doctoral education. It is important to understand that nurses who earn each of these doctorates may demonstrate all forms of scholarship. However, each program of study prepares students to excel in one or two categories of Boyer's model (Boyer, 1990).

The four domains are presented in the model in Fig. 5.1 and explained as follows:

- The Scholarship of Discovery: Discovery refers to the conduct of experiments or explorations that seek to develop new knowledge.
- The Scholarship of Integration: Integration refers to interactions across disciplines to develop collaborations and innovations.
- The Scholarship of Application: Application refers to the responsible application of knowledge that improves outcomes to benefit individuals and organizations.
- The Scholarship of Teaching and Learning: Teaching refers to valuing good theory and best practices to achieve optimal learning.

This chapter provides an overview of the PhD and DNP options and introduces several other doctoral degrees that may be of interest to nurses, depending on their career goals. Our emphasis is on ensuring you have a full understanding of the many options available so you can select a high-quality program that matches your goals. The purposes of this chapter are to:

- Provide an overview of terminal degrees in nursing (PhD and DNP);
- Describe the non-nursing doctorates commonly sought by nurses;
- Highlight questions for key stakeholders; and
- Identify other factors to consider.

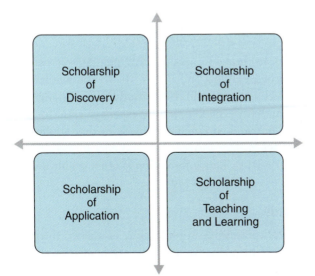

Fig. 5.1   Boyer's Four Categories of Scholarship (Boyer, 1990).

Overview of Terminal Degrees in Nursing

RESEARCH-FOCUSED DOCTORATE: DOCTOR OF PHILOSOPHY IN NURSING

Nurses who earn a PhD are groomed to advance nursing research and contribute to the development of new knowledge to support the discipline and practice of nursing (AACN, 1999, 2020, 2021c). Courses and experiences in these programs focus on theories, ways of knowing, the history of nursing science, quantitative and qualitative methods, analytics, ethics, and advocacy. Students who complete a PhD will have become experts in the area of concentration that is the focus of their research.

Students who pursue a research-intensive doctoral program will be required to develop a high degree of curiosity and self-direction. They will need to learn to embrace criticism. They must focus on achievement of long-term goals that include the conduct of original research, dissemination of findings, and securing grant funding to support a program of research. This is in high contrast to the educational experience in baccalaureate and master's level education. Research-intensive PhD programs foster development of the nurse as scientist, generally emphasizing depth over breadth of a phenomenon under study. Nurse scientists are often employed in academia. In fact, the PhD remains the preferred credential for those seeking faculty positions (NLN, 2021). https://www.nln.org/detail-pages/news/2022/01/12/nln-value-statement-on-workforce-demands-of-the-future-the-educational-imperative.

Career Opportunities for PhDs

More recently, PhD-prepared nurses are found contributing in essential roles across many sectors of healthcare beyond academia, such as professional organizations, health systems, government, and industry (Polomano et al., 2021). Careers outside academia require a workforce of nurse scientists able to bridge research, practice, and policy.

The AACN (2021b) lists 133 nursing PhD programs across the United States (including District of Columbia and Puerto Rico). You will have many factors to consider as you select your program. Evaluating PhD programs involves considering a school's or university's mission, faculty expertise, grant funding, research history and priorities, program curriculum, delivery method (online, hybrid, or direct contact hours via face-to-face instruction), and educational and technological resources (Jones et al., 2018). This information is often readily available on program websites.

Program of Study

Most programs offer coursework in philosophy of science, theory, ethics, statistics and quantitative research, qualitative methods, psychometrics, and multidisciplinary teams (team science). Some programs will offer additional emerging and priority areas of science informed by the National Institutes of Health (NIH), such as: omics (genomics, proteomics, metabolomics) and the microbiome, biobehavioral science, e-science/informatics, advanced methods, translational/implementation science, health technologies/point of care engineering, advancing health equity, and understanding social determinants of health (research priorities by the National Institute of Nursing Research [NINR] are found here: https://ninr.nih.gov/aboutninr/ninr-mission-and-strategic-plan).

Students seeking a research-intensive PhD could narrow their list of prospective schools by investigating NIH funding as one metric of research productivity. NIH is housed in the U.S. Department of Health and Human Services and is charged with advancing discoveries that improve health and save lives. Scientists, including nurse scientists, seek highly competitive funding from agencies such as the NIH. The Blue Ridge Institute for Medical Research lists schools of nursing, medicine, and dentistry, ranked by NIH funding: http://www.brimr.org/NIH_Awards/2020/) (Blue Ridge Institute for Medical Research, 2020). Students can best learn grantsmanship and the conduct of research by selecting a program whose infrastructure supports NIH funding and whose faculty have active and funded programs of research. As you make your decision, consider if you are able to relocate, as doing so can position you to work alongside experts in your area of interest and allow you to align your scholarship with a mature program of research (Jones et al., 2018).

Funding

The majority of funding for nursing and other scientific research is awarded through the NIH and NINR. These awards may be classified as: Program or Center ("P") grants (which provide funding for common, expert research, and exploratory topics); Training ("T") grants (which fund more specific, expert research); and awards for developing researchers ("K" awards) (National Institutes of Health, 2019). Research ("R") grants fund principal investigators (PI), and may offer additional training and financial support to PhD students working with the PI (NIH, 2019). Grants and funding may also come from private foundations (e.g., Robert Wood Johnson Foundation, Jonas, Gates Foundation) and professional organizations (e.g., American Nurses Association, SIGMA International Nursing Honor Society).

Fit

You will want to explore the faculty members' programs of research at each institution you consider. The more closely aligned your interests are with those research initiatives, the more your efforts will be advantaged by study in that program. You may not find a perfect agreement, but finding a close one is important. You may want to study with faculty who are investigating a particular disease process, clinical phenomenon, research methodology, or social challenge. In the long run, it is the goodness of fit between your interests and aspirations and those of the faculty that will help you be successful. Closely aligning your research interests with those of the program faculty will facilitate opportunities for mentorship, networking, and collaboration.

Options for Dissertations

Prospective students should inquire about the PhD dissertation types as they narrow their list of schools. There are two major types of PhD dissertations: traditional and manuscript options.

- The traditional dissertation is one large study conducted at the end of the required coursework that demonstrates the student's ability to apply all they have learned to the conduct of an original scientific inquiry. It is reported in a single five-chapter document and defended at the university with a panel of faculty who judge scholarship, rigor, authenticity, and results of the work.
- The second option requires the student to produce a set of manuscripts that may include an integrated review or state of the science paper, a methods paper, and a report of the work including the findings and results. This option advances the student's publication record.
- Both options position students for postdoctoral fellowships and faculty positions.

Questions for Key People

Once you have reviewed the websites of the programs that interest you, you will want to narrow the list of target schools to five or so. The questions shown in Boxes 5.1–5.6 could be asked of program faculty, leadership, staff, or students.

BOX 5.1 ■ Questions for Admissions Counselors

Questions for Admissions Counselors

1	When is your admission deadline?
2	How long does it generally take applicants to complete their application? Is there an application fee?
3	Do you use a computerized platform to receive applications? If so, does that influence my timeline in compiling my application?
4	Does your program require the GRE or other standardized examinations?
5	Are there any prerequisite courses such as graduate-level statistics?
6	If applying to an accelerated Baccalaureate-to-PhD or BSN-to-PhD, do I have the appropriate prerequisite degrees and courses?
7	Is my Grade Point Average (GPA) competitive with your applicant pool?
8	What is the cost of the program? What funding or financial aid opportunities are available?
9	Do you accept international students? Do they have specific requirements (i.e., residency, nursing licensure, English language proficiency)? Do I need an RN license from the state where the school is located?
10	Do you accept students who are not nurses?
11	Do you accept students who do not have an earned master's degree? If so, do I qualify for that track?
12	Are applicants required to complete an interview? Is this done in person?

GRE, Graduate Records Exam; *PhD,* Doctor of Philosophy.

BOX 5.2 ■ Questions for the Graduate or Research Dean

Questions for the Graduate or Research Dean

1. Is your university nonprofit or for-profit? Why should that matter to me?
2. Are there identified, signature science areas of the faculty?
3. Does your institution currently have grants such as T32 s, P20, P30 awards or a Clinical and Translational Science Award (CTSA) (https://ncats.nih.gov/ctsa/)? If not, how can I identify faculty who are currently collaborating within the school or with other researchers on campus?
4. How do you anticipate that faculty expertise and availability will evolve over the next 5 years?
5. How do you anticipate that federal research priorities will evolve over the next 5 years?
6. Do you have any broad career advice for me to become an independent scientist with sustained extramural funding?

BOX 5.3 ■ Questions for the PhD Program Director

Questions for the PhD Program Director

1. How many students are admitted to each cohort annually? How many students are currently in the program?
2. Historically, how many students complete the program in three years? In 4 years? In 5 or more years? Or do not complete?
3. What percentage of your students attend full-time?
4. Are there research/teaching assistant opportunities for students (for pay or tuition reduction) in your program?
5. How is the program delivered? Face-to-face, online synchronously or asynchronously, a hybrid combination with some students face-to-face and others connecting synchronously? Are classes "executive style," meaning that they meet 2–3 long days every few weeks? If the program has distance options, does my current state qualify to participate in your program? Do you anticipate the program delivery to change in the next 2–3 years?
6. Do you have an option for students to develop published manuscripts for a dissertation rather than a traditional dissertation? What are the trade-offs in writing manuscripts for publication rather than a traditional dissertation? At what point in the program do students need to decide which option is best for them?
7. What is the diversity in your current PhD students (e.g., race/ethnicity, first generation to college, rural/underserved, gender, veteran)? Same question for faculty.
8. What kind of jobs do your graduates have? Have your graduates taken post-doctoral positions?

PhD, Doctor of Philosophy.

BOX 5.4 ■ Questions for the PhD Admission's Committee Chair

Questions for the PhD Admission's Committee Chair

1. What do I need to know to submit a competitive application?
2. Do you have any faculty who match my area of interest? Be prepared to briefly describe your area.
3. How do I find the faculty's publications, grants, or other key information on the school's website?
4. What opportunities exist for taking courses outside the school of nursing or in an interprofessional scientific setting? Can I work with research faculty outside the School of Nursing?
5. Will you please introduce me to faculty at your school or other schools who match my area of interest?

PhD, Doctor of Philosophy.

BOX 5.5 ■ Questions for the Potential Faculty Member Matches (Advisor/Chair)

Questions for the Potential Faculty Member Matches (Advisor/Chair)

1. Are you currently accepting new doctoral students?
2. Based on your review of my application, do you think we have a research match? *(Be sure to read several recent publications by the faculty member and be prepared to ask broad questions about their research findings or future directions.)*
3. How many doctoral students and post-doctoral student committees do you currently chair?
4. Are you part of an interprofessional team of scientists? If so, what are each of your roles?
5. How do you negotiate authorship and dissemination opportunities?
6. What type of dissertation options are offered here (e.g., manuscript option or traditional)? How do you advise students in choosing a dissertation type?
7. Will you tell me about your experiences as a doctoral student and how that has shaped your approach to mentoring?
8. Would you consider giving my contact information to two of your current students or recent graduates so that I could talk to them about their doctoral experience?

BOX 5.6 ■ Questions for Current Doctoral Students and Alumni

Questions for Current Doctoral Students and Alumni

1. Who is/was your major advisor or dissertation chair?
2. How much access do/did you have to this faculty in terms of time and available data?
3. Do/did you publish or present at major scientific meetings with this faculty? Do/did they introduce you to key opinion leaders in the field?
4. How has this faculty promoted your independence as a scientist?
5. How have you handled any uncomfortable situations (e.g., changing advisors/chairs, changing research topics, differences in opinion between course faculty and advisors/chairs, unsuccessful in meeting a benchmark)? Please tell me about those.

BOX 5.6 ■ Questions for Current Doctoral Students and Alumni—cont'd
Questions for Current Doctoral Students and Alumni
6   How has your coursework promoted your independence as a scientist?
7   How much do/did you work as a registered nurse (for pay) during your PhD program?
8   Have you worked at the school as a teaching or research assistant?
9   What recommendations do you have for me regarding this program?

Note: Each school will have different structures or titles for faculty and staff. We suggest starting with the admissions counselor and identifying other key people in their organization. Resources in Chapter 10 will offer further guidance to organize your application for each program.

PRACTICE-FOCUSED NURSING DOCTORATE: DOCTOR OF NURSING PRACTICE

Nurses who earn a DNP are groomed to apply the best available evidence to optimize outcomes for individuals, populations, or systems (AACN, 2006). They tend to focus either on advanced nursing practice (Nurse Practitioners, Nurse Anesthetists, Nurse Midwives, and Clinical Nurse Specialists) or on leadership (in service or academe). These nurses will help shrink the 17-year gap between discovery (research) and impact (application) across all relevant settings. Like the PhD, DNPs become experts in the area of their focus. The difference is that their goal is to apply evidence to improve outcomes.

As you explore your options, you will find that this distinction is imperfect. Many PhD programs assert that their graduates are focused on improving outcomes in care as well. So, it is important to discuss in detail the program objectives and outcomes to ensure that you select the program that best meets your needs.

Students who pursue a practice doctorate will be required to develop a high degree of curiosity and self-direction. They will need to learn to embrace criticism and will need to identify a timely and relevant problem in their area of practice. They will need to focus on long-term goals, disciplined scholarship, and the conduct of a scholarly project. They will develop a full understanding of the needs of their teams with whom they work and the patients they serve, translate evidence into practice, conduct quality improvement, evaluate and improve programs, and achieve sustainability. As a DNP, you will be expected to disseminate findings in the facilities that host their work and more broadly to the profession. Moreover, you will be expected to repeat the cycles of innovation and improvement as a central component of your practice.

Fit

There are two categories of DNP programs, advanced practice nursing (APRN) focused and executive practice. The first prepares APRNs to practice at the top of their license. Courses and experiences in the APRN-focused programs include advanced pathophysiology, advanced pharmacology, and advanced physical assessment. The content in these courses builds upon coursework at the undergraduate level and is focused on the population of concern. One thousand hours of precepted clinical experiences help students develop the knowledge, skill, and judgment required for independent advanced practice. The second prepares nurses to lead teams and systems to achieve important change in complex and dynamic healthcare systems and other organizations.

Coursework

Coursework in both categories of DNP programs follows guidance from the AACN. The DNP Essentials published in 2006 provided the foundation for the early DNP curricula. New Essentials for Graduate Education in Nursing was published in 2021, and programs are working to revise curricula accordingly. This is important for you to understand because you will want to engage in a thoughtful discussion about the curricula you will follow during your selection process (AACN, 2021a). See Box 5.7 for the original DNP Essentials and Box 5.8 for the new Essentials for Graduate Education.

Career Opportunities for DNPs

DNPs can be found providing direct care to populations of patients who share common experiences and concerns. For example, DNP-Family Nurse Practitioners (FNPs) are seen in federally qualified health centers helping mitigate the impact of many social determinants. DNPs may provide care for very particular populations such as those with diabetes, heart diseases, transplant, cancers, sickle

---

BOX 5.7 ■ **Doctor of Nursing Practice Essentials**	
I	Scientific Underpinnings for Practice
II	Organizational and Systems Leadership for Quality Improvement and Systems Thinking
III	Clinical Scholarship and Analytical Methods for Evidence-Based Practice
IV	Information Systems/Technology and Patient Care Technology for the Improvement and Transformation of Health Care
V	Health Care Policy for Advocacy in Health Care
VI	Interprofessional Collaboration for Improving Patient and Population Health Outcomes
VII	Clinical Prevention and Population Health for Improving the Nation's Health
VIII	Advance Nursing Practice

American Association of Colleges of Nursing. DNP essentials; 2006. Retrieved from https://www.aacnnursing.org/DNP/DNP-Essentials.

BOX 5.8 ■ Essentials for Graduate Nursing Education

Essentials for Graduate Nursing Education 2021

I	Knowledge for Practice
II	Person-centered Care
III	Population Health
IV	Scholarship for Nursing Practice
V	Quality & Safety
VI	Interprofessional Partnerships
VII	Systems-Based Practice
VIII	Information and Healthcare Technologies
IX	Professionalism
X	Personal, Professional, and Leadership Development

American Association of Colleges of Nursing. The essentials: core competencies for professional nursing education; 2021b. Retrieved from https://www.aacnnursing.org/Portals/42/AcademicNursing/pdf/Essentials-2021.pdf.

---

cell disease, obesity, addiction, genetic syndromes, exposure to hazards, etc. The common denominator here is that DNPs become experts with a particular population and consistently use evidence and collaboration to achieve the best possible outcomes. They use data to evaluate those outcomes and test the impact of solutions derived of evidence. They advance the application of science in service of those in their care.

As of October 2020, 407 nursing schools across the nation (and District of Columbia) offer the DNP degree and an additional 106 are planning to launch new programs (AACN, 2022; https://www.aacnnursing.org/DNP/Fact-Sheet). In 2021, 381 programs offered post-master's options, and 280 offered post-baccalaureate options. Since the COVID-19 pandemic, applications to DNP programs have increased by 8.9% (AACN, 2021d).

The DNP practice-focused doctoral degree may be described as "direct" or "indirect" (AACN, 2015). A direct practice doctoral education has been traditionally linked to advanced practice registered nurse (APRN) roles (e.g., nurse practitioner, clinical nurse specialist, certified nurse midwife, certified registered nurse anesthetist), and have dedicated a significant portion of their curricula to patient care and development of clinical expertise (McCauley et al., 2020). AACN (2015) suggests that the DNP should be an entry-level requirement for APRNs, in parity with other healthcare colleagues (e.g., medicine [MD], pharmacy [PharmD], dentistry [DDS, DMD], psychology [PsyD], physical therapy [DPT], among others). More recently, the National Organization of Nurse Practitioner Faculties, which sets standards for nurse practitioner programs, made the commitment to move all entry-level nurse practitioner education to the DNP degree by 2025 (National Organization of Nurse Practitioner Faculties, 2018).

The DNP programs with an indirect practice focus are more commonly related to leadership in health systems and organization. These are often sought by prospective students considering a future in clinical administration or management, health policy, or informatics (AACN, 2015). Curricula focus upon systems-level processes and designs, multidisciplinary efforts to enhance health outcomes, and continuous evaluation and process improvement (Caffrey, 2020).

The impetus to a practice doctoral degree is supported by the increasing complexity of APRN practice and health systems, and the need for experts to advance nursing practice (AACN, 2015). One mixed-methods study of 29 nursing programs commissioned by AACN concluded that "the value of the added content of the DNP education is almost universally agreed upon" (Auerbach et al., 2015). DNP programs offer immersion into clinical and leadership sites for experiential learning; moreover, they help develop a DNP student's practice scholarship, fostering skills in evidence appraisal and synthesis, scientific-clinical translation, implementation and evaluation, multidisciplinary teams and collaboration, and data integration and dissemination (Armstrong & Lindell, 2020). Expectations are that employers will recognize the unique contributions of the DNP-prepared nurse as more DNP graduates enter the workforce.

Options for DNP Projects

DNP students are required to complete a final DNP project as evidence of mastery of the Essentials. The requirements for the DNP project vary to some degree between schools; however, all projects are required to produce an original deliverable that is intended to improve individual, community, and/or public health outcomes (AACN, 2021a). Importantly, DNP projects demonstrate student competencies that bridge evidence and practice, systems thinking, transformational leadership, change management, and interdisciplinary collaboration (Spencer, 2020).

According to AACN (2015) all DNP projects are expected to:

- Focus on a change that in-/directly impacts healthcare outcomes;
- Focus on systems (micro-, meso-, or macro-level) or population or aggregate;
- Implement strategies that are appropriate to a particular practice context and setting;
- Present a foundation in a detailed and sustainable plan that addresses financial, systems, policy, or other pragmatic realities;
- Demonstrate formative or summative evaluation of processes and/or outcomes;
- Describe significant contributions to clinical practice, systems change, and/or policy; and
- Provide a foundation for future practice scholarship.

Potential outcomes for DNP projects will vary according to a doctoral student's educational path (i.e., direct vs. indirect roles). Some schools, like Vanderbilt University, publish indices of projects by DNP graduates (Vanderbilt Univeristy, 2021; https://nursing.vanderbilt.edu/dnp/scholarlyproject.php).

Practice scholarship and outcomes also rely on curricula that provide solid foundations in methods for translation, quality improvement, change management, teamwork, and interprofessional collaboration as well as the resources, access to qualified faculty and mentors, and infrastructure needed to design and achieve systems improvement. Because the DNP is relatively new as compared to the PhD and EdD, the rigor and impact of DNP projects are the focus of significant oversight and there is an appetite for both evaluation and refinement.

Asking Specific Questions of Key Stakeholders

After reviewing information of DNP programs, curricula, and DNP projects at different schools via their websites, you will want to speak with representatives of the programs that hold your interest. Consider asking questions like the ones shown in Boxes 5.9–5.12.

BOX 5.9 ■ Questions for Admissions Counselors

Questions for Admissions Counselors

1. Do you offer prospective student orientation sessions to your DNP program(s)?
2. I found the following advanced practice specialties on your website: (e.g., Family Nurse Practitioner, Psychiatric/Mental Health Nurse Practitioner, Certified Nurse Midwifery, Pediatric Nurse Practitioner, Acute Care Nurse Practitioner, Nurse Executive). Do you offer any others?
3. What accreditation does your school hold? Is the DNP program accredited?
4. When is your application deadline? Is there an application fee?
5. How many students apply to my area of interest and how many are generally accepted?
6. When will my file be reviewed?
7. When will I know if I am offered an interview? If I am offered an interview, do I need to attend in person?
8. When will I be notified about admission status?
9. When will I know about my financial aid package?
10. How long does it generally take the school to process a completed application?
11. Do you use a computerized platform to receive applications? If so, does that influence my timeline in compiling my application?
12. Does your program require the Graduate Records Exam (GRE) or other standardized examinations? If so, which ones are required?
13. Are there any prerequisite courses such as graduate-level statistics?
14. If applying to a prelicensure-to-DNP or BSN-to-DNP, do I have the appropriate prerequisite degrees and courses?
15. Is my GPA competitive with your applicant pool?
16. What is the total cost of attendance in the program? (This information should be available on the web site.)
17. Do you accept international students?
18. Are there specific additional requirements for such students (residency, nursing licensure, English language proficiency)?
19. What else do I need to know to submit a competitive application?
20. Do I need an RN license from the state where the school is located?

DNP, Doctor of Nursing Practice.

BOX 5.10 ■ Questions for the DNP Program Director or Faculty Advisors

Questions for the DNP Program Director or Faculty Advisors

1   Is your university nonprofit or for-profit? How will that impact my experience?
2   How do you see the role of the DNP changing in the future?
3   How do employers in your area see the role of the DNP?
4   What are the unique features of your DNP program?
5   How many students are admitted to each cohort annually? How many students are currently in the program?
6   How many student projects does each advisor chair lead?
7   How long is the program for full time students?
8   What is average time from admission to graduation?
9   What percent of your students successfully complete the program?
10 Is there a part-time option? If so, how many of your students attend part time?
11 Are there research/teaching/practice assistant opportunities for students that help pay for tuition in your program?
12 How is the program delivered? 100% face-to-face, online asynchronously, a hybrid combination with some students face-to-face and others connecting synchronously from a distance, or some part online and some in-person at a specified site?
13 Are classes "executive style," meaning that they meet 2–3 long days every few weeks?
14 Do you anticipate the program delivery to change in the next 2–3 years?
15 If the program has distance options, does my current state qualify to participate in your program? (See National Council for State Authorization Reciprocity Agreements [NC-SARA].)
16 Are there opportunities to take courses or interact with nursing PhD students or non-nursing clinical doctoral students (e.g., MD, DDS, PharmD, DPT)?
17 What is the diversity in your current DNP students (e.g., race/ethnicity, first generation to college, rural/underserved, gender, veteran)?
18 What is the diversity in your current DNP faculty (e.g., race/ethnicity, first generation to college, rural/underserved, gender, veteran)?
19 What percentage of your faculty are DNP? PhD prepared?
20 What kind of jobs do your graduates have now?
21 Do you have requirements for the DNP project? How are your projects different from PhD research or undergraduate quality improvement/quality assurance projects?

DNP, Doctor of Nursing Practice; *PhD,* Doctor of Philosophy.

BOX 5.11 ■ Questions for the APRN Program Director in a Direct-Care Program

Questions for the APRN Program Director in a Direct-Care Program

1   Will I obtain a master's degree on my way to the DNP? If not, are there disadvantages to not having a master's degree?
2   Please tell me about your DNP projects.
3   If team projects are acceptable, what is an example of the independent role of each student?
4   Do students join ongoing projects, work independently, or in teams?
5   Can you give me some examples of recent projects completed by your students? Do you have a bank of completed projects I can view online or in the library?

BOX 5.11 ■ Questions for the APRN Program Director in a Direct-Care Program—cont'd

Questions for the APRN Program Director in a Direct-Care Program

6. What percentage of your faculty are nationally certified in their specialty and maintain a clinical practice?
7. What percentage of your faculty publish in peer-reviewed journals or present at professional conferences?
8. Do your students publish or present with faculty?
9. What national certification test do your graduates take? What is your pass rate for national certification?
10. Do I need to find my own clinical practice sites and/or clinical preceptors? How are clinical placements determined?
11. What is the total number of hours of clinical?
12. What are some examples of your clinical sites?
13. How much travel time should I expect for clinicals?
14. Do you provide virtual clinical (telehealth, e-health)?
15. Is it possible to do clinical rotations that will allow me to specialize in a population or setting (e.g., rural, veterans, gerontology, cardiology, school health)?
16. What recommendations can you give me to optimize my success in your program?

APRN, Advanced practice registered nurse; *DNP,* Doctor of Nursing Practice.

BOX 5.12 ■ Questions for Current Doctoral Students and Alumni

Questions for Current Doctoral Students and Alumni

1. How has your coursework and DNP project promoted your independence as a DNP prepared nurse?
2. How were you assigned to your project chair (the faculty overseeing your DNP project)?
3. How much access do/did you have to this faculty in terms of time and available data?
4. Do/did you publish or present at professional meetings with this faculty?
5. Do/did they introduce you to key opinion leaders in the field?
6. How has this faculty member promoted your independence as a doctorly prepared nurse poised to conduct and disseminate implementation science work?
7. How have you handled any uncomfortable situations (e.g., changing advisors/chairs, changing DNP project topics, differences in opinion between course faculty, preceptors, or other students, unsuccessful in meeting a program benchmark)?
8. How many hours a week do/did you work for pay during your DNP program?
9. How satisfied were you with your clinical site placements?
10. Did you orchestrate your clinical placements or were they secured and vetted by faculty? If the latter, did you have any opportunity to influence the choices? If you had to find your own clinical sites, please tell me about that process.
11. How would you suggest I prepare for an admissions interview?
12. What other recommendations do you have for me regarding this program?

DNP, Doctor of Nursing Practice.

Dual Doctorate: DNP and PhD

For nurses interested in becoming experts in both knowledge application and knowledge generation, the dual DNP and PhD in Nursing is appealing. Dual-degree programs combine course work, practicum experiences, and expectations for scholarship of the DNP and PhD programs to produce graduates whose competencies span both areas of expertise. These graduates will be counted upon to contribute to nursing knowledge that will be transferable and generalizable; lead and collaborate with scientific, academic, and practice teams according to research interests and goals; and influence evidence-based clinical, education, and policy initiatives (Cygan & Reed, 2019; Loescher et al., 2021). Similar dual programs are available in other health professions such as MD/PhD and DDS/PhD.

At least seven universities in the U.S. offer dual-doctorate programs with both post-baccalaureate and post-master's options. However, students may choose to complete two independent programs, often the DNP followed by the PhD. Within schools that offer graduates the DNP and PhD, in dually enrolled or individually enrolled programs, ample opportunities for team science and collaboration have great potential to integrate practice and research scholarships (Armstrong & Lindell, 2020). The prospective dual-doctorate nursing student must reflect upon *all* of the aforementioned considerations of the DNP *and* PhD, but also give attention to the time required to complete the degrees, funding and cost, and exceptional mentorship(s) (Cygan & Reed, 2019; Loescher et al., 2021; Sebach & Chunta, 2018). Completion of a dual-doctorate may depend upon whether enrollment in DNP and PhD curricula is simultaneous or consecutive, and overall access to data and healthcare systems, and often takes 5 to 7 years to complete.

Non-Nursing Doctorates

Some nurses choose to pursue doctorates outside of nursing, though this is less common as the PhD in Nursing and DNP become increasingly available. Nurses who earn professional doctorates outside our discipline may be uniquely prepared to influence policy, law and statute (JD), public and global health (DrPH), learning neuroscience and curricular development (EdD), and healthcare administration (DHA). Historically, nurses have also pursued the research doctorates (PhD) in other disciplines, including anthropology, organizational development, the hard sciences, education, or healthcare administration.

Table 5.1 provides a high-level summary of four non-nursing doctoral education options.

Other Factors to Consider

Regardless of your entry to practice education and the degree you chose to pursue before deciding to earn your doctorate, you have options. Historically, earning the

TABLE 5.1 ■ **Professional Non-Nursing Doctorates**

Degree	Selected Program Descriptions, Competencies or Outcomes
Doctor of Education (EdD)	An EdD, or Doctor of Education, in higher education, prepares students to teach or hold administrative roles at the postsecondary level. The EdD differs from the PhD in that the Doctor of Education is more oriented toward the practice of teaching with a deep and scholarly curriculum that supports a student's development and expertise in innovative curricula, the identification and analysis of organizational problems of teaching practice, and assembling diverse educational methods.
Doctor of Healthcare Administration (DHA) Or PhD in Administration-Health	The Doctor of Health Administration (DHA) program prepares students to fill a gap in health administration education. DHA graduates will be skilled in incorporating current technology in developing solutions to healthcare administration and leadership challenges, but not necessarily nursing care system challenges. Students who earn the DHA will demonstrate knowledge of healthcare finance, accounting, and general business principles in addressing the challenges of healthcare healthcare advocacy, or the highest levels of healthcare administration.
Doctor of Public Health (DrPH)	The Doctor of Public Health (DrPH) prepares its recipients for a career in advancing public health practice, leadership, research, teaching, or administration. DrPH graduates explore systems delivery that focuses on the human collective: epidemiology, biostatics, environmental and occupational health, public policy, nutrition, and maternal and child health. The curriculum of the DrPH prepares graduates with abilities to influence decision-making regarding policies to advance public and scientific knowledge to design and evaluate system-level and programmatic initiatives in multidisciplinary teams promoting public health outcomes and health equity.
Juris Doctor (JD)	A Juris Doctor degree (JD) provides graduates with an academic credential sufficient for training for entry into law practice. A JD graduate is guided in the knowledge and understanding of the law, legal research, problem-solving, legal writing and oral communications, and the numerous other professional skills needed for competent and ethical participation as a member of the legal profession.

https://www.usnews.com/education/best-graduate-schools; https://www.usnews.com/.

PhD has taken 7 to 10 years on average (2 to 3 years for a master's and then 4 to 7 years for the doctorate) (US News and World Report; www.usnews.org). The National Academy of Sciences and Robert Wood Johnson Foundation advocate for a far more expedient path in their *Future of Nursing Report* (2010). Thought leaders in these organizations strongly encourage programs to graduate students within

3 years after their master's degree and within 5 after their baccalaureate. Accomplishing this ambitious target promises to transform the workforce and healthcare. Accomplishing this goal presents significant challenges to nursing programs.

Achieving this paradigm shift is the reason this book was written. Smoothing entry to doctoral study where students select the best options for their goals and the best programs for their needs will go a long way to achieving the goals set by NAS and RWJ. The book you are reading was written in support of this goal: It is a target we intend to hit.

Summary

Be systematic in your search and patient in making your decision. Ultimately, selecting the right program for you will set you up for success and happiness as you enter the next phase of your career.

Bibliography

American Association of Colleges of Nursing. *Defining Scholarship for the Discipline of Nursing*. 1999. Available at: https://www.aacnnursing.org/news-information/position-statements-white-papers/defining-scholarship.

American Association of Colleges of Nursing. *DNP Essentials*. 2006. Available at: https://www.aacnnursing.org/DNP/DNP-Essentials.

American Association Colleges of Nursing. *The Doctor of Nursing Practice: Current Issues and Clarifying Recommendations Report from the Task Force on the Implementation of the DNP*. 2015. Available at: https://www.aacnnursing.org/Portals/42/News/White-Papers/DNP-Implementation-TF-Report-8-15.pdf.

American Association of Colleges of Nursing. *DNP Fact Sheet*. 2020. Available at: https://www.aacnnursing.org/DNP/Fact-Sheet.

American Association of Colleges of Nursing. *Doctor of Nursing Practice (DNP) Tool Kit*. 2021a. Available at: https://www.aacnnursing.org/DNP/Tool-Kit.

American Association of Colleges of Nursing. *The Essentials: Core Competencies for Professional Nursing Education*. 2021b. Available at: https://www.aacnnursing.org/Portals/42/AcademicNursing/pdf/Essentials-2021.pdf.

American Association of Colleges of Nursing. *PhD Education*. 2021c. Available at: https://www.aacnnursing.org/Nursing-Education-Programs/PhD-Education.

American Association of Colleges of Nursing. *Student Enrollment Surged in U.S. Schools of Nursing in 2020 Despite Challenges Presented by the Pandemic*. 2021d. Available at: https://www.aacnnursing.org/News-Information/Press-Releases/View/ArticleId/24802/2020-survey-data-student-enrollment.

Armstrong GE, Lindell L. The history and future of the DNP in nursing. In: Armstrong GE, Sables-Baus S, eds. *Leadership and Systems Improvement for the DNP*. New York, NY: Springer; 2020:3–22.

Association American of Colleges of Nursing. *DNP Fact Sheet*. 2022. Available at: https://www.aacnnursing.org/DNP/Fact-Sheet.

Auerbach DI, Martsolf GR, Pearson ML, et al. The DNP by 2015: a study of the institutional, political, and professional issues that facilitate or impede establishing a post-Baccalaureate Doctor of Nursing Practice Program. *Rand Health Q*. 2015;5(1):3.

Blue Ridge Institute for Medical Research. *Ranking Tables of NIH funding to US Medical Schools in 2020 as Compiled by Robert Roskoski Jr. and Tristram G. Parslow*. 2020. Available at: http://www.brimr.org/NIH_Awards/2020/.

Boyer E. *Scholarship Reconsidered: Priorities for the Professoriate*. Princeton, NJ: The Carnegie Foundation for the Advancement of Teaching; 1990.

Caffrey SJ. Leading process improvement. In: Armstrong GE, Sables-Baus S, eds. *Leadership and Systems Improvement for the DNP*. New York, NY: Springer; 2020:77-94.

Campaign for Action. *Welcome to the Future of Nursing: Campaign for Action Dashboard.* 2020. Available at: https://campaignforaction.org/wp-content/uploads/2019/07/r2_CCNA-0029_2019-Dashboard-Indicator-Updates_1-29-20.pdf.

Cygan HR, Reed M. DNP and PhD scholarship: making the case for collaboration. *J Prof Nurs.* 2019;35(5):353-357. Available at: https://doi.org/10.1016/j.profnurs.2019.03.002.

Jones KD, Baggs JG, Jones MR. Selecting US research-intensive doctoral programs in nursing: pragmatic questions for potential applicants. *J Prof Nurs.* 2018;34(4):296-299. doi:10.1016/j.profnurs.2017.11.005.

Loescher LJ, Love R, Badger T. Breaking new ground? The dual (PhD-DNP) doctoral degree in nursing. *J Prof Nurs.* 2021;37(2):429-434. doi:10.1016/j.profnurs.2020.05.001.

McCauley LA, Broome ME, Frazier L, et al. Doctor of nursing practice (DNP) degree in the United States: reflecting, readjusting, and getting back on track. *Nurs Outlook.* 2020;68(4):494-503. doi:10.1016/j.outlook.2020.03.008.

National Institutes of Health. *2023 Virtual NIH Grants Conference: Funding, Processes, & Policies.* 2019. Available at: https://grants.nih.gov/grants/oer.htm.

National League for Nursing. *Values Statement on Workforce Demands of the Future: The Educational Imperative.* 2021. Available at: https://www.nln.org/detail-pages/news/2022/01/12/nln-value-statement-on-workforce-demands-of-the-future-the-educational-imperative

National Organization of Nurse Practitioner Faculties. *NONPF DNP Statement May 2018.* 2018. Available at: https://www.nonpf.org/news/400012/NONPF-DNP-Statement-May-2018.htm.

Polomano RC, Giordano NA, Miyamoto S, et al. Emerging roles for research intensive PhD prepared nurses: beyond faculty positions. *J Prof Nurs.* 2021;37(1):235-240. doi:10.1016/j.profnurs.2020.09.002.

Sebach AM, Chunta KS. Exploring the experiences of DNP-prepared nurses enrolled in a DNP-to-PhD pathway program. *Nurs Educ Perspect.* 2018;39(5):302-304. doi:10.1097/01.Nep.0000000000000382.

Shapiro D, Ryu M, Huie F, et al. *Completing College 2019 National Report (Signature Report 18).* Herndon, VA: National Student Clearinghouse Research Center; 2019.

Spencer T. The DNP project—the essentials. In: Armstrong GE, Sables-Baus S, eds. *Leadership and Systems Improvement for the DNP.* New York, NY: Springer; 2020:221-250.

Vanderbilt School of Nursing. *Doctor of Nursing Practice program.* 2021. Available at: https://nursing.vanderbilt.edu/dnp/scholarlyproject.php.

CHAPTER 6

Clarifying Your Aspirations

Stacia M. Hays, DNP, APRN, CPNP, CCTC, CNE, FAANP

The ones who are crazy enough to think they can change the world are the ones who do.

—Steve Jobs

Choosing a path to a doctoral nursing degree can appear daunting at first. Essential first steps in the process include identifying where you are now, what you enjoy, and what you can envision your personal and professional self focusing on in the future. With literally hundreds of accredited schools of nursing to choose from, matching your career goals with a program offering high-quality faculty, resources to support you and your learning styles, and a mission that aligns with your nursing passion will lead to a rewarding and successful doctoral educational outcome.

This chapter will explore the roles and purposes of both the research doctorate (Doctor of Philosophy [PhD]) and practice doctorate (Doctor of Nursing Practice [DNP]). Additionally, it will help you decipher the variety of educational delivery options and identify markers of quality programs best suited to your learning needs and professional goals.

The purpose of this chapter is to:

- Provide guidance on identifying the degree option best suited to your personal and professional aspirations
- Explain the differences between the PhD and DNP credentials
- Discuss the components of each type of doctoral program
- Help navigate the variety of doctoral program delivery options
- Identify critical indicators that define high-quality programs

Your Personal and Professional Goals

- As an experienced nurse working in oncology, you see the effects of depression after cancer treatment on patients and families, leading to inactivity and poor quality of life. You want to understand why this happens so you can design an intervention to make an improvement in patient care and outcomes.

- You have gained experience as a neonatal ICU nurse. Through your work, you have recognized that little is known about optimal nutrition for extremely preterm infants. You have a passion to study and explore this problem.
- It is the end of another busy day in the clinic. As a nurse practitioner (NP), you look back at the positive impact you had on the new mother who was diagnosed with post-partum depression by utilizing the Post-Partum Depression Screening tool. Due to the identification of depression, she is receiving timely and appropriate therapy. The bonding between the infant and mother is apparent, and both are thriving.
- You have just left the board meeting of the hospital in which you work. Registered Nurse (RN) turnover numbers were above national statistics. As a nurse executive, your knowledge, experience, and expertise in this area have led to changes based on current knowledge that has reduced turnover and improved job satisfaction. As a result, RN turnover decreased by 20% over the past year.

To which of the above scenarios are you drawn? If you said the first two, then perhaps a research focus doctorate, the PhD, should be your path. If you chose the third and fourth, then perhaps a practice doctorate, the DNP, is right for you. Before we discuss the doctoral paths for nursing, consider:

- where you are now in your personal life,
- where you are now in your professional life, and
- where you want to be in your professional life (your goals).

Beginning your path to doctoral education requires time, motivation, and self-reflection. One way to take time and reflect on your future is to journal. The thoughts and stories you share in your journal can be helpful in clarifying who you are now and who, what, and where you want to be in the future. Are you passionate about improving patient care and outcomes? If so, then the doctoral path is definitely for you! The first step on this journey is to examine your time commitments (and constraints) and how you envision your career trajectory. Before deciding to pursue doctoral education, consider the time you are willing, and able, to put toward coursework and study; ask yourself if you are self-motivated to study and commit to a schedule. As a general rule, for every 1 hour of a course, the expectations are to be spending 2 to 3 hours outside of class time for study and additional work (US Department of Education, 2008). This means a 3-credit course will require a minimum of 6 hours of time outside of class per week, in addition to the 3 hours of class time. Is this time you are willing to set aside for your success? Consider your current job: will the hours or workdays be flexible with notice? Is your manager supportive of you furthering your education? Do you have supportive family or friends who can help with some of your other responsibilities, such as childcare, or cooking dinner, for example? It is important to identify early potential challenges so you can plan accordingly. Chapter 11, Time Management, provides a variety of resources for time management.

Consider your current professional position and experience. Do you identify areas for improvement at your workplace? Have you seen issues with "the system" where your experiences can innovate to lead change? Are you eager to take what the research says "works" and move it into your facility? These clinically focused questions will likely lead you to select the DNP.

Are you asking "how" or "why" of health, illness, and outcomes? What are the best treatments for providing optimal nutrition to extremely preterm infants? How does the family influence the end-of-life decision making of patients with a terminal illness? How will the COVID vaccine improve outcomes of patients of underrepresented minorities following booster shots? The nursing PhD, the "nurse researcher," will study and propose new discoveries that can be used to devise novel solutions to problems such as how to manage illness and its treatment to support patients toward leading meaningful and productive lives (American Association of Colleges of Nursing [AACN], 2021a). To answer these questions, one must have knowledge and skills in the theoretical, methodological, and analytic approaches to the discovery and application of new knowledge in nursing and healthcare. Taking inventory of your current workplace interests and strengths will guide you to the doctoral program that is right for you.

Nursing is a profession with almost limitless career possibilities and opportunities in a variety of settings and specializations. In considering your professional goals, look back at the scenarios at the beginning of this chapter. Is your goal to address the complex needs of the health system and lead change in clinical settings, either as an advanced practice nurse or executive? Perhaps your passion is to move and change policy related to healthcare. Are you excited about looking for new information, building new understandings and new facts? At the end of the day, what provides satisfaction and pride in your work, demonstrates your impact on care, and motivates you to do it again tomorrow? Your ability to clearly articulate your goals will be critical when applying to any doctoral program (more about this in Chapter 10). As you consider your pathway, an early step is to seek out two or three PhD- and DNP-prepared nurses to discuss their journeys toward their doctorate degrees. They can offer insight and support as to the *why* and *how* of their particular degree and specialty area.

Expectations of a Doctoral Student

Health systems in the United States and worldwide are evolving at an unprecedented rate. Not only are systems becoming increasingly complex, but caring for those within the system requires the ability to navigate advanced technology and the dynamic clinical expertise and leadership that doctoral education provides. Future directions of healthcare include a growing emphasis on cost constraints and value-based reimbursement, a wider lens on population health, rapid care delivery innovation, and changing demands of the healthcare workforce (Rubino et al., 2020). These trends highlight the need for increasing the number of nurses prepared as leaders in clinical practice and research.

As a student enrolled in a doctoral program, you are considered one of those leaders and will be challenged to contribute to the nursing profession. You will be expected to build upon the knowledge, skills, and expertise developed in previous educational programs and professional experiences. You will be required to read extensively, write in a scholarly manner, present to colleagues and other professionals (including legislators), and challenge the status quo based on current evidence (Valiga & Thornlow, 2018). Doctoral learning will require self-motivation and personal initiative, while independently seeking out resources through faculty and peer guidance. Interactions with faculty, peers, and other disciplines are expected to be professional and collaborative. These expectations may sound daunting, but they actually reflect the significance with which a doctorally prepared scholar is viewed. Doctoral education is an opportunity to gain significant influence in your career field that can help you become a powerful agent for change.

To Doctor of Philosophy or Doctor of Nursing Practice? That Is the Question

It is common for prospective students to struggle with the decision to attain either a nursing PhD degree or DNP degree. The goal of all doctoral programs in nursing is a "scholarly approach to the discipline and commitment to the advancement of the profession" (AACN, 2006, p. 3). However, the differences in these programs are both the type of preparation and the area of expertise conferred (Chism, 2019). Prior to 2004, choices were limited to research-focused doctorate degrees such as the PhD and Doctor of Nursing Science (DNSc), among a few others. This changed in 2005 when the National Academy of Sciences report titled *Advancing the Nation's Health Needs: NIH Research Training Programs* called for nursing to develop a non-research practice doctorate similar to medicine (MD), dentistry (DDS), pharmacy (PharmD), and law (JD) in order to "prepare expert practitioners who can also serve as clinical faculty" (see Chapter 5) (AACN, 2020). Prior to choosing a doctoral pathway, it is important to fully understand how PhD and DNP programs differ in their objectives, components, and outcomes. Understanding curriculum and its impact on practice before deciding on a doctoral degree will guide your decision and make your choice clear. Table 6.1 provides an overview of PhD and DNP degrees.

The Nursing Doctor of Philosophy Degree

PhD programs prepare nurses to conduct research focused on developing new knowledge that will drive improvements in patient care and outcomes. PhD-prepared

TABLE 6.1 ■ Comparison of Doctor of Philosophy and Doctor of Nursing Practice

	PhD in Nursing	DNP
Focus	Nursing Research	Nursing Practice
Objective	Prepare nurse scientists to develop new knowledge for the science and practice of nursing; design and conduct research to answer a nursing and related clinical and healthcare questions or test a hypothesis	Create nursing leaders in healthcare, populations, and communities; translation and integration of evidence (research) into practice
Curriculum Focus	Research design and methodology, philosophy of science, statistics, grant writing	Clinical practice, healthcare leadership
Impact on Practice	Generates new knowledge for clinical practice and adds to knowledge base	Assesses, implements, and improves processes, programs, and systems to improve patient and organizational outcomes
Clinical Hours	None	1000 minimum, with additional for scholarly project
Scholarly Project	No	Yes: Quality Improvement or Evidence-Based Practice focus
Dissertation	Yes: An intense mentored research experience with a faculty investigator with an established funded program of research	No
Point of Entry	BSN or related nursing master's degree	BSN or master's degree. Certification may be required
Program Length	3–5 years full-time study	BSN-DNP 3–5 years full-time study; more if course load is reduced Post-Masters DNP 1–3 years; more if course load is reduced.
Funding	Varies from program to program	Varies from program to program
Employment Opportunities	Nurse scientists prepared for a career in research, academia or other research-intensive environments focused on the development of new knowledge and the design of interventions to advance nursing and healthcare	Nurse leaders including advanced practice nurses and administrators prepared to implement clinical innovation and knowledge translation to benefit individuals, populations, organizations, and communities

DNP, Doctor of Nursing Practice; *PhD,* Doctor of Philosophy.

nurses focus their original research on particular areas, or themes, of interest to them that are relevant and timely. These nurse researchers carry out clinical research in a variety of areas. Some examples include trajectories of chronic care such as those related to cancer, aspects of psychiatric and mental health disorders, wellness issues such as smoking cessation, and health policy. Through conducting research and leading interdisciplinary research teams, the PhD nurse builds a more robust body of knowledge that can be expected to add to current practice science to support all aspects of care within a variety of healthcare disciplines (Neal-Boylan, 2020). Nurse scientists are expected to disseminate work in peer-reviewed journals and with national and international presentations. Researchers in many settings are often expected to secure grant funding for their research, and it is not uncommon for a portion of their salary to be generated from this funding support as well. PhD-prepared nurses can be found in a variety of settings, including academia, industry, healthcare agencies, hospitals, and policy arenas.

DOCTOR OF PHILOSOPHY CURRICULA

All nursing PhD curricula require similar core courses. These include advanced research methods, focus on quantitative and qualitative research, statistics, philosophy of science, and theory development. The PhD program requires commitment but can offer flexibility related to full or part-time study. Typically, a PhD requires:

- Investing 3 to 5 years, depending on full- or part-time study
- Creating a viable research proposal
- Conducting research
- Propose an original scientific investigtion based on a deep understanding of all related knowledge and science
- Demonstrating understanding and application of the core principles through a "Qualifying Exam"
- Defending a completed research project (the "Defense") with an oral presentation to your PhD committee and other experts in your research area (Nursing Times, 2020).

ADMISSION REQUIREMENTS AND FINANCIAL ASPECTS OF OBTAINING A DOCTOR OF PHILOSOPHY

There are two main points of entry for the PhD. In the past, most nursing PhD programs were open to those holding master's degrees in nursing or a related field. Today many schools offer BSN-to-PhD programs where students proceed directly from the entry to nursing practice education into the highest level of nursing education.

The admission requirements vary, but generally the application packet requires transcripts from all previous schools attended, GRE results (which are increasingly becoming optional), a personal statement or essay, established proficiency in the

English language, and letters of recommendation (AACN, 2021a) (for information on the application process, see Chapter 10).

Many schools offer stipends or tuition support for PhD students, as well as scholarship opportunities. Financial support may be obtained through competitive academic and research awards (AACN, 2010). There may be part-time job opportunities to serve as a research or teaching assistant to decrease the cost of tuition. This information may be posted on the program website, but if not, inquire with the admissions office.

THE DOCTOR OF PHILOSOPHY DISSERTATION

The PhD dissertation is a comprehensive and highly structured process that generates new knowledge and results in production of document summarizing independent student-led research completed during the program. The dissertation is a scholarly work that synthesizes the problem statement, background, significance, literature, hypotheses, methods, measures, data, analytics, evaluation, results, conclusions, and implications of the work (Graves et al., 2018).

The Doctor of Nursing Practice Degree

Nursing has responded to the changing demands and complexity with the development of a practice-focused doctorate, the DNP degree (Chism, 2019). This highest level of educational preparation is the terminal degree for advanced practice nursing in order to support the highest knowledge and practice expertise to assure high-quality patient outcomes (AACN, 2020).

DNP programs are designed to prepare nurse leaders as experts in their respective areas of practice prepared to lead system-wide, evidence-based changes to improve health (Chism, 2019). This is achieved through a concentration in advanced practice nursing (APRN) or nurse executive leadership. DNP-prepared nurses are addressing healthcare dilemmas in areas of clinical practice, health policy and advocacy, health systems leadership, academia, and informational technology, among others (Valiga & Thornlow, 2018). DNP scholarship generates innovative practices and processes in settings, systems, or populations (Chism, 2019).

What truly distinguishes the DNP from the PhD is the disciplined approach to selecting trustworthy research findings and develop in change management plans that facilitate effective uptake of the research in clinical settings and evaluate the impact of the efforts. This is achieved through the application of evidence-based practice (EBP) and quality improvement (QI) processes and initiatives. In EBP, evidence is applied in clinical practice settings. In QI, clinical practices are evaluated and modified based on outcomes. EBP and QI processes work together for meaningful translation and implementation of evidence to develop and improve processes and outcomes for individuals, communities, and systems.

The DNP is an expert at identifying problems in practice settings, critiquing the evidence, selecting trustworthy strategies suited to the particular practice environment, planning and implementing practice changes, assessing and evaluating outcomes, and adjusting processes to achieve sustainable change. The translation and implementation of evidence serve to develop and improve processes and outcomes for individuals, communities, and systems.

As you can see, the DNP degree is appropriate for nurses from a variety of backgrounds who want to gain knowledge and advance their expertise as in clinical practice, implementation of EBP, QI initiatives, health policy, and other areas. DNP-prepared nurses can be found in a variety of settings, including academia, industry, healthcare agencies, hospitals, and policy arenas.

DOCTOR OF NURSING PRACTICE CURRICULA

All DNP curricula build upon the master's in nursing programs through coursework in QI, and systems leadership. Courses also include statistics, ethics, and theories related to the clinical setting. In 2006, the American Association of Colleges of Nursing (AACN) implemented the Essentials of Doctoral Education for Advanced Nursing Practice. In 2021, AACN initiated a revision of the Essentials. Until approved, the current seven essentials remain the foundational outcome competencies for graduates of all DNP programs (AACN, 2021b-essentials) Table 6.2 presents the original DNP Essentials and the revised Domains for Graduate Nursing Education.

TABLE 6.2 ■ **Comparison of Original DNP Essentials with New Essentials for Graduate Nursing Education**

	Essentials for Graduate Nursing Education 2022	DNP Essentials 2006
I	Knowledge for Practice	Scientific underpinnings for practice
II	Person-centered Care	Organizational and Systems Leadership for Quality Improvement and Systems Thinking
III	Population Health	Clinical Scholarship and Analytical Methods for Evidence-Based Practice
IV	Scholarship for Nursing Practice	Information Systems-Technology and Patient-Care Technology for the Improvement and Transformation of Healthcare
V	Quality & Safety	Health Care Policy for Advocacy in Health Care
VI	Interprofessional Partnerships	Interprofessional Collaboration for Improving Patient and Population Health Outcomes
VII	Systems-Based Practice	Advanced Nursing Practice
VIII	Information and Healthcare Technologies	
IX	Professionalism	
X	Personal, Professional, and Leadership Development	

Just as in the PhD program, the DNP program requires commitment but can be flexible related to full- or part-time study. Typically, a DNP requires:

- Investing 1 to 3 years, depending on full- or part-time study
- Demonstrating understanding and application of the Essentials for Graduate Nursing Education through successful course work and DNP Scholarly Project
- Creating a viable practice-based scholarly proposal
- Completing a practice-based Scholarly Project
- Disseminating the results of the Scholarly Project.

DOCTOR OF NURSING PRACTICE SCHOLARLY PROJECT

Unique to the DNP is the scholarly project. The project aim is to improve care outcomes through evidence-based or QI initiatives while demonstrating understanding and application of the Essential for Graduate Nursing Education (AACN, 2020).

Components of the DNP scholarly project include:

- Generating a problem statement
- Critiquing the evidence
- Implementing an evidence-based or QI project that impacts care and supports a practice setting
- Evaluating outcomes, and adjusting processes to achieve sustainable change.
- Disseminating results

ADMISSION REQUIREMENTS AND FINANCIAL ASPECTS OF OBTAINING A DOCTOR OF NURSING PRACTICE

Although stipends are not commonly offered for DNP students, federal grant monies are available through the Title VIII Nursing Workforce Reauthorization Act of 2019 (Congress.gov). Funding amounts and requirements change frequently but can be accessed through the .gov website. Many professional organizations offer scholarships to their student members based on need, scholarly project, and other deliverables. Chapter 10 offers numerous financial strategies and resources that support doctoral students on this educational journey. Finally, never hesitate to reach out to the selected program's admissions office for more information.

Table 6.3 provides examples of the kinds of problems and challenges PhD and DNPs will address in their scholarship and throughout their careers.

Selecting a Quality Program

Choosing a quality program that meets your needs can take some time. Your search should include:

- Identification of accredited nursing schools with degree options
- Certification exam pass rates
- Delivery format (brick and mortar, online, or hybrid)

TABLE 6.3 ■ **Comparison of Doctor of Philosophy and Doctor of Nursing Practice Approaches**

Problem	PhD	DNP
Communication issues and adverse events that occur after patients are admitted from the recovery room	Development and validation of a new hand-off reporting tool.	Implementation of formal hand-off reporting.
Factors that influence 30-day unplanned readmissions in adults with heart failure	Prospective or retrospective study to identify factors.	Hospital-wide process improvement initiative to prevent or mitigate factors contributing to readmission.
Controllable influences on coronary artery disease	Research to identify association between vitamin D levels, blood pressure, and depression in adults with coronary artery disease.	Implementation of order sets incorporating vitamin D dosing and depression screening in adults with coronary artery disease in the primary care setting.
Quality of life in those with chronic renal failure	Measuring and improving quality of lives for adults living with chronic renal failure.	Utilization of the quality-of-life tool, incorporating activities that have been demonstrating to improve quality of life in adults with chronic renal failure.
RN turnover rates in the hospital setting	Studies identifying factors that influence RN job satisfaction.	Implementation of a clinical ladder to support the development and expertise of RNs in the hospital setting.

DNP, Doctor of Nursing Practice; *PhD*, Doctor of Philosophy; *RN*, registered nurse.

- Course load and time to degree completion
- Faculty to student ratio
- Faculty outcomes demonstrating expertise and success such as manuscripts, textbooks, presentations, professional leadership activities
- Clinical faculty practicing in their specialty
- For those pursuing a PhD: are there faculty whose research agendas align with your interests
- For those pursuing a DNP: are there sufficient faculty with current clinical expertise in your preferred focus area?

Once you have chosen your doctoral track, the next step is to look for a doctoral program that is nationally accredited. Accreditation is important, as it ensures programs adhere to common standards of quality, identifies that faculty and staff are involved in institutional evaluation and planning, and criteria for professional licensure and certification are upheld. Schools that are accredited also have national certification exams that meet or exceed national rates (NursingCAS, 2018). The primary nursing accrediting organizations are the AACN's Commission on Collegiate Nursing Education (CCNE), the Accreditation Commission for Education in Nursing (ACEN), or the National League for Nursing's Commission for Nursing Education and Accreditation (CNEA). Several APRN specialties (Nurse Anesthesia and Midwifery, for example) have additional accrediting organizations that indicate the highest-quality program accreditation (see Chapter 1).

Attending an accredited institution is important for several reasons. Only those institutions that are accredited are eligible for federal financial aid. Therefore, if you require federal financial aid, you must attend an accredited institution (see Chapter 9 for in-depth financial considerations and direction). Additionally, if the need arises to change schools, earned credits to date are more likely to be eligible for transfer. Finally, students who have graduated from an accredited school are more competitive in the job market, since employers are aware the school is upholding national standards (NursingCAS, 2018). Accredited nursing programs post their accreditation status on their websites; however, the most up-to-date information can be found on the above-mentioned accrediting institutions' websites.

Education delivery has changed over the past several years and nursing schools are evolving to meet the needs of today's students. Many schools are moving from all in-person, brick-and-mortar classrooms to delivering course content through online modalities. Many provide a combination of both methods, called "hybrid." Consider your initial reflection at the beginning of this chapter. If time constraints are of concern, a fully online program may best suit your needs rather than attending classes in person with a required schedule. In this format, courses are structured on an electronic learning (E-learning) platform that can be accessed at any time while due dates for assignments are standardized for all students. These are also called "asynchronous" courses. A fully online program demands exceptional discipline and time management to delve into self-directed modules that are characteristic of this delivery system. Prior to committing to fully online courses, you may want to try out the approach through massive online open courses (MOOCs) from companies such as Coursera (coursera.org) to see if it meets your needs and to get a feel for the expectations of online learning. Finally, be aware there may be program requirements for occasional live and/or in-person components such as seminars and experiences that require on-campus participation beyond the online courses. Be sure to inquire about these components when performing your searches.

Faculty are a vital part of your educational success. Ask about student-faculty ratios in both classroom and clinical practice courses. Other helpful questions:

- How many mentees are typical for research faculty and clinical faculty?
- Do students collaborate with faculty on projects or are they individually designed?
- Are student-faculty publications supported?

- Is there an opportunity for students to participate in faculty-led research, scholarship, or professional activities? (Chapter 5 provides a list of example activities.)

One of the most important responsibilities, and rewarding aspects, of doctoral education for both students and faculty is the mentoring relationships that support professional growth. The opportunity to collaborate with faculty on projects, manuscripts, and presentations builds confidence and magnifies your future as an up-and-coming expert in the field. A respectful, encouraging professor-student relationship is a gateway to professional and nursing organizations' membership and leadership opportunities. These memberships are vital to enhancing personal growth, expanding knowledge and professional development, and finding support for shared goals and support for change. Professional association memberships provide opportunities to assemble with experts in your area of focus, as well as develop relationships with colleagues throughout the world. As a nurse researcher, these relationships lead to essential interprofessional collaborations for building and disseminating your research. As a clinical expert, membership in professional organizations is essential to maintaining up-to-date knowledge while empowering your ability and confidence to change practice based on current clinical evidence. To this end, we encourage you to explore the school's website and professor biographies to discover their professional activities and dedication to the advancement of the nursing profession.

There are many components that define a quality program. Choosing one that meets your personal and professional goals is important to your academic success. Before finalizing your decision, take the time to explore the options. Consider attending virtual or live open houses and visiting the school to meet with faculty and current students to better understand the program, its support for students, and to discuss delivery options. The information available to you is vast; browse the internet for nursing schools, read online reviews from current and former students, and ask for input from those whom you trust to help guide your decision. Do your homework and you will be confident that you have chosen the right school for you.

Summary

Choosing the best doctoral path may feel overwhelming. The process takes time, dedication, and personal reflection to ensure your choice best fits your personal and professional goals. Truly knowing your passion and your plan for impact is key to making the process a positive one.

Understand that doctoral education is not only a way to advance in your nursing career; it also empowers you to contribute your clinical expertise, knowledge, and joy of nursing to improve and move healthcare, systems, and policies forward. The credentials of a doctorate degree do not make you an esteemed NP, executive leader, or researcher. The doctoral degree develops leadership skills and builds your expertise as a change agent so that what you bring to the table expands high-quality care and the profession of nursing.

Both the PhD and DNP improve outcomes and advance the profession of nursing, so consider your options mindfully, utilize available resources, and investigate opportunities for impact. Completing a doctoral program in nursing is an amazing achievement, and being prepared for your new role will make this achievement even better!

Bibliography

American Association of Colleges of Nursing. *The Essentials of Doctoral Education for Advanced Nursing Practice.* 2006. Available at: https://www.aacnnursing.org/Portals/42/Publications/DNPEssentials.pdf.

American Association of Colleges of Nursing. *The Research-Focused Doctoral Programs in Nursing: Pathways to Excellence.* 2010. Available at: https://www.aacnnursing.org/Portals/42/Publications/PhDPosition.pdf.

American Association of Colleges of Nursing. *DNP Fact Sheet.* 2020. Available at: https://www.aacnnursing.org/DNP/Fact-Sheet/.

American Association of Colleges of Nursing. *PhD Education.* 2021a. Available at: https://www.aacnnursing.org/Nursing-Education-Programs/PhD-Education.

American Association of Colleges of Nursing. *AACN Essentials.* 2021b. Available at: https://www.aacnnursing.org/AACN-Essentials.

Chism LA. *The Doctor of Nursing Practice: A Guidebook for Role Development and Professional Issues* 4th ed. Jones and Bartlett Learning; 2019. https://www.jblearning.com/.

Congress.gov. *Title VIII Nursing Workforce Reauthorization Act of 2019.* 2019. Available at: https://www.congress.gov/bill/116th-congress/house-bill/728.

Graves NM, Postma J, Katz JR, et al. A national survey examining manuscript dissertation formats among nursing PhD programs in the United States. *J Nurs Scholarsh.* 2018;50(3):314-323. Available at: https://doi:10.1111/jnu.12374.

National Academy of Sciences. *Advancing the Nation's Health Needs.* 2005. Available at: https://researchtraining.nih.gov/sites/default/files/pdf/nas_report_2005.pdf.

Neal-Boylan L. PhD or DNP? That is the question [Editorial]. *J Nurse Pract.* 2020;16(2):A5-A6. Available at: https:doi.org/10.1016/j.nurpra.2019.11.015.

NursingCAS. *What's the Deal with Accreditation.* March 12, 2018. Available at: https://nursingcas.org/whats-the-deal-with-accreditation/.

Nursing Times. *The Challenges and Benefits of Undertaking a Nursing PhD.* February 17, 2020. Available at: https://www.nursingtimes.net/roles/clinical-research-nurses/the-challenges-and-benefits-of-undertaking-a-nursing-phd-17-02-2020/.

Rubino LG, Esparza SJ, Reid Cassiakos YS. *New Leadership for Today's Health Care Professionals: Concepts and Cases* 2nd ed. Jones and Bartlett Learning; 2020. https://www.jblearning.com/.

U.S. Department of Education. *Structure of the US Education System.* 2008. Available at: www2.ed.gov/about/offices/list/ous/international/usnei/us/credits.doc.

Valiga TM, Thornlow D. What to consider when choosing a graduate nursing program. *Nursing.* 2018;48(1):11-14. doi:10.1097/01.NURSE.0000527614.67902.8e.

CHAPTER 7

Common Impediments to Success

Jennifer A. Korkosz, DNP, NP, WHNP-BC, APRN

Exploring Yesterday's and Today's Most Common Barriers

Fear makes come true that which one is afraid of.

—Victor Frankl

As you have been traveling through this text to explore the history of the doctoral nursing journey, the authors have clearly outlined the call for highly educated and scientifically cutting-edge nurse clinicians, researchers, educators, and policy leaders.

By this time in the text, you have considered your personal and professional career goals, strongly evaluated your choice of doctoral degree, and selected programs that address your needs and expectations. As you set out on your journey and map the plan for best strategies to accomplish this challenge, we hear your concerns on how to get this done. Anxieties such as *"I cannot afford this!"* or perhaps: *"As amazing as I know I could be with this degree; I don't have time for this right now in my life."* Maybe you feel like this: *"There is no one I know who I can relate too, and will this degree really make a difference."* Furthermore, you may have a combination of these. Please keep in mind, you are NOT ALONE. This chapter goes straight at these common barriers and provides evidence-based tactics to deploy throughout your doctoral education journey. Due to the deep reach of most of these impediments, we will direct you to chapters in the text that offer more comprehensive approaches to support your success.

The barriers to pursuing doctoral education have been the same for quite a long time, keeping nurses from taking critical first steps toward their doctoral pursuits for almost as long as the growth and establishment of the doctoral degree in nursing itself. Barriers to successful entry to, and progress through, doctoral education have remained with us since the 1950s. Kurt Lewin termed a Force Field Analysis where there are driving forces (factors that encourage the change) and restraining forces (factors that discourage the change). For change to occur, the driving forces must overpower restraining forces. Cathro provides a helpful

TABLE 7.1 ■ Evidence-Based Driving and Restraining Forces in Pursuit of Doctoral

Driving Forces	Restraining Forces	Chapter of Text
Interest in pursuing graduate studies	Lack of available programs with a focus in nursing education	2: The Story of the Doctoral Prepared Nurse 3: Looking to the Future of the Doctoral Prepared Nurse 4: Reflection on Challenges 5. Understanding the Degree Options 6: Clarifying Your Aspirations 13: Determining Good Fit
Financial Assistance	Financial costs—tuition, time off work/lost salary, decreased salary when moving from clinical practice to education	9: Understanding and Managing Expenses
Flexible program delivery options	Work responsibilities that may limit time and access to graduate studies	4: Reflection on Challenges 5: Clarifying Your Options 13. Determining Good Fit
Mentoring	Lack of available mentors	8: Mentors
Time constraints	Recognize the importance	11: Using Time Wisely & Well
Family support and responsibilities		7: Common Impediments to Success 13: Determining Good Fit

Modified from Cathro H. Pursuing graduate studies in nursing education: Driving and restraining forces. *Online J Issues Nurs.* 2011;16(3):7. doi:10.3912\0jin.VOL16NO03ppt02.

analysis of driving and restraining forces in relation to pursuit of doctoral education in nursing (2011). In Table 7.1, we take this one step further and identify the chapters in this text that provide guidance to manage and overcome the restraining forces.

This chapter introduces and places these long-standing, well-documented barriers into two categories: internal and external factors. Though not every barrier will resonate with every reader of this text, many are relatable and may haunt and complicate the doctoral journey you are ready to conquer. We will describe proven strategies for helping nurses navigate and overcome these barriers nimbly, confidently, and optimistically.

INTERNAL STRUCTURES

"The worse danger we face is being paralyzed by doubt and fears."

—PRESIDENT HARRY S. TRUMAN

Internal structures are those that well up inside our heads and hearts and can paralyze us at so many points. They include disorganization, fear of failure, imposter syndrome, and lack of self-confidence. These are barriers set by an individual's self-perception of one's own ability to accomplish and achieve the goal. Let's explore and debunk.

Disorganization

Disorganization is defined as "lacking coherence, a system, or guiding central agency" (https://www.merriam-webster.com/dictionary/disorganized). When you feel disorganized, you may know what needs to get done, but you may not be able to figure out how to start, what supplies may be necessary, or even how to find the supplies you need. Some people find that lists or organizers (either electronic or hard copy) work best for them to stay on task. Deciding on a system and then following through with using it are necessary, initially. It does not mean that you will stick with that plan forever, but getting into the habit and practicing will help identify approaches that are best for you. Organizational skills are needed to get all the pieces of your application together. Chapter 10 outlines and offers strategies on steps to put into action to meet deadlines. Many of these same skills and strategies can be refined and easily molded to be a successful doctoral program graduate.

Fear of Failure

The fear of failure is not at all uncommon and in fact is predominant in our lives, as Angela Duckworth mentioned in her *New York Times* best-seller, *Grit: The Power of Passion and Perseverance.* Many of us are afraid to persevere. Afraid to fail because of the humiliation and the shame. We appreciate your fear of failure. You are not alone, and strategies exist to help you conquer your fears.

Burnette and Evans (2016) ask us to imagine a vaccine to prevent failure—nothing but smooth sailing, no grief, no agony of defeat. But that vaccine isn't here just yet, and until it comes along, it's up to you to learn and grow from the lessons that failure offers, make progress, reframe your perspectives, and build your own immunity to failure. Consider flipping the script on the "success good, failure bad" mantra that you have likely grown up with and challenge yourself to minimize the failure-negative feelings that surround and burden your life.

Try the reframing activity in Box 7.1.

The hockey Hall of Famer Wayne Gretzky said it best: "You miss 100% of the shots you don't take" (Brown, 2014). It is a matter of starting. Not letting fear take over and rule the next step. There will never be a time that is 100% right to start a program or begin a new challenge, but if you do not start, then you are 100% guaranteed to never finish.

BOX 7.1 ■ Reframing Activity

Dysfunctional Belief: We judge our life by the outcome.
Reframe: Life is a process, not an outcome.
_____

From Burnette B, Evans D. *Designing Your Life*. Knopf Publisher; 2016: 184.

Imposter Syndrome

That feeling of "this should be someone else, not me" is pervasive when a role is new. The old job, duties, and responsibilities are comfortable. Being thrown into new ones without that background experience can create discomfort and even an identity crisis. Change is a risk, and excellent returns come with significant risk. Having worked hard to get to this point, you deserve to enjoy the new challenges that lie ahead. No one will expect you to know every bit of related information or apply every different thing you are learning, but doctoral scholars know their resources and use them well. Whether scholarly references or reliable, trusted people, you have a resource to access. Working with a trusted mentor to bounce ideas off is a scholarly and wise approach to identifying the best path and picking up your confidence (see Chapter 8).

Self-Confidence

Self-esteem and self-confidence influence our daily lives, and their absence is known to stifle outward dreams, future performance, and mental health. Individuals with a good sense of self-esteem are proud of themselves and their accomplishments. They tend to be happier and find more creative ways to design their lives more flexibly. Confident people attract other like-minded people to their circle, so they nourish one another and motivate achievements. One place to begin exploring self-esteem building blocks is with "The Science of Well-Being," a free online Coursera program from Yale University. Another approach for building confidence is celebrating the small wins for completing each task or project you take on. The small pieces combine into a significant venture, and along the way, self-confidence can grow. For example, the confidence that arises from finishing the components of your application will propel you into the next component of the application process and, in turn, build confidence.

Fear of Standardized Testing

Taylor and Terhaar (2018) and Granner and Ayoola (2021) emphasize that standardized testing skills often required by doctoral programs can become a barrier to moving ahead. The most current literature reveals that Graduate Record Examination (GRE) and other testing scores may not be predictive of doctoral success, and many doctoral programs around the country are dropping the GRE requirement (https://dailyiowan. com/2020/11/13/the-trend-of-universities-dropping-gre-requirements-post-covid/). Since the COVID pandemic, data show that across the board, doctoral programs in the neurosciences, biological sciences, psychology, and nursing are dropping the GRE requirement. Academic leadership in this area is concerned that these testing mechanisms are hindering program diversity and inclusion, in addition to not being as strong a predictor of doctoral student success as was once believed (https://www. prepscholar.com/gre/blog/no-gre-required-graduate-school/).

With that in mind, please do not shy away from a doctoral program that aligns with your area of interest, introduces you to accomplished faculty, and provides resources to support your journey, just because of a GRE or other standardized exam requirement.

Here is what you do. Make a plan and take it one step at a time. Take a class, practice, discuss, analyze whatever you can get your hands on. Sit down with your mentor and find out what strategies worked well for them and how they "ate their elephant." Mentors can help form an accountability plan for studying and keep you on target (https:// mygreexampreparation.com/best-way-to-prep-for-gre/). Try these steps:

- Prepare a study plan with 1-,2-,3-month schedule (https://mygreexampreparation. com/best-way-to-prep-for-gre/)
- Take a free online course: (Coursera)
- Online testing preparation programs may be expensive; plan your budget and seek out a variety of options within your budget (Try Magoosh) (see Chapter 9)
- Buy a study guide book and do 25 questions a night—**in other words, practice!**
- And to stay on target and hold yourself accountable,
  - Use resources in Part 4: Toolkit GRE study schedule resource (https:// mygreexampreparation.com/free-gre-prep/)
- Self-care and routine sleep schedules have been shown most effective in addressing internal anxiety regarding standardized test taking.
- Meet with a text anxiety specialist—while most students won't need one, if you find that your mastery of the material can't shine because you are paralyzed in the face of the real exam, working with a specialist may help you get through the roadblock that is holding you back.
- Focus on calmness, not scores. Math and verbal aren't the only areas you need to study. Staying calm, keeping your mental focus, and honing the ability to work quickly and effectively in mental "crisis" mode, instead of hurried and frazzled in "panic" mode, is a skill to build.

EXTERNAL

You just have to make up your own damn mind…

—THE ORACLE, *THE MATRIX*

The external factors that can deter pursuing an advanced degree or completing a program already started can be just as daunting as the internal structures. They are not significantly different for nursing students as compared to students in other concentration areas and have historically been consistent.

Family Responsibilities

What makes a nursing doctoral student different is that most nurses work full time while taking courses part time. This can lead to a complicated balance of time and responsibilities, especially when family needs are factored into the work and school/class schedule. An understanding support system of friends and families has been shown to help doctoral students. As Volkert et al. (2018) noted, if the support of friends and family decreases, the intent to leave a program of study increases. Higher educational institutions are increasingly aware of and responsive to the various family constellations of the students they serve. Frequent, transparent communication, well-structured time management skills (see Chapter 11), and working collaboratively with your social network help manage expectations and should occur before the application is submitted. Seeking assistance from social support and family on specific tasks and educating family members on the doctoral student experience can help keep your doctoral journey on target.

Making sure to have dedicated quality time on the calendar, in short-term and long-term chunks, gives everyone a touch of family time to look forward to. Sometimes, decisions are difficult, and trade-offs are necessary. Attending family activities and events will take time away from assignments, and tough choices must be made. Consider making these choices together with the people impacted. For instance, asking a child, "Would you rather I come to your soccer game today or Tuesday?" gives family/friends ownership of the options, increases the quality of the time spent together, and makes attendance at selected events even more special.

Access to Funding

Finances are one of the top four reasons individuals either fall out of the doctoral program they are enrolled in or likely do not begin the application process. Because finances are a significant barrier, Chapter 9 explains relevant financial policies, scholarship opportunities, and addresses other money-related concerns. Many resources are available and can make a difference in the bottom line of your tuition bill. However, no one will knock on the door and hand you the money you need for tuition, fees, books, and all the other related expenses. You have to seek the support. The first place to start is the Human Resources department at your workplace, then the Financial Aid Office at the (potential) doctoral program. Explore the support you might qualify for and how to apply for assistance.

Another great resource is the American Association of Colleges of Nursing financial aid and scholarships page (https://www.aacnnursing.org/Students/Financial-Aid).

There are scholarships, resources, and even more search assistance links on that page. The options are impressive.

One fiscally responsible option that can hold a tremendous amount of weight is military service. There are programs within the armed forces for certification and specialty training, plus opportunities to seek formal education and graduate degrees. The significant benefit of military service is that it can be the student's job to go to school. So, not only is tuition paid for, but the student can earn regular compensation for their rank and time in service. Of course, after graduation, there is an obligation to serve for a set period (it depends on how long the schooling takes), but there is no worry about finding a job—it is there waiting!

See Chapter 9 for a broad perspective on financial planning and strategies for managing your money.

Time

Having a time management plan and practicing the many skills offered in Chapter 11 is the best way to ensure application submission and programmatic success when all the balls being juggled feel like they are going faster and faster. Additionally, numerous tools and resources are offered in Part 4 of this text.

Summary

Life's challenges are not supposed to paralyze you; they are supposed to help you discover who you are.

—BERNICE JOHNSON REAGIN

The significant, long-standing barriers to entering nursing doctoral education include the following:
- Financial constraints
- Job and family responsibilities
- Concerns about the ability to be successful
- Low self-confidence.

You may have others that are not touched upon in this chapter. What we want you to take away from this chapter is that it is possible to mitigate the barriers that lie ahead and not be paralyzed by the challenge of pursuing doctoral education. We want to share that in no uncertain terms: YOU CAN DO THIS. Taking things one step at a time, being flexible, and being open and welcoming for each of the experiences along the doctoral highway will contribute to building a mightier and more resourceful you. The journey may not look the way you have planned or envisioned that is all right. Be open to each challenge and be proud of the ever-expanding nursing knowledge and scholarly confidence that are blooming inside. All the steps on this journey are essential to becoming the doctoral-prepared nurse that nursing and society are desperately need.

Bibliography

Brown PB. *'You Miss 100% of the Shots You Don't Take.'* You Need to Start Shooting at Your Goals. Forbes (January 12). 2014. Available at: https://www.forbes.com/sites/actiontrumpseverything/2014/01/12/you-miss-100-of-the-shots-you-dont-take-so-start-shooting-at-your-goal/?sh=5037564a6a40.

Burnette B, Evans D. *Designing Your Life*. Knopf Publisher; 2016:184.

Granner JR, Ayoola AB. Barriers for BSN students to pursue a PhD in nursing and recommendations to address them: a scoping review. *Nurs Outlook*. 2021;69(6):1101-1115.

Taylor LA, Terhaar MF Mitigating. barriers to doctoral Education. *Nurs Educ Perspect*. 2018;39(5):285–290. doi:10.1097\01NEP0000000000000386.

Volkert D, Candela L, Bernacki M. Student motivation, stressors, and intent to leave nursing doctoral study: a national study using path analysis. *Nurse Educ Today*. 2018;61:210-215.

Williams JK, Sicard K, Lundstrom A, Hart S. Overcoming barriers to PhD education in nursing. *J Nurs Educ*. 2021;60(7):400–403.

CHAPTER 8

Mentoring for the Next Generation of Nurse Scholars

Versie Johnson-Mallard, PhD ■ Paula Alexander-Delpech,
BSN, MSN, PhD, PMHNP-BC ■ Marcia Parker, EdD ■
Cassandre Jean-Antoine, PhD, RN, NEA-BC

A mentor is someone who allows you to see the hope inside yourself.
—Oprah Winfrey

The Mentor: What It Is and Why Do We Need It?

Throughout this text, we strive to stimulate excitement and build momentum for your professional future. All roads (and the literature) tell us that your best chance in reaching greater professional and personal growth and career success will involve a mentor. Mentoring is essential for expanding our generational cultural perspectives, strengthening leadership and clinical skills, and guiding individuals toward better decision making for overall personal and professional growth. It is the secret ingredient for preparing the future nursing generation.[1-5] As discussed in previous chapters, the authors believe that your ability to advance the art of caring and the science of nursing will require doctoral education. This chapter on mentoring intends to help you see the capability and the hope inside yourself to make that happen.

Mentors help individuals navigate the process by demystifying the procedures needed to support the ambition for graduate and doctoral education. Mentoring provides an experienced guide to direct the process of navigating graduate education. Mentors are primary agents for socialization, the bridge between the students and their doctoral education.[1-8] Therefore, much of what occurs before, during, and after one's doctoral education is the ability to socialize to the practice.

Socialization is a complex concept that involves a process of interaction, development, and adaptation.[1-8] The role of socialization includes igniting a sense of belonging and forming professional identities during all interactions. A mentor that role models caring is an important professional value garnered from mentorship, followed by the action of activism for the mentee's success.[1-8]

Mentors for future and current graduate students portray a crucial role in helping students navigate graduate education and transition to professional connections. The role of mentor is dynamic in the mentor-mentee relationship and should change to adapt to the needs of the individuals. Much of the mentee's experiences as a doctoral student depend on the relationship garnered by the mentor's intentional/formal role modeling. The mentor roles can be that of an expert, advocate, cheerleader, enforcer, confidant, teacher, or friend.[1,2,6-16]

INTENTIONAL/FORMAL MENTORING

Mullen and Klimaitis describe a mentor as a competent and trustworthy person who consciously accepts personal responsibility for the growth and development of another person.[17] Mentoring is essential for personal and professional growth, and the term is dynamic depending on discipline, organization, gender, age, culture, or other factors. No matter the traits, mentoring is intended to create a climate of trust and support, and provide guidance.[17-19] The following are likely outcomes from the *intentional* mentor-mentee relationship (Box 8.1):

1. Identifying needs and expectations
2. Recognizing individuals who can meet needs the best
3. Connecting with someone who can help you identify strengths
4. Linking with someone who is vested in your professional growth
5. Trusting someone to help you minimize your weaknesses

Tip 1: Seek connections that create a climate of trust and feelings of comfort with shared experiences.[20]

The mentor-mentee dyad is a unique partnership that does not happen spontaneously; it requires preparation and thought and intentionality. It is important to consider what type of characteristic is desired for the building of this valuable partnership. The role of individuals mentoring students toward a doctoral education is specific to guiding an individual into the graduate student role, from navigating the application process to completion of their doctoral studies to helping them select a professional-track, postdoctoral study. Accordingly, mentoring could fall under several different paradigms: (1) traditional, (2) coach, (3) sponsor, and (4) connector (Fig. 8.1).[21]

BOX 8.1 ■ Purpose of Mentoring

1. Identifies needs
2. Recognizes needs
3. Connects with individuals who can identify your strengths
4. Links with individuals dedicated to your professional growth
5. Trust in helping you strengthen your weakness

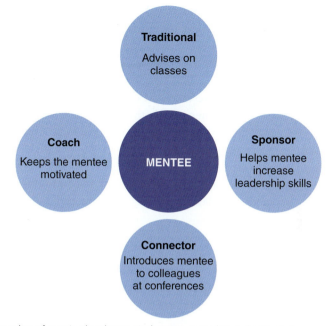

Fig. 8.1 Examples of mentor involvement. A nurse pursuing a doctoral degree may have multiple mentors throughout their journey. There is no specific order for when a particular type of mentor may join the student's team.

THE TRADITIONAL MENTOR

Traditional mentors can be viewed as a way of taking on the role of protecting the mentee. The mentor sees the result of the partnership as their responsibility, like that of the parent. Respect and trust are important tenets of this traditional relationship. The goal of the traditional mentor is to make sure that the mentee acquires the skill and knowledge necessary to be successful. An example of a traditional mentor could be a high school or college academic advisor. For instance, an academic advisor's role is prescriptive; they will provide mentoring based on a set plan to ensure that the mentee acquires the skill and knowledge needed to be successful. They answer simple and concrete questions as to steps the mentee needs to take to achieve a specific goal.

THE COACH MENTOR

The coach as a mentor inspires and motivates the mentee in the way the mentee directs. The mentee lays the foundation and leads in this model. The mentee brings to the table experience and knowledge but may require periodic push/motivation. The coach supports the mentee at every level of their becoming. Unlike the traditional mentor, the coach is hands off and provides support to the mentee in the form of motivation and a push when needed. The coach mentor is the most essential of all the different mentors. A new doctoral student may be assigned a faculty chair/advisor experienced in the student's area of research interest. The coach avails themselves for questions or guidance as the student moves through the graduate curriculum. The coach mentor may have expertise in a specific research methodology or research area needed for a specific semester. An added advantage of a coach mentor is that the mentoring can be done one-on-one or in a small group. For instance, as a doctoral student, several of my fellow classmates were using a particular theory for our dissertation. We as a group wrote to the theorist who coached us as a group on their theory. In contrast to the traditional mentor, the coach mentor is nondirective and focuses on making sure the mentee is learning new skills through self-reflection and self-awareness.

THE SPONSOR MENTOR

This mentoring role is distinctive in the partnership. The sponsor mentor takes on the responsibility of expertise in a chosen field. The sponsor mentor uses their influence to help propel the mentee. In this mentor-mentee relationship, it is important that the mentor is cognizant of their influence and is intentional about their approach to increasing the mentee's presence in the field. A sponsor mentor can use their influence to open opportunities for the mentee. Sponsor mentors often serve on executive boards at the national level; a nurse leader is often an advocate for the profession. The sponsor plays a key role in translational mentoring, helping scholars build leadership skills that are used at the bedside, at the bench, or in the board room. The process of the supportive mentor is ongoing throughout the graduate education process and into the professional arena, contributing to the continuous development of the protégée. The sponsor mentor is experienced with advanced knowledge, guiding the protégé on making informed education and career choices. Similar to the traditional mentor, the sponsor mentor is committed to teach, learn, counsel, and, hopefully, befriend the protégée, leading to a lasting and effective professional relationship.[22]

THE CONNECTOR MENTOR

Just as the word implies, the connector mentor's role is to connect their mentees to resources. The connector mentor is an expert networker with an array of contacts. They help their mentees by introducing them to key stakeholders. They may or may not be the head of their organizations; however, they know the formal and informal leaders and how to introduce them. A connector gets you into a network, such as LinkedIn, or introduces you to others at a professional conference. Of all the different types of mentors, the connector mentor is the one who brings to the profession the ability to create a pipeline of future leaders into their network.

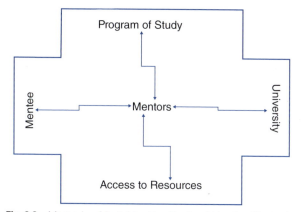

Fig. 8.2　Mentoring Model for Pre-Doctoral Nursing Students.

Connectors tend to be at the pinnacle of their career. I once had an academic mentor who invited me to attend a national conference; at the conference, they not only knew a majority of the attendees, but they also took the time to introduce me, a "doctoral student," to a plethora of the conference attendees. More specifically, they made a special emphasis to introduce me to experts in our area of study. Today, several years after my doctoral studies, I am still in touch with a few of the people I was introduced to at that conference. Like the traditional mentor, the connector mentor is well connected and shares their expertise across networks (Fig. 8.2).

BE OPEN TO MENTORING, EVEN WHEN YOU LEAST EXPECT IT

There are many benefits to informal and intentional/formal mentors. One of your earlier informal mentors may have been a parent, a neighbor, a coach, or casual acquaintance. This person may have never known that they influenced you or contributed to a feeling or goal. When asked how important it is to be a mentor, famed cartoonist Jules Feiffer once noted that he hadn't realized his mentoring abilities until he began teaching, and that it was his ability to establish a classroom environment of openness and inclusivity that positively affected and changed the career direction of the students. The role of mentor helped Feiffer appreciate his many gifts and the impact he had on others' active pursuit of life's goals and dreams. I shared the following lived experience with my dissertation mentor years after completing my dissertation studies under her mentorship:

"I didn't choose my faculty mentor. Instead, I received a letter from the College of Nursing stating who they selected to guide and support me during the next four years. Once I knew her name, I did what any inquisitive student would do—I Googled her. Based on my extensive internet search, it looked like my mentor's research interest included women's health, reproductive health promotion, sexually transmitted infection prevention, and Human Pappilloma Virus screening and prevention. On the other hand, I wanted to explore nursing leadership and management. What in the world did we have in common? How did they pair us? I was curious how this relationship would work if we didn't share the same focus in nursing.

It didn't take long to see that it was an ideal match. We didn't have to share the same methodologies or interests for her to be my Academic Advisor. What she was able to offer me was invaluable. She knew how to maneuver in a PhD program—she did it before. She knew what it was like to be an underrepresented minority—she looked like me. And she knew how to get me to the finish line—thank God. My mentor will send me random texts or brief emails to check on me even after graduating. She recently invited me to collaborate on a book chapter about mentorship (the one you're reading!). She is genuinely invested in my career after the PhD program. And for that, I am grateful.

My advice to the doctoral nursing student in search of a mentor is to be open. Do not limit your options, whether it's your responsibility to seek a mentor or your mentor is appointed to you. You never know who will take you to the next level."

Tip 2: Mentor in the academic space can be synonymous with doctoral advisor, doctoral mentor, dissertation director/chair, and doctoral supervisor, bringing to the partnership knowledge, skills, experience, and connection with the responsibility of active mentorship.

Mentoring Across the Profession of Nursing

The practice of mentoring is influenced by trust, motivation, and vision. Mentoring across the profession of nursing comes with mutual benefits.[15,17-20,23] The demystified process of doctoral education from preapplication to independent scholars is an end goal of the mentor/mentee partnership. Yet, with the well-documented current and future faculty shortage, fewer students are finding their way to the bench to conduct research, the podium as an academician, and the practice setting as expert clinicians.

The leading nursing organizations and associations, such as the National League for Nursing (NLN), the American Association of Colleges of Nursing (AACN), and the Robert Wood Johnson Foundation (RWJF), have predicted the snowball effect of lack of students in doctoral programs of nursing (see Chapter 1). A lack of doctoral students snowballs into a limited number of qualified doctorally prepared nursing faculty, perpetuating limiting access of nursing students in both undergraduate and doctoral programs across the nation, highlighting the snowballing effect on the national nursing shortage. Nowhere is this phenomenon more evident than in the tens of thousands of qualified applicants to nursing programs being denied admission around the country. Most distressing is the decrease in completion rates from graduate nursing programs from around the nation due to registered nursing delaying degree completion to work at the beside due to the impact of COVID-19.[18]

COMMITMENT TO CAREER GOALS AND AWARENESS OF CAREER PATHWAYS

Benner's Novice to Expert model encourages the idea that a novice nurse should seek to develop clinical skills, interprofessional healthcare culture skills, and the confidence to prioritize and organize patient care from a well-developed foundation found in the tertiary care setting (i.e., Medical-Surgical tertiary care).[22] Contemporary learning models preferred by many recent new graduate nurses include mentoring at hirer to specialty units not requiring or expecting pre–Med Surg experience, expecting mentoring from experienced nurses with content knowledge and skills.[5] In addition, hospitals offer nurse residency programs to support and mentor newly licensed registered nurses (RNs), mentoring models designed to navigate the transition to specialty units.[24]

Tip 3: Newer models of learning encourage hiring novice nurses into specialty units that offer well-crafted nurse residency and mentoring models designed to support newly licensed registered nurses' navigation into specialty units.

Career mentorship of novice RNs to beyond bedside nursing, both in and outside of acute care settings, offers a plethora of career options (Table 8.1). There are multiple career paths and opportunities in nursing, irrespective of years of experience.

The success of the novice nurse is enhanced with intentional mentoring, promoting support for learning difficult concepts. RNs receiving intentional mentoring early in their career are likely to move more directly from undergraduate studies to a doctoral program.

Many research questions are grounded in work experiences and the workplace environment. Practicing nurses from all areas of healthcare are likely to seek out

TABLE 8.1 ■ **Nurse Options**

Nurse Leader/Executives	Infection Control
Nurse Educator/Academician	Quality Management
Nurse Researcher/Scientist	Nurse Coordinator
Nurse Practitioner	Nursing Informatics
Clinical Nurse Specialist	Occupational Health
Nurse Midwife	Case Manager
Infection Control	Forensic Nurse
Quality Management	Flight Nurse
Telehealth Nurse	School Nurse

answers to dynamic clinical questions through scientific inquiry earlier in their careers. There is no specific career pathway for nurses with doctoral degrees, because the opportunities are endless. Nurses with terminal degrees can serve as nurse executives, nurse scientists, and nurse academicians. Let's explore some of the many options for a nurse with a doctorate degree (see Table 8.1), many of which are listed on several professional websites such as the American Nurses Foundation, Wolters Kluwer, and the American Nurses Association.

NURSE EXECUTIVES

A nurse who is mentored to nurture their leadership skills can play a critical role in a healthcare organization's business in the quality and safety of service delivery.[25] A nurse executive is part of the leadership team and holds the highest level of nursing decision-making and contribution in a healthcare organization.[25] Nurse executives have different titles in various organizations (see Table 8.1). Some title examples include Chief Nursing Officer (CNO), Chief Nurse Executive, Director of Nursing, Vice President of Patient Care Services, Vice President of Nursing, and Patient Care Administrator, all potential mentors to colleagues, staff, students, and patients.

According to the American Organization of Nurse Executives (AONE) and the Robert Wood Johnson Foundation (RWJ), nurse leaders should have at least a master's degree, and nurses at the highest levels of executive leadership are encouraged to seek educational preparation at the doctoral level.[26] Similarly, nurse leaders interviewed state, "In university-based hospitals, the CNO with a doctoral degree has the formal leadership skills and knowledge to command the authority to fulfill their role in this environment" (Shaffer, p. 295).[27] However, a nurse leader with the most experience is not always the most effective mentor. The most effective mentor shares traits of availing self, availing time, and appreciating two-way communication between those with or without years of experience.[27] Leadership positions outside the hospital environment can also include nurse scientists and nurse educators.

NURSE SCIENTIST

Nurse scientists are educated to create, conduct, and teach research, and are necessary in improving patient care as well as investigate issues that may affect the nursing profession and patient outcomes. Nurse researchers are scientists with influence. An influential nurse scientist plays a vital role in the quality and safety of service delivery and helps shape national policies and create new nursing knowledge.[18,26,28] With a doctorate degree in nursing, nurse scientists conduct independent research, generate new knowledge, and establish new ways to achieve high-quality care.[28] Nurse researchers work in academia, in a clinical setting, or both. Some positions allow the nurse scientist to work part time in a healthcare organization and part time in a college of nursing with "presence noted in both the health care environment and the academic setting" (p. 299).[28] This shared academic clinical setting model allows the researcher to function as mentor, while translating research into practice.[28] In either setting, the Nurse Researcher helps develop the science, guide the discipline, and mentor the next generation of nurses.[28,29]

NURSE ACADEMICIANS

The nation's current nursing shortage is reflected in the nursing faculty shortage. The current shortage is predicted to worsen in a few years; one-third of current faculty are predicted to retire by 2025, 44% of whom hold research-focused doctorates.[30] Due to the scarcity of nurse academicians, it is estimated that 50% of current PhD students are already in faculty roles and at least half of DNP graduates seek faculty roles.[31] According to the American Association of Colleges of Nursing (AACN), most of the current vacancies (89.7%) in schools of nursing are faculty positions requiring or preferring a doctoral degree.[18] The profession has available nurse academic position openings across the nation for DNP and PhD nurses to serve as mentors to future nurses.[18]

Graduate education at the doctoral level can be less difficult to navigate with intentional mentoring.[23,32] Seeking mentoring, actively and strategically, has a role in demystifying the process. Intentional mentoring to individuals seeking a nurse science-focused degree is a major step toward decreasing the faculty shortage and clinical shortage.[23,32] We mentor to guide nurses to doctoral programs to explore the many different opportunities and career pathways in nursing with an end goal of sustaining a fulfilling nursing career (Table 8.2).[23,32]

Tip 4: List what is most important to you in your next role, review HR's job description, determine if it's the right role for you, and ask if you can shadow for a day.

TABLE 8.2 ■ **Traits and Objectives of Mentoring**

Traits	Objective
Trust	Build confidence early in the relationship
Motivation	Inspire effective two-way communication
Initiatives/vision	Develop mutual goals with aligning expectations
Respect for DEI	Exhibit admiration for diversity, equity, and inclusion
Advice	Actively listen and respond ethically and professionally
Demystification	Foster professional development and independence

DEI, Diversity, Equity, and Inclusion.

Adapted from Cohen NH. The journey of the principles of adult mentoring inventory. *Adult Learn.* 2003;14(1):4–7.

Securing a Mentor

Securing a mentor to help guide individuals to the infinite opportunities the profession of nursing avails requires being intentional when securing a mentor with the passion, skills, and desire to guide individuals into a rich career path in nursing.[18,23,32] Securing a mentor can be a daunting experience made even more challenging when one is not intentional and not equipped to recognize the unwritten rules and expectations. The importance of a role-modeling pre formal graduate school application has limited documentation. Thus, developing a guide to securing a mentor is to inform the process of navigating graduate education at the doctoral level.[23,33-36] Within this context, historically marginalized, minorities, and first-generation students find themselves navigating unique sets of roadblocks.[33-36] Some students' confidence in self and their ability to secure a mentor can be impacted by experiences of racism, low social economic status, biases, and stereotypes.[37] Further, if a mentor is not readily available within one's immediate surroundings, it can be difficult to recognize what mentorship might entail.[a]

Several elements should be considered when selecting a mentor, including the element of trust. Trust is key for both mentor and mentee. Students may receive suggested mentors by family, friends, or colleagues who have previously experienced mentorship from a trusted individual, whether it is an arranged connection or network or one that a student initiated independently. Consistently it is reported that effective career pursuits are developed through engagement, modelling, and feedback from those who are viewed as trusted in decision-making positions.[b] Mentors who show themselves as realistic, transparent, and approachable are the most effective mentors.[38] Moreover, those who demonstrate an openness to listening, particularly to the unique perspective of historically marginalized students, may experience a deeper benefit from the mentor-mentee relationship themselves.[9]

Mentorship is an incredibly important concept for all nurses, yet the historically marginalized and first-generation graduate students are likely the most vulnerable when pursuit of doctoral education is a goal. Mentors that embrace Diversity, Equity, and Inclusion (DEI) efforts to diversify nursing doctoral programs will surely help alleviate the nurse faculty shortage. For this reason, this chapter focuses on students in guiding the next generation of nurse scholars to identify mentors that have skills to help the student navigate the doctoral educational journey.

Diversity, Equity, Inclusion-Based Mentoring

In 2018, a 2-year-old girl became famous for staring at a portrait of First Lady Michelle Obama at the National Portrait Gallery in Washington, DC. For

---

[a]References 18, 22, 26, 27, 32, 34, 36.
[b]References 18, 22, 23, 26, 27, 32–36.

many, the picture suggested a little girl admiring someone who looked like her. The picture may have for the little girl symbolized possibility and hope. It also showed that representation matters. Finding a mentor can be challenging, especially for individuals seeking same-race and/or same-sex mentor-mentee dyads.

In addition to the lack of mentors in general, it is even more difficult to find minority mentors for those seeking same-race mentors. Those seeking same-race mentors may find opportunities by joining national ethnic professional nursing organizations. Ethnic nursing organizations include the Asian American Pacific Islander Nursing Association (AAPINA), National Association of Hispanic Nurses (NAHN), National Black Nurses Association (NBNA), Philippine Nurses Association of America PNAA, and the National Alaska Native American Indian Nurses Association (NANAINA). Respect for diversity, equality, equity, and inclusion (DEEI) in providing strategic navigational skills for the nursing doctoral program journey appears to be underresourced and requires strategic and intentional mentoring.[15,17-19,23] A lack of minority mentor representation could have a significant role in lack of retention and success for reaching education and career goals. Intentional mentoring with DEEI on the radar may translate to behaviors that are supportive. Mentors trained in DEEI are crucial and more equipped to provide guidance and advice on navigating bias spaces that are perceived as not welcoming based on gender, race and ethnicity, degree earned, specialty, profession, and more.

Once the decision is made to make an application to a doctoral program, who can minorities go to for guidance? A qualitative study examined the perceptions of minority nurses in leadership in the United States. An interesting yet perhaps controversial finding from the research was that same-race mentoring is essential for professional success.[10] Similarly, other studies have reported that a structured mentorship program matching minority nurse leaders with same-sex and race was viewed as a safe space to discuss diversity and career advancement from experienced senior leaders within the organization.[9-13,37,38] These study findings further support the benefits of having experienced minority leaders mentor minority nurses. Further study findings support a lack of same-race mentorship can be a perceived barrier to education and career advancement.[6,9-13] The Institute of Medicine's ([IOM], currently the National Academy of Medicine) *Future of Nursing Report* sets a clear priority to transform the next generation of nurses by providing nurse mentoring programs and opportunities to lead.[33] The IOM's report elaborates that active mentoring requires training, and that DEI is important.[33] The Robert Wood Johnson Nurse Faculty Scholar's and Future of Nursing Scholars programs were built on the concept of networking to form mentor-mentee training and include DEI as a role in mentoring.[16,33] Both programs provided mentors from diverse backgrounds to serve as mentors to PhD students in nursing and academic mentoring to nurses new to the faculty role. Diversity provides differing perspectives with goals of supporting retention and elevating the profession.

In an integrative literature review, researchers examined perceived barriers to mentoring in general and minorities specifically in health-related research. Ransdell et al. found that the major barriers to mentoring were a lack of time and finding work-life balance.[20] However, the most frequently mentioned institutional barrier to mentoring was a lack of individuals willing to serve as mentors.[20] According to the study, "Mentors may be less willing to participate if they are not receiving workload credit for mentoring or if the experience is not mutually beneficial" (p. 28).[20]

Historically, there is a lack of minority mentors in nursing. With that said, racial or gender pairing isn't always necessary for successful mentoring to occur. Exposure to differing race, backgrounds, and gender could increase social trust. The results in one study found that "perceptions of similarity with their mentor were the dominant factor influencing the quality of mentoring—not demographic similarity" (p. 14).[16] In this example, perceptions of similarity included shared values and a shared outlook. Similarly, in another study, students felt having a mentor of one's own gender or race was somewhat important for success; but, according to another study in terms of academic outcomes, matching by gender or race made no difference in outcomes.[10] Based on these findings, nurse scholars may benefit from mentors who may or may not share the same gender, race, or social background but share similar viewpoints and interests. Diversity in race, gender, ethnicity, or thought should not influence the development of trust. Diversity as defined, perceived, or requested by the graduate student should not be dismissed if building a successful mentor-mentee relationship is the end goal. The "go to" mentor may vary as professional growth occurs. Mentors should challenge the student to think in novel ways, engage in challenging areas of study, and embrace diversity in all forms.

Navigating the Application Process

Chapter 10 provides a thorough examination of the specific steps needed to navigate the application process for graduate education. Research findings have shown that to navigate the graduate school application process successfully, students must adopt paradigms such as resilience, openness, and a firm sense of academic identity.[35] Some of these paradigms are formed early through life experiences, whereas others are nurtured through intentional mentorship. The following section provides insight on these paradigms and the important role that networking and mentorship may play in recognizing as well as developing these concepts.

RESILIENCE

Multiple authors attest to the influence of resilience on a student's development process.[13,14,16] The value of resilience is elevated for graduate students as they cope with academic challenges that place them in numerous "first situations" that lead to potential discomfort or anxiety (p. 126).[1] Being a first-generation graduate student, having no one with personal experience to guide you through the application process can be a nonstarter for some students. According to Stephens, mentors can serve as one of several protective factors that underscore the confidence needed to push through challenging circumstances and decreasing anxiety that could play out as fear of the unknown. Mentors can enhance resilience skills by helping students moderate how they react to anxiety by highlighting behaviors such as seeking help early and by working actively with mentors.[8]

Tip 5: Ask questions aimed at clarifying perceptions, positive or negative, regarding personal ability to develop resilience.[15]

Throughout stages of the application process, you may have past experiences from undergraduate work to draw upon. The ability to foster resilience will empower you to pivot with confidence through unfamiliar circumstances of making your application to graduate school. Participants in a recent study reported using resilience to navigate financial barriers and family illness to become successful graduate students.[35] As a testament to their character, these students utilized resilience to navigate unfamiliar circumstances. Mentors drawing upon past experiences with difficult situations during graduate school used stories to encourage and empower resilience in others.[7] These stories were received as good examples of translation of lived experiences used to support and motivate. Resilience can be especially helpful for those applying to programs at the graduate level who are first-generation students or facing financial hardships. Resilience is the ability to navigate academic challenges through networks and the confidence to access preparatory programs that may enhance coping skills for learning difficult academic courses.[35] Moreover, mentors can work with students to persevere and demonstrate an academic "pattern of growth," providing further strength to their application and evidence before committee review (p. 130).[1]

Tip 6: Offer personal thoughts, storytelling, and genuine sharing of experience and feelings to emphasize the value of learning from unsuccessful or difficult experiences (as trial and error and self-correction, and not as growth-limiting "failures").[15]

OPENNESS

Mentors play an incredibly important role in helping you become open to learning and seeking new experiences with confidence. Openness to broader experiences can facilitate understanding of the various forms of academic ways of learning. Openness to participating in student organizations, including those outside of one's own comfort zone, may help demonstrate an openness to learning about traditions other than one's own. Openness can be exhibited by enrolling in elective courses outside of one's major, to broaden your perspective and view of the world.[35] Gurin et al. reports that experiences out of an individual's comfort zone may increase an individual's openness to the value of learning about other groups, which is important for those pursuing graduate education.[2]

For illustration, studies have shown that students who are surrounded by substantial cross-racial interactions have a greater sense of openness to diversity, a key trait in developing nurses of the 21st century.[2] Further, students who can travel or study outside of their home country can further expand their perspective, assisting in both their choice of graduate school and the impact they can have on future patients.[35] Mentees who experience and can articulate the importance of global learning, exposure to diversity, and civic engagement may secure a competitive advantage when presenting their graduate education.[3] Likewise, mentors who have lived any of these perception-altering experiences can help shed light on their impact and potential for future growth.

Tip 7: Pose hypothetical questions to expand individual views.[15]

SENSE OF ACADEMIC IDENTITY

Academic identity, or academic mindset, has been expressed as the key belief or psychology of a student regarding their academic ability and success.[4,12] Closely aligned with the concept of resilience, a strong sense of academic identity helps students perceive setbacks as temporary, something they can overcome. Parker, for example, explored the experiences of multiple students who overcame challenges with standardized tests required for admission into a particular health professions school.[35] After initially receiving a less than optimal score, one student reestablished her sense of self-confidence and sought out a mentor who offered suggestions on preparing for standardized tests. Mentors who are actively engaged and transparent in sharing strategies that are tried and true to their journey can help build or rebuild self-confidence.[4,13,38]

Self-actualization may look like the ability to identify challenges and plan strategies to overcome. Academic identity may help students think critically and make decisions toward self-correction, such as to retake classes in which they initially struggled or use the opportunity in a different learning environment to determine what they could have done differently. Nursing mentors can increase mentee confidence by engaging in dialogue, and actively listening around approaches to self-correction.[12]

Tip 8: Offer personal thoughts and genuine feelings to emphasize the value of learning from unsuccessful or difficult experiences (as trial and error and self-correction and not as growth-limiting "failures").[2]

Mentor-Mentee Relationship

According to the National Academies of Sciences, Engineering, and Medicine, mentorship has two primary conceptual components: "science" and "mentorship." Science is defined as "the intellectual and practical activity encompassing the systematic study of structures and behaviors through observation, experiment, and theory."[33] Mentorship as a professional working alliance in which individuals work together over time to support the personal and professional growth, development, and success of the relational partners through the provision of career and psychosocial support is the goal of the relationship. This chapter reinforces the mentor-mentee relationship beyond a relationship in which a mentor and mentee are simply assigned to one another as part of an organizationally supported program. Mentoring is an intentional method of engaging effectively to meet the needs of the individuals. Mentoring is a collaborative relationship informed by building an alliance based on intentionality, trust, and shared responsibility for the interaction in mutual, purposeful relationship building toward an effective and shared beneficial interaction. The relationship should be intentional to garner long-term associations, which refers to a coordinated method of engagement to an effective mentor-mentee connection. Mentoring in the traditional form of pairing an expert with a novice, master-apprentice or patron-protégé relationship has been challenged as a modern approach.[5] A more modern approach moves beyond the hierarchical tone of traditional mentoring and focuses on creating equal partnerships that result in reciprocal benefit.

Summary

Our overall goal in this chapter is to demystify mentoring. As stated at the beginning and throughout the chapter, the relationship between mentor and mentees is reciprocal. Both the mentor and the mentee must be willing to be vulnerable in the relationship. The mentor should think about what is best for the mentee and not themselves. A willing mentor must be ready to give credit to the mentee, embrace DEI, and allow the mentee to branch out, despite the threat of failing or succeeding above and beyond the mentor. Also, the mentor should be ready to have difficult conversations with their mentee and be available for the mentee. On the other hand, the mentee is responsible for choosing their mentor wisely, being willing to listen and consider suggestions, meeting deadlines, and, finally, not losing sight of the relationship's goal.

CHAPTER 9

Understanding and Managing Expenses: Financing Your Education

Laura A. Taylor, PhD, RN, ANEF, FAAN ■ Mary F. Terhaar, PhD, RN, ANEF, FAAN

> *Education is the most powerful weapon you can use to change the world.*
>
> —Nelson Mandela

Dr. Nelson Mandela referred to education as transformative and powerful: He did not say it would be cheap. In fact, the cost of higher education can be breathtaking, even intimidating. In our workshops with nurses like yourself, who are contemplating doctoral study, concern about money is universal. You will undoubtedly want to give this careful thought, and we have assembled information to help you do that. We want you to be prepared to have several meaningful conversations about money as you approach your decision to pursue your doctorate.

Once you read this chapter, you will be able to:

- Discuss the factors driving expense in higher education,
- Explore the total cost of the education you seek,
- Evaluate and compare the expense associated with the programs you are considering,
- Engage in a direct and informed conversation with a financial aid officer about the support that might be available to you,
- Explore other options for funding, and
- Identify the important steps you can take to position yourself to be eligible for funding.

The Cost of Higher Education

The cost of education at elite private colleges has reached $80,000 to $90,000 and even public college tuition has reached $30,000 (in-state residents) to $50,000 (out-of-state residents) per year (Levine, 2022). Colleges and universities are required by law to disclose costs of attendance, including tuition, fees, room and board, books, as well as other related and foreseeable expenses (Higher Education Act, 2018). Reading these figures can lead to sticker shock.

Some propose that net cost would be a more useful measure to report and consider. The *net cost of education* would include the sum of the tuition paid to the university, the work students contribute in partial payment for education (think research assistantships and teaching assistantships), plus payments made directly to the college by federal programs, gifts, or endowments (Levine, 2022). Parsing the expenses this way can help you understand what your out-of-pocket costs will be in relation to the total expense associated with the education you seek (Fig. 9.1).

The Cost of the Degree You Seek

To really understand the cost of the education you seek, it is useful to consider the tuition charged, the length of the program, the completion rate, and the support available to defray your expenses. Every one of these metrics should be available to you as you make your decision. It is helpful to consult the program web pages and federal reports and ask questions directly of the faculty and administration of the programs you are considering. It is particularly helpful to build a spreadsheet to help you clearly see and understand the data. This will help you make your decision confidently with eyes wide open.

The Department of Education provides data about the debt burden carried by students in the United States. You can expect to see those figures updated regularly, and that information can help establish the context for the debt you are considering carrying. Graduates from professional doctoral programs carry the highest debt, approaching $200,000 in 2016. Those who have earned research doctorates carry less debt, slightly more than $100,000 in the same year.

You will want to ask the admissions staff, finance officer, or program director about the debt load of their graduates on program completion. According to national data available to you, you can compare that figure to the average debt load of other students earning a similar terminal degree. This will inform your decision (Fig. 9.2).

Completion is another important consideration and perhaps not something you would have considered before reading this chapter. Not all students who enter doctoral study will go on to complete or graduate. So, it is important to understand the percentage of students who complete a program you are considering. Fig. 9.3 illustrates the variability in program completion according to the type of degree offered.

You can see that a program that leaves students with less debt but produces a lower percentage of graduates may not be a bargain. A program that is more expensive and has a higher completion rate may impress you as worth the investment.

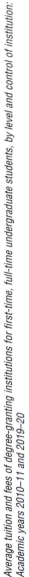

Average tuition and fees of degree-granting institutions for first-time, full-time undergraduate students, by level and control of institution: Academic years 2010–11 and 2019–20

[In constant 2019–20 dollars]

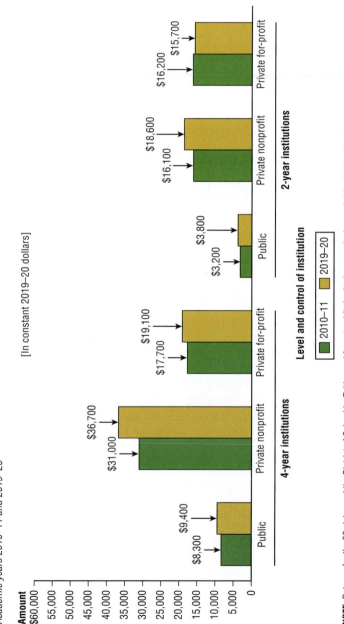

NOTE: Data are for the 50 states and the District of Columbia. Tuition and fees at public institutions are the lower of either in-district or in-state tuition and fees. Excludes students who previously attended another postsecondary institution or who began their studies on a part-time basis. Data are weighted by the number of students at the institution who were awarded Title IV aid. Title IV aid includes grant aid, work-study aid, and loan aid. Constant dollars are based on the Consumer Price Index, prepared by the Bureau of Labor Statistics, U.S. Department of Labor, adjusted to an academic-year basis.

Fig. 9.1   Cost of higher education.

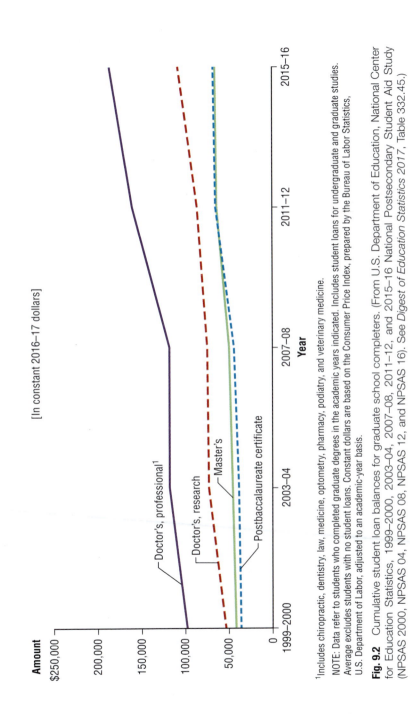

[In constant 2016–17 dollars]

Fig. 9.2 Cumulative student loan balances for graduate school completers. (From U.S. Department of Education, National Center for Education Statistics, 1999–2000, 2003–04, 2007–08, 2011–12, and 2015–16 National Postsecondary Student Aid Study (NPSAS 2000, NPSAS 04, NPSAS 08, NPSAS 12, and NPSAS 16). See *Digest of Education Statistics 2017*, Table 332.45.)

[1]Includes chiropractic, dentistry, law, medicine, optometry, pharmacy, podiatry, and veterinary medicine.

NOTE: Data refer to students who completed graduate degrees in the academic years indicated. Includes student loans for undergraduate and graduate studies. Average excludes students with no student loans. Constant dollars are based on the Consumer Price Index, prepared by the Bureau of Labor Statistics, U.S. Department of Labor, adjusted to an academic-year basis.

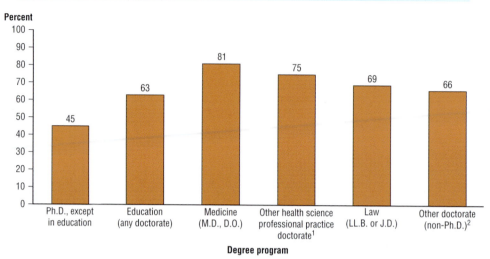

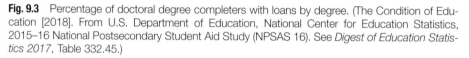

[1]Includes chiropractic, dentistry, optometry, pharmacy, podiatry, and veterinary medicine.
[2]Includes science or engineering, psychology, business or public administration, fine arts, theology, and other.
NOTE: Data refer to students who completed graduate degrees in 2015–16. Includes student loans for undergraduate and graduate studies.

Fig. 9.3 Percentage of doctoral degree completers with loans by degree. (The Condition of Education [2018]. From U.S. Department of Education, National Center for Education Statistics, 2015–16 National Postsecondary Student Aid Study (NPSAS 16). See *Digest of Education Statistics 2017*, Table 332.45.)

In the end, doctoral education is an investment of time and money, and the choice to take both on is yours to make. Nearly two-thirds of graduates from public and private nonprofit colleges leave school carrying student loan debt, and you should expect to carry debt too (The Institute for College Access & Success, 2018). On average, 76% of students graduating from nursing programs at any level carry debt, and on average, that debt is $100k (aacn.org; https://www.aacnnursing.org/Portals/42/Policy/PDF/Debt_Report.pdf).

- The average Bachelor of Science in Nursing (BSN) to Doctor of Nursing Practice (DNP) curriculum is 60 to 80 credit hours and requires 3 to 5 years to complete; tuition runs $40,000 to $70,000 per year.
- A post-master's DNP program averages 35 to 50 credit hours and requires 2 years to complete. When you factor in the expense of the graduate degree and the years to earn it, the cost and duration are quite similar to the BSN to DNP in the end (aacn.org; https://www.aacnnursing.org/Portals/42/Policy/PDF/Debt_Report.pdf).
- The average Doctor of Philosophy (PhD) program costs $30,000 per year and requires 6 years to complete. Students incur a total cost of $180,000 (https://www.beyondphdcoaching.com/academic-career/how-much-does-a-phd-cost/).

These upfront costs are startling at first, and we understand the anxiety that such debt will induce. Only you can decide the overall impact of taking on doctoral

Degree Earned	Percent of Graduates Carrying Loans
Master's	71%
Practice Doctorate	67%
Research Doctorate	48%

NOTE: AACN Debt Report 2017.

Fig. 9.4 Percentage of Graduates Carrying Debt at Graduation from each Program of Study. (From AACN Debt Report 2017.)

education—it is an exceptionally individual decision. We offer the tools to guide and inform the decision and make it with confidence. The experts at Wharton Business School, University of Pennsylvania, have created an online Post-Graduate Education Return on Investment (ROI) calculator. We strongly encourage you to explore the data of the financial experts (https://online.wharton.upenn.edu/blog/education-roi-calculator/) (Fig. 9.4).

Expense Associated With the Programs You Are Considering

Understanding the length of the program, the total costs, and the likelihood that you will carry debt helps to inform your decisions (https://nursejournal.org/resources/how-much-does-nursing-school-cost/). Fig. 9.5 provides a reference for the percentage of students carrying loans for each graduate and terminal degree.

Program & Degree	Ranking	Fit with Career Goals	Fit with Faculty	Total Credits	Cost per Credit	Years to Completion	Completion Rate	Fees	Total Tuition	Scholarships Available	TA & RA Opportunities	Additional Costs	Other Considerations

Fig. 9.5 Data summary to inform program selection.

Your Conversation With the Financial Aid Team

Financial aid officers are there to help. The majority of funding to support doctoral study is available through their office in the school of nursing (American Association of Colleges of Nursing [AACN], 2022). So, you want to reach out, make contact, and learn about your options. I suggest you make an appointment and do your homework in advance.

For many of us, talking about money is uncomfortable. Financial aid officers are good at these conversations and can be tremendously helpful. Their mission is to connect students with available funds so you and the school can be successful. Before that conversation, you can do a few things to prepare.

You will want to be prepared to discuss the *net cost of education*. Such a focused conversation will help you learn the total tuition, fees, and related expenses that will be paid to the university; the work you can contribute to defray the total cost (research assistantships and teaching assistantships); and any funds that may be paid directly to the college to support your education (from federal programs, gifts, or endowments). Discussing these three buckets of expenses and funds can help you understand and plan to cover the total expense associated with your doctoral education.

Considering the Expense of Different Programs

We have already explained in Chapters 5 and 6 the different types of doctoral programs, DNP, PhD, Education Doctorate (EdD), Doctor of Public Health (DPH), etc. We have presented program components you want to consider in making your decision, such as remote and face-to-face options. The expenses will vary. So, as you make your decision, it will be helpful to track those details along with expenses to make a fully informed decision about which program is best for you.

We offer the worksheet in Fig. 9.5 to help you track your options and the associated expenses.

Financial Aid Definitions

The process of getting financial aid can be unfamiliar and confusing. Like nursing and healthcare, the world of finance has its own language. One barrier is not understanding that language and using it precisely. It is important to understand the difference between a loan and a scholarship or a grant and a financial aid package. Here are some terms you might encounter during your explorations (https://www.allnursingschools.com/financial-aid/).

- **Financial Aid Package:** This term describes all of the financial help given to a student. Your package could include multiple types of loans, grants, and scholarships, depending on your eligibility.

- **Financial Need:** The difference between the amount you are expected to be able to pay and the amount your chosen school or program costs. So, if the estimated amount you can pay for school is $3000 a year and your program costs $10,000, your financial need would be $7000.
- **Interest:** The fee you pay for using borrowed money. It is applied to loans at a percentage rate determined by the lender.
- **Scholarship:** Money awarded **based on achievement or accomplishment**. Scholarships can come from private organizations, schools, the government, or other groups. The amount of money provided by a scholarship will depend on the group and the individual student. For example, a scholarship from a church or nonprofit may cover $500 worth of general expenses. In contrast, a school-based scholarship may cover thousands of dollars but apply only to tuition.
- **Grants** are money given to pay for school or other expenses. Grants are **generally need based**. You might qualify for a grant if you are below a certain income level or meet other financial requirements.
- **Federal Loan** is a loan granted by the federal government to pay for education. These loans are need based and part of a financial aid package. They generally have lower interest rates than private loans, making them appealing. Most federal loans **do not require a credit check or a co-signer.**
- **A private loan** is a loan granted by banks and other financial institutions. Unlike a federal loan, these loans will have **credit and financial requirements**. You might need a co-signer if you do not have good credit, and you will likely be charged a higher interest rate.
- **Application:** For some scholarships, you need to fill out additional applications on top of the application to the program and the Free Application for Federal Student Aid (FAFSA) form. These applications might ask for transcripts, essays, resumes, letters of recommendation, or other information. Such documents help to determine the individuals best qualified to receive the award. It is well worth the work to seek the funds.
- **Qualification:** All financial aid has a qualification process. Qualifiers can provide information about your credit score, income, tax records, or previous schooling.

Necessary Steps You Can Take to Position Yourself to Be Eligible for Funding

The first thing to do is complete your FAFSA form (https://studentaid.gov/h/apply-for-aid/fafsa). Many nurses entering doctoral study think they will be ineligible for funding. You may recall from your undergraduate experience that the distribution of funds was based heavily on financial need. Furthermore, you may think that you do not meet the threshold for need because you are employed. In 2021, 32% of eligible students failed to complete the form, but failing to complete the FAFSA is a big and expensive mistake. *"If you don't complete the FAFSA, you're not in line for that aid"* (https://www.forbes.com/advisor/student-loans/fafsa-mistakes-to-avoid/).

The FAFSA form becomes available EVERY YEAR on October 1, and according to *Forbes*, there are 14 costly mistakes that millions of students make every year (Box 9.1).

It is important to understand that there are different funding sources for doctoral study, and you cannot know them all. So, we strongly encourage you to do everything you can to ensure that you will be considered eligible for any funding stream. Consideration for the majority of those funds and often for eligibility to receive funds that come in the form of gifts and endowments begins with the FAFSA

BOX 9.1 ■ Costly Mistakes to FASFA Completion

Avoid These Costly Mistakes

1. Not filling out the FAFSA Form.
2. Forgetting your Login/Application Information—take time to file your login number; it is the same every year.
3. Filing an incomplete form—Do not leave any blank spaces; pay attention to emails from the Department of Education.
4. Assuming you missed the FAFSA filing deadline, many states and colleges set priority deadlines. You must submit the FAFSA form to be considered for the aid programs they administer. There is also a federal deadline each academic year (https://studentaid.gov/h/apply-for-aid/fafsa#deadlines).
5. Not naming every school you are considering. List all schools you are considering in your list. You are allowed up to 10, and you can change them up after further review. Some states want you to list the state schools first.
6. Not watching how your school ranks on your list. Some states will provide funds only for the top three schools on your list. Make sure your list aligns with your most favored program.
7. Not filling out the form early enough. The longer you wait, the less money there is available. The form opens October 1 every year.
8. Not filling out the other scholarship and grant applications. Many schools have additional forms that need to be completed. Look into this!
9. Not filling out the FAFSA EVERY YEAR. Enough said.
10. Filling out FAFSA after you filled out Annual Income Tax. This requirement has recently changed, and now you can list prior income tax filings. So DO NOT WAIT.
11. Thinking there are age requirements. Nope. Even senior citizens can get financial aid. Married, active-duty military, with children: Everyone qualifies.
12. Thinking there are income requirements. Yes, for Pell grants (exceptional financial need), but no income requirements otherwise.
13. Not filling out the Special Circumstances Form after submitting the FAFSA—with the pandemic and economic hardships experienced nationwide, there are ways to reevaluate your financial aid package.
14. Not asking for help when you need it. Many financial aid prep companies will charge a steep fee to help families fill out the FAFSA, but there is a lot of free help.

FAFSA, Free Application for Federal Student Aid.

NOTE: You can contact the Federal Student Aid Information Center at (800) 433-3243, and/or your college's financial aid office, if you have questions.

form. Regardless of the funding source, you will need to complete the FAFSA if you wish to be considered. The form can be found online at http://www.fafsa.ed.gov.

The next thing to do is think about what you would like to learn from your conversation with the financial assistance officer. You want to treat this meeting seriously and plan your questions in advance. Some questions you might like to ask are:

- What financial support is available to students like me?
- Do you have research assistant opportunities?
- Do you offer teaching assistant opportunities?
- What amount of loans can I stake on?
- Do you have external funding for doctoral students, and am I eligible?
- Do you have gifts and endowments for which I might be eligible?
- Do you have Nurse Faculty Loan Program funds available, and am I eligible?
- Are there any state funds available to support me as I earn this doctorate?
- Are there any local funds available to support me as I earn this doctorate?
- Is there anything you would recommend I do to increase the likelihood that I might be considered for funding?

Selecting questions like this can help you get the conversation going. You can use some of this language to help you form your own question and be prepared to make the most of your time with the expert on staff at the school and program you are considering. Keep in mind, the amount you borrow now will affect your budget for years after you graduate or leave school. Before you sign a loan agreement, you want to understand the total you expect to borrow throughout college and how much you will owe each month in the future.

Other Options for Funding

There are also federal funds for which you can apply directly to the Bureau of Health Professions.

- The Nurse Faculty Loan Program requires you to teach for up to 3 years after graduation. In return, it will pay as much as 85% of your tuition.
- The Nurse Loan Program requires you to practice for up to 3 years after graduation in a healthcare facility designated as experiencing a critical shortage. The program will pay as much as 85% of your tuition.
- Faculty Loan Repayment Program forgives loans for individuals from disadvantaged backgrounds who teach for 2 or more years in designated schools for health professionals.
- Scholarships for Disadvantaged Students are awarded based on financial need to full-time students from disadvantaged backgrounds.
- Indian Health Service Loan Repayment Program. The Federal Indian Health Service awards up to $40,000 in loan repayment to clinicians who commit to 2 years of service in healthcare facilities serving American Indian and Alaska Native communities. A wide range of professions can qualify, from advanced

practice nurses to physical therapists (with a master's or doctoral degree) to licensed acupuncturists.

- Centers for Disease Control and Prevention (CDC) Epidemic Intelligence Service Program. This 2-year postgraduate fellowship is an opportunity for physicians, nurses, veterinarians, pharmacists, and more to investigate epidemiologic outbreaks, natural disasters, or other public health issues for the CDC. You may be assigned to a state or local office or the CDC headquarters.
- Health Professional Scholarship Program (HPSP) offers financial assistance to students receiving education or training in a direct or indirect healthcare services discipline and assists in providing an adequate supply of personnel for the U.S. Department of Veterans Affairs (VA). Scholarships are determined and published for Veterans Administration workforce needs.
- Other scholarships are available to full-time nursing students who will practice for 2 or more years in healthcare facilities designated as experiencing a critical shortage of nurses.

Still More Ways to Subsidize Your Education

Generally speaking, more students earning their DNP will remain employed throughout their education. If that describes your plans, then you will want to explore tuition benefits from your employer.

- Some offer benefits that pay your tuition as you go, and in that way you can keep your debt down. Often there is a ceiling for the number of credits you can carry. Understanding the terms of such plans will be key to selecting your program and planning your course of study.
- Some offer reimbursement, which compensates you for tuition you have paid for courses you have successfully completed. Commonly, these programs require a grade of B or better and may have stipulations as to the type of degree or area of concentration you may pursue.
- Some offer loans that you can pay back with a year or more of service for each year of study.

Some programs offer paid assistantships. These are commonly less attractive to DNP students who find they can earn good wages in practice while they pursue their programs of study. Assistantships tend to be more attractive to PhD students because the work is on campus or in the labs or communities where they are studying. Even more importantly, these positions are commonly affiliated with or funded through the same faculty serving as research or professional mentors to PhD students. It is important to explore opportunities for such assistantships as part of the interview and decision-making process. These opportunities tend to be reliable, flexible, and closely aligned with programs of study and can be particularly helpful to any doctoral student.

Some of the most robust and up-to-date information you can find for financing your graduate nursing education is located at Forbes. Who knows money better?

Here are the April 2022 BEST Options for Graduate Loans (https://www.forbes.com/advisor/student-loans/best-graduate-student-loans/).

1. **Federal Direct Unsubsidized Loans:** They are the best overall deal, and the fixed interest rate is one of the lowest available. This loan IS NOT credit based and does not require a co-signer. All eligible graduate borrowers qualify and receive the same rate regardless of credit history. There are numerous income-driven repayment options and other protections NOT available on private personal loans.

2. **Federal Graduate PLUS Loan.** These offer higher limits than Federal Direct Unsubsidized Loans, many repayment options, and low-interest rates. However, because of the higher loan amounts, credit checks are required. The student must be enrolled in school part time and not have an adverse credit history.

A number of private banks and state offerings are also available, and we encourage you to explore those, including PNC Bank, Discover, and Prodigy Finance, to name a few.

Building a Budget for Your Doctoral Pursuits

The same financial planning skills that will help you be a successful doctoral student and graduate are skills many of us are not accustomed to navigating. As we noted earlier in the chapter, talk of money is both uncomfortable and essential to our success. Developing the skills and comfort to approach such conversations will prove essential to finding the money you need and realizing your goals. It will take time for you as it does for every other doctoral student.

The skills you build now in preparation for this doctoral journey will set you up for a lifetime of financial accomplishment. Mapping out a budget will better prepare you to meet the demands of your current and future expenses. It can also help you to anticipate and manage the significant, irregular expenses you are likely to incur (e.g., car repairs, travel, veterinarian bills, large appliances that go on the blitz), and much more.

Once you know what expenses to expect and what money you will have coming in, create a budget using these steps (https://www.forbes.com/advisor/student-loans/build-a-college-budget/).

1. **Calculate monthly where the money is coming from and where it is going**
   Add up the available money from different sources, and figure out where your money is coming from and where it is going. Explore your income and savings, scholarships, grants, and student loans.

2. **List all of your expenses**
   Make a list of all your school-related expenses, including tuition, rent, groceries, insurance, utilities, and textbooks. Ideally, a little extra money should be available after paying fixed expenses to cover additional costs or emergencies. The fixed costs are just the tip of the iceberg: cell phone, car insurance,

health insurance, gas expenses, rent, mortgage. It would be best to track at least a month's worth of spending to see where your pocket money is going (more flexible expenses). Keep receipts, and review your debit and credit card statements, looking for extra fees and making sure there are no unauthorized purchases.

3. **Identify areas to cut back on**

   If money is tight—or you are looking to minimize the need for student loans—look for areas where you can cut back. Even minor adjustments can pay off over 4 or more years of school.

   For example, let's say you currently subscribe to three streaming services for entertainment at $10 each. You will save $20 per month—$240 per year and $960 over 4 years by canceling all but one. A little extra planning (5 minutes to brew coffee versus $6.00 three times/week for a pricey latte) will save you quite a bit of money.

   Other things you can do to reduce your expenses include:

   - Get a roommate to split housing and utility costs
   - Make a budget! Use the tool Building a Budget in Six Easy Steps (Found in the Tools section).
   - Cook meals at home and meal preparation with basic meals made in bulk
   - Go to grocery store with a grocery list, and do not go to the store hungry
   - Do not buy couture coffee (Coffee calculator)
   - Minimize convenience purchases (fast food and coffee takeaway)
   - Rent textbooks instead of buying them (rent.com)
   - Downgrade your cell phone plan

4. **Think about goals**

   Think about your educational and financial goals when creating your college student budget. For example, you may want to study abroad for a semester or buy a car once you graduate. Set aside a little money each month to have the cash you need to make your dreams a reality.

5. **Monthly check-in**

   After creating a budget, make sure you check it often. It is a good idea to review your budget weekly or monthly to help you stay on track. You can minimize excess spending and stay within your limits by making it a habit.

6. **Set aside savings**

   Add a line to your budget for savings. It is critical to have an emergency fund if you get sick or something unexpected happens. Finally, by developing solid financial habits in graduate school, you will likely use them for the rest of your life. (Your future self will thank you!)

   Just like you set a budget for spending, you should also set a budget for how much you would like to save. Set a goal of committing to saving a percentage of your monthly paycheck. Over time, it will allow you to get in the habit of always putting something away.

7. Minimize reliance on credit cards

Addressing ways to pay off your credit cards can begin the year before you begin school. One evidence-based approach is called the debt snowball or debt avalanche method. With this approach you can help chop down your debt. You pay more on the debt with the lowest balance each month while paying the minimum on the rest of your debt. Once that is paid off, you apply what you were paying on that card to the debt with the next lowest balance.

8. Make budgeting easier for yourself

The last essential graduate school budgeting tip is to get rid of the temptation to spend money whenever possible. If your weakness is ordering stuff online, it may be wise to use a site blocker during periods you know you should not be spending money. The first great tip is to minimize impulse buying. If stopping impulse buying altogether is not realistic, consider adding it to your budget. Designate a set amount each week or month, and keep your impulse buying below that amount (Nurse Journal, 2022).

Second, to best stay within your spending limit when you go out, bring only a set amount of cash to pay instead of a credit card, to limit your spending.

Summary

Obstacles don't have to stop you.
If you run into a wall, don't turn around and give up.
Figure out how to climb it, go through it, or work around it.

—MICHAEL JORDAN

From our work with nurses contemplating doctoral education, we have learned that finding a way to fund that education is a top priority for almost everyone. We strongly encourage you to situate that concern in context. Contemplating any big stretch goal (and earning a doctorate is certainly a stretch goal) invites any reasonable person to consider those things that might become threats to our success. So, identifying the threat to managing finances is reasonable and prudent. Your charge is not to stop there but to use that threat assessment to generate an action plan.

Funding your education can appear to be Michael Jordan's wall. Our intent in this chapter is to help you develop a plan to work your way over it, around it, or through it. We intend to help you focus not only on the expense of education but the ways you can manage those expenses, subsidize your education, avoid making decisions that lead you to take on more debt than necessary, and remind you to keep your goals in focus on the return you can expect from this investment.

We get it. Pursuing a doctoral degree will cost a lot of money. We understand the challenges that you must consider as you ponder the importance of doctoral education to your future self. It is overwhelming, to say the least, and we want you to know that we hear the groans and woes of your inner planning self. "Wait, I have a mortgage, credit cards, and kids and life."

Still, we challenge you to envision a future in which you are a doctorally prepared nurse. We cannot even fully list the many opportunities that will become available here because we are only just beginning to understand the contributions of nursing to practice, research, education, informatics, genomics, and policy. The nursing positions nowadays were not even identified in years past. By earning a doctoral degree, you leverage to pivot quickly and be responsive to the future of our healthcare delivery and educational system—to have the talent and the capability to affect significant practical changes in how healthcare is delivered.

Reading this chapter, you have learned about the language of tuition, loans, and funding. You have learned about FASFA, budgeting, and support available to you through employers and faculty. You have discovered the kinds of questions you can ask to help you make informed decisions with confidence, and you have learned to consider the financial aid officers among your best friends and allies.

Bibliography

American Association of Colleges of Nursing. *Financing Graduate Nursing Education: The Numbers Behind the Degree*. 2017. Available at: https://www.aacnnursing.org/Portals/42/Policy/PDF/Debt_Report.pdf.

American Association of Colleges of Nursing. *Your Guide to Graduate Nursing Programs*. 2022. Available at: https://www.aacnnursing.org/Portals/42/Publications/Brochures/GradStudentsBrochure.pdf.

The Condition of Education Trends in Student Loan Debt for Graduate School Completers. 2018. Available at: https://nces.ed.gov/programs/coe/pdf/coe_tub.pdf. Accessed April 13, 2022.

H.R. 4508, the PROSPER Act: Proposed Reauthorization of the Higher Education Act. 2018. Available at: https://files.eric.ed.gov/fulltext/ED593626.pdf.

The Institute for College Access & Success. *Student Debt and the Class of 2018*. The 14th Annual Report. 2018. Available at: https://ticas.org/wp-content/uploads/2019/09/classof2018.pdf.

Institute of Educational Sciences. *College Affordability Views and College Enrollment*. 2022. Available at: https://nces.ed.gov/pubs2022/2022057.pdf. Accessed April 13, 2022.

Levine P. *The College Cost Conundrum: College is Cheaper Than Students and Their Families Think*. The Chronicle of Higher Education; 2022. Available at: https://www.chronicle.com/article/the-college-cost-conundrum.

National Center for Education Statistics. *Tuition and Fees of Degree-Granting Institutions*. 2022. Available at: https://nces.ed.gov/fastfacts/display.asp?id=76. Accessed April 13, 2022.

Nurse Journal. *How Much does Nursing School Cost?* 2022. Available at: https://nursejournal.org/resources/how-much-does-nursing-school-cost/.

United States Department of Education. Federal Student Aid. Creating Your Budget. Accessed February 7, 2023. https://studentaid.gov/resources/prepare-for-college/students/budgeting/creating-your-budget

CHAPTER 10

Presenting a Strong and Authentic Application

Laura A. Taylor, PhD, RN, ANEF, FAAN

Let us never consider ourselves finished nurses… We must be learning all of our lives.
—Florence Nightingale

Your application is the program faculty's first objective encounter with you. A strategic, calculated approach is essential, because this document will evidence what you value and what you have achieved and will reflect your attention to detail. This chapter will outline the process and components of the application, highlighting the many intricacies of a doctoral application, and will offer a few simple rules to help your application stand out among the many reviewed.

Schools of nursing receive hundreds of applications every year: far more than the number of spaces available for admissions and certainly more than there are faculty to support. The faculty and staff who are charged with making admissions decisions seek to find applicants who are a good fit for their program and are likely to be successful. Reviewers do not want to eliminate people: they want to find the very best. Your challenge is to present an application that gives those reviewers confidence that you will be successful as a doctoral student and that you are just the person that they will be proud to claim as an alumnus.

The purpose of this chapter is to:

- decode the application as a narrative
- provide some guidance to help you avoid common problems
- encourage you to take the risk of presenting your best, authentic self.

Application as Narrative

Your application is the most important story you have told (yet). It is a document that introduces you to the team charged with making admissions decisions. The admissions process is competitive, but it is not adversarial. Faculty want to find the very best students for their programs. They want to find students who can be successful, and following directions is essential to success in doctoral study. That is why it is so important that you read carefully and eliminate errors. When an applicant does not follow the directions and does not proofread the application package, the reviewers will not likely move the application forward. They are likely to not give one of the few admissions slots to a person who does not seem to be committed to, or capable of, preparing a strong application package (Farrington, 2019).

So…

A FEW SIMPLE RULES FOR WRITING YOUR APPLICATION

Before we discuss the substance of your application, let's identify a few simple, yet important rules.

- Follow the directions.
- Provide all the information requested.
- Help the reviewers know who you are, what is important to you, and why you are the perfect fit for their program.
- Be sure your application is error free.

Getting Organized

The key to a successful application process is disciplined organization. It might seem like common sense, but it is imperative to cover organization processes and emphasize the importance of carefully following directions to ensure your application is complete. Here is why. A disproportionately large number of applications are declined because of something that has nothing to do with the knowledge or passion of the applicant, but merely poor organization skills and failure to follow the directions (*Forbes*, https://www.forbes.com/sites/robertfarrington/2019/08/29/why-your-college-application-was-rejected/?sh=2383a668513f; Taylor & Terhaar, 2018). Without a consistent, organized approach to your application process, you risk infractions such as failing to answer all the questions on the application or, ultimately, failing to complete the entire application by the due date.

Being orderly minimizes stress and increases your overall productivity. Creating a logical infrastructure to the application processes allows for easy retrieval of necessary files and needed documents. Each doctoral programs' application demands similar deliverables, such as transcripts, recommendations, and essays, and therefore having common folders for the common elements seems a reasonable approach (Weiner, 2013). A streamlined central document file system, also known as "directory tree," to track applications, due dates, and other requirements, can keep you organized and on target for a timely submission (https://www.forbes.com/sites/robertfarrington) (Fig. 10.1).

You will want to construct a mechanism to track the completed steps and those that still need to be finalized. Approaches to getting this done are many, and we encourage you to choose an approach that is easy to document and track and is best for you. For those who prefer nonelectronic methods of planning and tracking deadlines, try a paper day calendar scheduler or a dry-erase board. Lifehacks

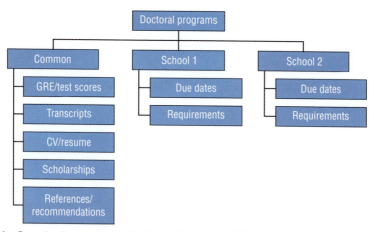

Fig. 10.1   Sample directory tree. *CV*, Curriculum vitae; *GRE,* Graduate Record Examination.

(lifehacks.org) offers an annual review on best new electronic calendar apps and scheduling products currently on the market, available on both Android and Apple products.

Speaking of staying on target, at the end of the chapter we have crafted a 12-month pre-application submission calendar (the entire purpose of this text) that includes best practice time frames for assuring that your doctoral application submission is timely, accurate, and successful. First we will identify the most common components of the doctoral application and offer evidenced-based strategies for completing each component with confidence.

GRADUATE RECORD EXAMINATION SCORES

If the thought of taking the Graduate Record Examination (GRE), or any other standardized test, promotes gastrointestinal reflux, do not despair! You are not alone, and there are numerous H2 antagonists available to provide rapid relief. More importantly, universities and colleges around the country are reading the data highlighting the lack of effectiveness of standardized testing on predicting doctoral candidate success and are reporting a tremendous increase in admissions numbers and diversity across their student populations with the removal of required standardized testing. "We saw tremendous gains in college admissions for disenfranchised students during this year," bringing "true equity and progress for students" (Hoover, 2021).

Today, graduate programs are incorporating a more balanced application experience for applicants, known as "Wholistic Admissions." This approach includes a "constellation of characteristics" that can be found in the confluence of letters of recommendation, essay and purpose statements, interviews, and college transcripts (reflecting GPA) and is viewed as a very welcomed trend in graduate and doctoral education (Benderly, 2017).

This trend can have a calming effect on applicant anxiety across future applicants. However, DO NOT cross a program off your prospective program list because of a GRE requirement. With this approach, you decline yourself! We realize that standardized testing anxiety is real, but do not let it stop you from applying to the program of your dreams. Here are some tips to prevailing over GRE anxiety.

1. Some doctoral programs guide you toward successful test preparation resources and practice tests, with both free and fee-based options (see Chapter 33).
2. Programs often share the average score for the most recently admitted/matriculated cohort. It may also be on the website in the application page.
3. There are numerous review books available.
4. Organizations around the country offer excellent test preparation options, including Education Testing Systems (ETS) with a Powerprep practice site (https://www.ets.org/gre/revised_general/prepare/powerprep/) and Magoosh (https://gre.magoosh.com/) and Coursera (coursera.org). You can find these resources in Chapter 33.
5. If you need to achieve a specific score, you may need to take the exam multiple times. Determine a target score and how many times you are willing to retake the exam. Resources such as Varsity Tutors (https://www.varsitytutors.com/gre-practice-tests) and Mometrix (https://www.mometrix.com/academy/gre-quantitative-practice-test/) allow you to gauge the level of preparation needed on an individual level, thereby creating personal data and preparation plans.

Keep in mind that GREs scores and other standardized testing scores are only one small piece of the application process. Average or even subpar scores can be complemented with exceptional letters of recommendation in combination with error-free essay and purpose statement writing that highlights your leadership, team-building skills, and scholarly potential.

TRANSCRIPTS AND COURSE REQUIREMENTS

Securing all prior undergraduate and graduate transcripts and, occasionally, high school transcripts will take time. Today, college and university registrar offices offer online accessibility for ordering transcripts. There may be a nominal fee, and it may take up to 3 to 4 weeks to arrive by United States Postal Service (USPS). As transcripts are received, place them carefully in the directory tree for ease of access across program applications. Be sure to seek clarity from the admissions office if you have questions. Do not make assumptions and risk submitting a package that is incomplete.

A common requirement for doctoral programs is a graduate-level science course taken within the past 5 years. Closely review the level (graduate or undergraduate) and type (basic science, skills) being requested. An undergraduate nutrition course will surely let you down when jumping into advanced graduate anatomy and physiology and ultimately may disqualify the application. This is a tremendous opportunity to reintroduce yourself to the graduate-level education environment and explore the newest technology learning platforms that colleges and universities are integrating into their programs. Taken as a whole, this heightens your potential for success.

If you are concerned about a transcript that reveals a less than optimal undergraduate performance in a course or semester or two, we have some advice. First, this is where your ability to demonstrate growth in learning and dedication to improving can be highly evident in your success with the required graduate-level science course. Second, engage in some active preempting of admissions committee's questions with a purpose statement or essay acknowledging these challenges of undergraduate life and misguided youthful oblivion and how they have given way to incredible personal and professional development. Seal the deal by ensuring each component of the application is precisely crafted and submitted without error.

Building a Professional Resumé and Curriculum Vitae

Submitting an updated resumé and curriculum vitae (CV) is a common request of doctoral programs and requires paying close attention to the specifics such as word or page limit, font type and size, and formatting. Craft a resumé template beforehand, place it in your directory tree, and change out the information based on the program (https://thisgirlknowsit.com/how-to-organize-your-scholarship-binder/). Follow these basic tips in building a professional document.

Tip #1 Tailor the CV/resumé to the school of choice.

If the program is asking for a resumé or CV, the admissions committee is examining your past education and work experiences. They are looking for a correlation between your achievements and how you see the future. By carefully reviewing the website of the nursing program, you can see what the program is requesting and make sure you qualify for the program. Registered nurse anesthesia (RNA) programs demand at least 1800 hours of intensive care unit hours and Critical Care Registered Nurse (CCRN) certification. Make note of the program requirements, objectives, and relevant mission or vision statements, and be sure to align these with your resumé essays and purpose statements.

Tip #2 Showcase professional achievements and awards.

Highlighting an array of experiences, including internships, and professional certifications, underlines how you have continued to seek out contributing to the nursing profession. Course work and professional conferences attended demonstrate your dedication to professional development. List professional organizations and memberships, which further demonstrate additional breadth of your drive for professional nursing. List your publications and presentations or posters you have achieved to further underscore your leadership potential.

Tip # 3 Clear, concise, explicit (CCE).

The CV or resumé should be clear, concise and explicit, well formatted, and free of typos and grammatical errors. The resumé reflects you. It should be polished and well coordinated.

WRITING SKILLS

Doctoral faculty are not expecting applicants to enter as prolific scholarly authors, yet writing skills are showcased throughout the doctoral application. Admissions committees rely on clarity in your writing to learn your story, and well-crafted writing conveys confidence that the applicant will be a successful doctoral graduate. Dr. Deborah Trautman, Chief Executive Officer (CEO) of AACN, uses a key phrase in optimal writing: "Be clear, concise, and explicit in your communications. CCE" (Deborah Trautman, personal communication, January 20, 2019). The foundation of scholarly dissemination in doctoral work is crisp, logical writing.

Purpose statements, essays, scholarship letters, cover letters, and resumés demand fundamental writing skills (Russell-Pinson & Harris, 2019). A CCE application offers insights into your foundational skills and showcases your ability to build connections between thoughts and ideas, all the while using correct punctuation with proper grammar. Without CCE, your authentic message becomes murky, or could even get lost, thereby lessening your chances for a successful admission.

STRATEGIES TO BUILD YOUR CONFIDENCE IN WRITING

Most nurses report being more comfortable with "charting by exception" as compared with writing a complete sentence with a noun, a verb, and perhaps even adjectives. This section offers strategies to build skills in stringing multiple sentences together. Here are a few easy, inexpensive tactics to strengthen your writing, and many more are offered in Chapter 12 on Writing by Dr. Kim Currie.

Journal: Journaling every day helps get thoughts on paper. The more one writes, the less one focuses on writing as a threat. A gratitude journal not only has been shown to brighten your inner being, but thoughts being strung together repeatedly in daily journaling have been shown to strengthen writing fluidity (Burnett & Evans, 2016).

Just Read: The editor of the National Association of Clinical Nurse Specialists (NACNS) journal, Dr. Janet Fulton, once said, "You write what you read" (personal communication, March 10, 2019). So, read. Read an article every day. It can be an article on an application on your phone, a newspaper article, your facility newsletter, or email newsletters from your professional organization.

FREE RESOURCES TO SHAPE SKILLS

Websites: Websites are available to help you recraft a sentence and offer ways to strengthen punctuation and grammar. WritersWrite.com is fun to check out for punctuation and grammar hints. Lynn Truss is author of *Eats, Shoots & Leaves* (https://www.writerswrite.co.za/punctuation-for-beginners-what-is-punctuation/), a blog that is engaging and offers easy fixes to boost skills.

Check out **Coursera** (resource available in Chapter 33), free courses from renowned national and international faculty and programs. The courses very often include homework assignments and, most importantly, the opportunity receive quality feedback. Here are just a few offered across varying schedules.

Good with Words
https://www.coursera.org/specializations/good-with-words
Writing About Yourself!
https://www.coursera.org/specializations/memoir-personal-essay
Writing - Editing Structure
https://www.coursera.org/learn/writing-editing-structure
Stanford University's PhD program offers a free online course called Writing for the Sciences. The link is https://www.coursera.org/learn/sciwrite.

Community College: Check out your local community college (CC). Sign up for a refresher English course. CCs are usually inexpensive (comparatively) and allow you to ease back into the work and dust off distant writing skill sets.

Alumni Associations/Undergraduate Institution: Many colleges and university alumni associations support alum with a career center or learning lab to build and review applications, resumés, and a CV.

PURPOSE STATEMENT AND ESSAYS

A CCE essay and purpose statement explaining your area of interest assist admissions committees in unifying program offerings with your future work. This includes identifying the perfect complement of faculty mentoring, university resources, and outside community partners that can support your program of study (Gonzalez & Finnell, 2021). Writing convincingly makes it unmistakably clear why and how this doctoral program aligns with your future professional career goals. Admissions reviewers should be able to clearly identify the applicant's understanding of the importance and relevance of the proposed healthcare challenge discussed in the essay. Finally, a thoughtful, well-crafted essay and purpose statement help build a well-defined case on how you will be a phenomenal asset to the selected program (https://www.accepted.com/grad/application, retrieved May 2021).

When it comes to answering requested essays and short-answer components of the application, read carefully. Adherence to word and character count limits provides insights on your ability to read carefully and follow the guidance offered. Using "Word Count" and "Character Count" in your word processing software will ensure you stay within the required parameters.

CITATION MANAGEMENT

The format for citations may be clarified in the application. The consistency of the citations throughout the application is a must. Purdue Owl is a free resource available by Purdue University and offers citation management support and direction in either American Psychology Association (APA) or Modern Language Association (MLA) (https://owl.purdue.edu/search.html). APA offers free tutorials and online services including recorded webinars to help refresh your memory (https://apastyle.apa.org/instructional-aids/tutorials-webinars).

EDITING ASSISTANCE

Basic word editors (spelling and thesaurus) will look for spelling errors but not necessarily for context errors. Three common and easily accessible at-home editing options are Microsoft Word Editor, Microsoft Word 365, and Grammarly. Microsoft Word Editor does include a useful word count and character-counting function, a find-and-replace-text function (useful if you are using similar essays for different schools), spelling, and thesaurus. Microsoft Word 365 has some updated mechanisms as well. Take time to review the options (Microsoft Soft Support, https://support.microsoft.com/en-us/office/microsoft-editor-checks-grammar-and-more-in-documents-mail-and-the-web-91ecbe1b-d021-4e9e-a82e-abc4cd7163d7).

Grammarly is also extremely helpful (Grammarly.com; free install). Grammarly will assist with comma placement, context of words: *Their on the hill is a dear.* **Their** and **dear** are spelled correctly, but they are incorrect in this context. In addition, Grammarly hates passive voice. More about "voice" in your writing is discussed in Chapter 12. In summary, when writing the personal statement and essays, use active voice. Active voice means that the subject of the sentence is doing the action.

Passive: While applying (action verb) to doctoral programs, Susan (subject) began to get exhausted.

Active: Susan (subject) got exhausted while applying (action) to doctoral programs.

A critical review of not only your essays and purpose statement but the entire application packet is without a doubt one of the most important bits of advice we can offer. Ask a trusted friend or colleague to review your application. These individuals are well positioned to offer universal feedback, see broader themes, and offer direction for greater continuity. Be open, courteous, and receptive to seeking ways to strengthen and clarify your work. Receiving direct and constructive feedback is a major life skill in doctoral education. Do not get discouraged if it takes three or more revisions. Finally, be sure to acknowledge the efforts of every reviewer with a small token of appreciation and keep them apprised of your successful admission.

The Interview(s)

The interview is the stage of the application where program faculty, intrigued with what you have presented on the documents submitted, offer an invitation to interview. It indicates that the program wants to learn more about you, your interests, and your scholarly potential. One significant purpose of the interview is ensuring that you, the interviewee, can express an understanding of the degree being sought. This will be front and center during your interview (Jones et al., 2017). An interview is your opportunity to complete the story of you and to express intelligence, knowledge, confidence, flexibility and adaptability, professionalism, persistence, and passion to be a doctoral student and future alum of their program (Box 10.1).

The two major components to a doctoral program interview include the logistics of the process (online or in-person) and the substance of the interview.

LOGISTICS FOR THE ONLINE INTERVIEW

1. Know the platform of the online interview. Request a practice session especially if you have never used the video platform.
2. Double check the lighting (video conferencing) and camera angle. Fill your face with light. Keep the camera at head on or eye level. Use a stack of books or a table to elevate the camera. You do not want to offer an unflattering view up or down.
3. Look professional from head to toe (video and face to face). Our recent pandemic made the "Zoom call" a new Webster dictionary–approved term, and if Zoom is the interview approach, we suggest being clothed as if for an in-person interview. Check out the Indeed Editorial Team (2021) (https://www.indeed.com/career-advice/interviewing/how-to-dress-for-a-job-interview) and Chronicles of Higher Education to gather more best-dressed tips for your interview.

BOX 10.1 ■ What a Programmatic Interview Will Reveal About You[a]

Do you understand the program you are applying for?
- Ability to communicate
- Ability to deescalate and address conflict
- Ability to think about next steps/future
- Readiness to learn
- Ability to answer questions

Did you research the program you are applying for?
- Reasonable expectations
- Flexible, adaptable
- Problem solver

[a]https://www.resume-now.com/job-resources/interviews/job-interviews-20-things-an-interviewer-looks-for-during-an-interview.

---

4. Be careful of a messy background or anything distracting. Do not have an unmade untidy bed in the background, and do not allow the cat or gecko to run across your keyboard.

5. Video conference with a friend, and have him or her send a screen shot of what he or she sees. This helps you consider your online presence and identify where to focus your gaze.

6. Best practices suggest being at least 5 to 10 minutes early for either an online or in-person interview. Make sure all wires and connections do what they are supposed to do: connect (https://www.careeraddict.com/interview-arrive).

    a. Makeup is a huge benefit, especially in video conferencing. Consider the following points to counteract the "lighting" challenges many experience during video conferencing. (How to look good on video calls: https://www.youtube.com/watch?v=ACNGhPKnmok)

    b. Men and women both benefit from makeup or a little pressed powder to keep glare and shine to a minimum.

    c. The lighting for a video conference is very different than an for an in-person meeting. Experts suggest if you do wear makeup, put it on while looking into the camera of the video platform. What looks orange or overbronzed in person makes you look healthy and full of good color to those on the video call.

    d. Most video platforms allow you to "soften" the camera and autocorrect for low light (see settings of the video conference platform). Certain platforms will allow a "camera check" before turning your camera on. Take advantage of that option to make sure you are looking sharp and ready to take on doctoral education.

    e. Consider trimming your beard or mustache prior to the video conference.

7. To prepare for the face to face, follow many of the same steps mentioned above.

    a. Like #5, be aware of your gaze, and when face to face, maintain eye contact.

    b. Be 5 minutes early for the in-person meeting.

THE SUBSTANCE OF THE INTERVIEW

The selection of faculty in attendance during either an online or in-person interview is based on the information provided in your application. These faculty in attendance are most likely those assigned to mentor and advise you through the program (Jones et al., 2017). Request the names of the members of the interview committee. Never underestimate the importance of exploring the program website and seeking out information about these individuals. This showcases your ability to connect faculty scholarship with your interests and sends the signal that you dedicated time to explore how the program, the curriculum, and faculty will impact your doctoral journey.

There are questions commonly discussed during a doctoral interview (Table 10.1). An interview allows you to share stories of teamwork, communication tactics both

TABLE 10.1 ■ **Common Questions and Their Associated Themes**

Common Questions	What They Are Looking for in Your Answer
Tell us about a project that was very successful. What was it about that team/work/project that helped it go in such a positive direction?	Teamwork and project outcomes
What was your role in a project that didn't go so well, and what do you believe was the major contributing factor to the team?	Ability to understand best approaches to making a team function well
How would your colleagues describe you and your leadership style?	Leadership style, emotional intelligence of best practices in guiding teammates
How would your colleagues describe your strengths? Or challenges?	Are you a strong, consistent, reliable member of the team
Can you tell us about a time that you received critical feedback that was difficult to hear? How did you feel and what did you take away? How did you incorporate the feedback into your plan of care?	Ability to incorporate feedback and move forward with self-improvement
Share a time when you had to give critical feedback to a colleague. How did that go, and how might you do it differently next time?	Professional skills in communication; receptiveness to feedback
What makes a strong team? What would your colleagues say is your trigger for getting upset with a situation? What is the question you want to answer?	Awareness of positive teamwork and leadership style needed for cohesive work. Understanding of the degree
Is there a member of our faculty that speaks to your area of interest and why?	Research interest and alignment
What emerging and priority areas of science have caught your interest?	Awareness of nursing science and its contribution to healthcare
Why is this program good for you? Why now?	Thoughtful consideration of life's challenges and future directions and potential to navigate obstacles when presented
Tell us about some of the best books you have read or movies you have watched.	By interviewing you, the department is also trying to get a sense of who you are as a person (and as a potential colleague). They might ask general questions about your experiences, your taste in books, your undergrad experience, etc.—just to start a conversation. Be yourself.

good and bad situations, leadership challenges and successes, interprofessional collaborations, and your ability to move forward and learn from difficult feedback.

Reflect on key experiences in your career with story highlights and thematic strings that can be woven to showcase multiple layers of your professional leadership and perspectives toward a healthcare situation and your drive to explore more with your doctoral education. Connecting lessons learned to your future doctoral journey will contribute to a successful interview.

A wonderful preparatory tool is to have a mock interview with two or three colleagues to guide you during an online or face to face interview. Direct the mock interview team to ask the questions in Table 10.1 in a random fashion and to offer honest feedback on areas such as communication, clarity, body language, and ability to stay on point.

References

Read the directions for each program carefully to ensure your reference selections match the requirements. The specific number of references, qualities of the references (education level or position), and the format of the reference letter is unique to each program. These program-specific details can be outlined in your directory tree file. Seek out individuals you have worked with directly for a meaningful amount of time, as well as those who can speak to your specific strengths. The reference should be able to describe how these strengths will serve you well in a doctoral program and the benefits of the chosen institution for your professional growth.

In some cases, a required reference must be a direct supervisor. If your working relationship with this individual is turbulent at best, it is imperative to ensure that your other references are well positioned to focus attention on your scholarly potential and leadership skills.

REACHING OUT FOR REFERENCES

The following are some approaches to asking a favorite professor or colleague from prior work experience to be a reference. First, always contact the individual before submitting his or her name into the online application (https://www.indeed.com/career-advice/career-development/recommendation-for-graduate-school, retrieved May 2021). Explore your alma mater website and faculty listings, use LinkedIn, Google Scholar, or search in *PubMed or CINAHL* to find current publications. The institutions of employment for the corresponding authors are often cited in the publications.

Craft an email such as the one in Fig. 10.2. Share a short remembrance to guide the recipient to the purpose of your acquaintance.

- Offer a brief explanation on why you are reaching out.
- Share an important lessoned learned or invaluable pearl of wisdom that you gained from them.

Dear Dr. Taylor,

Eight years ago, I had the pleasure of having you as my academic adviser and professor. I clearly remember your voice in the pathophysiology class during a lecture on liver disease. You commented jokingly that a man needs to love you not with all his heart, but with his liver. Good times....

My acceptance to the BS to MSN program at XX School of Nursing was the culmination of several years of hard work and dedication. I started the nursing program in 2012, as a single mother to a two-year-old child. During that time, I balanced the obligations of an intensive accelerated BSN program and the responsibilities of motherhood. I ended up working in the ORs at a level one trauma center and later worked as an OR nurse at XX Medical Center. Working for both of these prominent institutions has enabled the growth of my nursing skills.

I reached out to you in April asking for a letter of recommendation for the XX Family Nurse Practitioner program and you kindly agreed to write me a letter. At this point in my life, I am more passionate and assured about my profession and the person I want to become and would like to know if you are still able to write me a letter.

I have attached my goal statement for your reference. Thank you very much for your kindness in writing me a letter of recommendation to support my application for the M.S. Family Nurse Practitioner program. A reference request will be emailed to you from NursingCAS. Your time and effort are greatly appreciated.

Sincerely,

Grateful Future Nursing Scholar

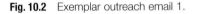

Fig. 10.2   Exemplar outreach email 1.

- Note the clinical acumen that made an impression on you.
- Share the accomplishments you have earned since working with them. This allows the individual to write a distinctive letter that aligns you and your work with the credentials and opportunities afforded by the program.

PROVIDING GUIDANCE FOR ACADEMIC OR PROFESSIONAL REFERENCE

These are very busy professionals, willing to move this request forward for you, so let's offer support to get the job done easily and done well. Proivde the following relevant information to make it easier for the individual to craft the letter and to get it completed accurately and in a timely fashion (Box 10.2.)

Today's universities use robust online forms that are very beneficial for getting references completed and submitted on time. Online reference letters from the Nursing Centralized Application System (NCAS) are quantitative in nature with Likert scale–like questions. There are opportunities in many online forms for the reference to offer qualitative support in the form of a letter/PDF or free text. Furthermore, it is

---

BOX 10.2 ■ Items to Offer for References

Letter of Reference Logistics

1. The university, college, program name
2. The statement of purpose
3. Research/work/leadership highlights
4. Awards and honors received
5. Resumé/curriculum vitae (CV)
6. Submission deadline
7. Instructions for submitting the letter
8. Your contact information

Scholarly Skills and Strengths to Highlight in the Reference Letter

1. Ability to lead colleagues
2. Enthusiasm for the work and the patients
3. Motivation and dependability
4. Trustworthiness getting jobs and projects done and done well
5. Decision-making skills and ability to take charge of volatile situations that demand leadership,
6. Ability to work with and across transdisciplinary teams and invite others
7. Ability to build cohesive complimentary teams
8. Ability to accept both constructive and positive feedback
9. Attentive listener
10. Incorporates positive change in self
11. Prior projects that showcase leadership

---

not uncommon for the reference to ask for you to a draft a letter of recommendation to amplify professional growth, teamwork, and scholarly potential. Accommodate them with a letter that you have built using the qualities in Box 10.2.

Please take note: When providing a draft letter and summary of your career for multiple references, remember to emphasize a different project or care quality in each letter. As mentioned earlier, these are busy individuals, and they may not offer additional verbiage to the letter you provide, thereby submitting the letter you drafted. Admissions committees have reported receiving the same letter of recommendation from different references. This is not helpful for you. The following are some steps to take to build your own personal reference letter and get it submitted on time.

THE LETTER

1. When beginning your story, try substituting your name with someone famous like Mary Poppins or Tom Hanks, and then start writing. It is easier to write positively about someone other than yourself. This tactic helps alleviate the discomfort, because Mary Poppins is practically perfect in every way. Choose a positive image.
2. Build the professional journey chronologically. This helps demonstrate growth as a nursing professional.

3. Describe a project or care delivery improvement you have been involved with that not only involved interprofessional collaborative work but that you led or co-led, and note how it inspired you to seek the advanced degree at this time.

4. Highlight critical experiences or questions that directly led to more unanswered questions. These questions are driving you back to school so that you can strengthen your understanding of successful teams, systems change, and discover the answers to the unique healthcare questions.

Provide the requested reference a comfortable way to decline because admissions committees report that receiving less than glowing recommendations can do more harm than good (https://www.indeed.com/career-advice/career-development/recommendation-for-graduate-school, retrieved May 2021). Be clear in your outreach to a potential reference. "Do you feel you can write a letter that addresses and highlights my strengths of organization and scholarly potential?" Here your reference can easily bow out if they are not able to write a strong, recommendation. Never forget to send a thank-you note to anyone who provided a letter, and be sure to apprise all references of your success in admissions.

REMINDERS FOR BUSY PROFESSIONALS

Send occasional reminders to help these generous individuals remember their commitment. Keep a notebook or a file in your directory tree on all potential references. A time frame of 4 to 6 weeks to complete the reference process is ample. Leave yourself 2 weeks before the due date because people get busy.

A CALENDAR TO PLAN YOUR APPLICATION JOURNEY

As you start this journey, it can become very difficult to stay organized and on target with your goal. An effective content calendar will keep you from missing meetings, appointments, and due dates. As in the title of this book, optimal consideration of your doctoral pursuits should begin about 6 to 12 months before the due date of the application. Many program applications are due November through February for the following Summer or Fall admission. Exploring nursing programs is easier now than ever before if you use the American Association of Colleges of Nursing (AACN) website to help identify accredited programs around the country (https://www.aacnnursing.org/Students/Find-a-Nursing-Program). A well-crafted calendar will save you time and energy. Below we "chunk out" the year before you apply with clear steps to successfully submit your best application. Table 10.2 shows a sample calendar you can use to track the stages of your applications.

Six to 12 Months Out

- Begin a new journal where you will write down what topic or area you want to explore; the location of the university (in or out of state); your favorite learning delivery modality (distributive learning only, face to face, hybrid); and favorite

TABLE 10.2 ■ **Sample Table to Track Your Application Progress**

Requirements	School of Nursing DNP/PhD	School of Nursing PhD
Essay	300 Words with prompt question	700 Characters with prompt question
Start Outline	6/1	6/1
Review by Outside Colleague	Requested Dr. Taylor 10/25	Requested Dr. Bob 10/25
Goal Date	11/20	11/20
Status	In progress	In progress
Recommendation requirements:	2 recommenders	3 recommenders
Recommender #1:	Professor Holmes	Professor Nightingale
Recommender #1 status:	requested 9/1	requested 9/1
Recommender #2:	Professor Sprout	Professor Chickpea
Recommender #2 status:	received by school 10/15	received by school 10/18
Recommender #3:	n/a	Professor Taylor
Recommender #3 status:	n/a	requested 9/2
Status:	currently editing	started draft
GRE requirements:	Regular GRE, Holistic Admissions	GRE Optional Wholistic Admissions
Test dates	6/1	6/1
Status:	test taken; scores sent	both tests taken; scores sent
Advanced Science Requirement	Graduate Level Science within 5 years	Graduate Level Science within 5 years: Anatomy, Pathophysiology recommended
Status	Completed 5/01	Pathophysiology
Grade	A	B+
Transcript Requirements:	College, AD program, LPN Program	College, AA Program Only
Transcript status:	Received 10/15	Requested 9/15
Application Form:	Due 12/15	Due 12/31
Goal date:	complete 11/20	complete 12/1
Application Fee	$150	$175

AD, Associate Degree; *DNP*, Doctor of Nursing Practice; *GRE*, Graduate Record Examination; *LPN*, License Practical Nurse; *PhD*, Doctor of Philosophy.

articles, colleagues, and healthcare experts whom you want to contact as you start this journey for direction or feedback.

- Explore programs, and make a list of pros and cons. Identify factors that are most important for you. Use the link to AACN to figure out where you want to explore (https://www.aacnnursing.org/Students/Find-a-Nursing-Program).
- List program requirements, and decide how you will tackle them: GREs, references, transcripts, essays, CV/resumé.
- Begin seeking resources to build confidence in writing (Coursera, Stanford, CCs).
- Attend program Open Houses and other outreach events for programs you are interested in.
- Find a mentor who will support you on this journey, perhaps a potential faculty mentor for your research proposal before formally applying. This approach can help to clarify the alignment of your research interests with the best program (Stanfil et al., 2019).

Four to 6 Months

- List requirements for each program in the folder, and decide how you will tackle them
- Set up appointments to take standardized tests
- Purposely reach out to program faculty via email or phone call
- Read program applications very carefully and begin to outline essays.

Two to 3 Months

- Continue to outline your essays.
- Reach out to individuals who will be strong potential references for letters of recommendation (see Box 10.2).
- Initiate transcript retrieval.

One to 2 Months

- Mock interview with trusted colleagues who can offer strong constructive feedback
- Application review by colleagues
- Keep working on essays

Two to 4 Weeks

- Make sure that recommendations and transcripts have been submitted
- Proofread the application
- Submit When Ready. Plan for 2 weeks before so that any items that are missing or had not been received can be acquired before due date (McMammon, 2017; https://www.prepscholar.com/gre/blog/when-to-apply-for-grad-school/).

Summary

Submitting a doctoral application is a process that calls for dedicated time to ensure that you have included all the required documentation and all the deadlines have been met. Getting into a doctoral program demands detailed preparation and thoughtful consideration of your career to date and heartfelt reflection on how this educational endeavor will elevate you and your future contributions to nursing and healthcare science. The programs receive many applications, and you want yours to shine and rise above the rest. The application is the first impression you will make on the university and the admissions committee. By understanding the interconnectedness of each component of the application and its reflection of your professional vision of who will become and how you will contribute to the future, you will be putting your best foot forward.

Bibliography

American Association of Colleges of Nursing. Find a Nursing Program. 2021. Available at: https://www.aacnnursing.org/Students/Find-a-Nursing-Program.

Benderly BL. *GREs don't predict grad school success. What does?* Taken for Granted Column. 2017. doi:10.1126/science.caredit.a1700046.

Burnett B, Evans D. *Designing Your Life: How to Build a Well-Lived, Joyful Life.* Knopf; 2016.

Farrington R. *5 Mistakes That Could Get Your Graduate Application Rejected.* Forbes Advisor; 2019. Available at: https://www.forbes.com/sites/robertfarrington/2019/08/29/why-your-college-application-was-rejected/?sh=2383a668513f.

Gonzalez Y, Finnell DS. Promoting and supporting a doctor of nursing practice program of scholarship. *J Nurs Educ.* 2021;59(9):526-530. doi:10.3928/01484834-20200817-10.

Hoover E. (2021). *Georgia's Public Universities will Reinstate ACT/SAT Requirement.* Chronical of Higher Education; 2021. Available at: https://www.chronicle.com/article/georgias-public-universities-will-reinstate-act-sat-requirement.

How to Look Good on Video Calls/Zoom Face Time Skype. Bloggers Secrets. How to Look Good on Video Calls. Available at: https://www.youtube.com/watch?v=ACNGhPKnmok.

Indeed Editorial Team. *How to Request a Letter of Recommendation for Graduate School.* May 20, 2021. Available at: https://www.indeed.com/career-advice/career-development/recommendation-for-graduate-school. Retrieved May, 2021.

Jones KD, Baggs JG, Jones MR. Selecting US research-intensive doctoral programs in nursing: pragmatic questions for potential applicants. *J Prof Nurs.* 2018;34(4):296-299. Available at: https://doi.org/10.1016/j.profnurs.2017.11.005.

McMammon E. *When to Apply to Graduate School: 4 Key Considerations. GRE Prep Online Guides and Tips.* 2017. Available at: https://www.prepscholar.com/gre/blog/when-to-apply-for-grad-school/.

Russell-Pinson L, Harris ML. Anguish and anxiety, stress and strain: attending to writers' stress in the dissertation process. *J Second Lang Writ.* 2019;43:63-71. doi:10.1016/j.jslw.2017.11.005.

Stanfil AG, Aycock D, Dionne-Odom JN, Rosa WE. Strategies and resources for increasing the PhD pipeline and producing independent nurse scientists. *J Nurs Scholarsh.* 2019;51(6):717-726. doi:10.1111/jnu.12524.

Taylor LA, Terhaar MF. Mitigating barriers to doctoral education for nurses. *Nurs Educ Perspect.* 2018;39(5):285-290. doi:10.1097/01.NEP.0000000000000386.

Weiner OD. How should we be selecting our graduate students. *Mol Biol Cell.* 2013;25:429-430.

CHAPTER 11

Using Timely Wisely and Well

Laura A. Taylor, PhD, RN, ANEF, FAAN

Lack of direction, not lack of time, is the problem. We all have twenty-four-hour days.
—Zig Ziglar

This chapter will describe strategies to conquer time, manage distractions, and work to your strengths in preparation for and progress through doctoral education. It will help align strengths, goals, priorities, and actions and will link to the tools presented in Part 4 of this text.

For busy men and women raising families, owning businesses, and working full-time jobs, the decision to return to school, much less structuring a school application, can seem overwhelming and impossible. Yet every day we read stories of folks who overcame these daunting obstacles and other stability-threatening barriers to earn a degree. These stories of remarkable challenges conquered can do one of two things: either inspire you (which I must imagine is their intent) or backfire and lead you to think you can never make it happen.

We are here to let you know that each of us has the skills, the mindset, the inquisitive spirit, and the wherewithal to make this happen. This chapter offers today's best strategies to make the most of your 24 hours, be kind to yourself, and let it go when you don't.

Considering the Doctoral Education Decision Demands Thought and Perseverance

THE DECISION IS TIME INTENSIVE

One of the most important things (MITs) you will want to consider before embarking on a course of study for a doctorate is your spirit and level of motivation to persevere (Cassuto, 2013).

When you decide to pursue an advanced degree, it is essential to consider the tremendous commitment of both money and time that will be required. Finances are presented in Chapter 9. In this chapter, we will delve into the time management skills you can apply to this life-changing decision.

This chapter presents evidence-based time management skills that will complement any doctoral student's journey. These aids include approaches to help you:

- conquer the ever-present time suckers such as procrastination, and
- address thorough goal development setting,
- offer keen distraction steering tactics.

All will facilitate one's ability to stay focused and achieve your doctoral program's degree ambition.

Becoming a Master of Your Time

By deciding to earn a doctoral degree you have chosen the path of greatest resistance. We mean that you have garnered the inner fortitude to take on a challenge that less than 2% of the 3.8 million nurses worldwide have accomplished. Therefore, negative forces are set against this conquest because the journey seems wrought with challenges and obstacles. The road to a doctoral degree resembles a small road or hiking trail with branches and vines growing over it. You know it is open for walking, but there are jagged rocks that haven't been cleared, and you will need dedicated time not only to walk the path but also to clear the way. Time is precious and at a premium, as we are afforded only 24 hours daily. A thoughtful understanding of how, where, and with whom you choose to share this precious commodity will be instrumental to your success in these high-stakes, high-stress conditions of doctoral education.

Time is never more precious than when you balance working full time and earning a degree. Amabile from Harvard explains, "The single most important component for your well-being is making progress on meaningful work. But first track your behaviors" (Amabile, 1999). One of the greatest services that as a future student you can do is to identify current habits and develop an understanding of how you truly spend your time.

Experts agree the best way to begin better time management is simply to keep a planner and WRITE IT DOWN. Use a scheduler, Day-Timer, or an app. You have to keep track of where you are supposed to go and who you are supposed to meet. Unload the data instead of trying to keep it all in your head. You need that mental space for more important information. Jim Rohn, author and life coach, explains how he writes everything down:

I jump in the limo to head for the airport. The driver says, "What airline?" And I say, "I'll have to look" because I don't store it in my head. Maybe I'm kind of freaky like that. Rather than keep all this stuff loaded in my head, I just find a convenient place to put it where it's all available. Keep your head open for bigger projects than what airline.

JIM ROHN, 2014, GUIDE TO TIME MANAGEMENT

Try it for 1 week: WRITE IT DOWN! This feasibility study will revolutionize your approach and help you achieve your goals. Gathering 1 week's worth of data about time-spending offers the opportunity to change how you spend your time. Covey's easy-to-use four-quadrant time management grid (Table 11.1) is a simple tracking tool that you can use to explore just how you are using your time at this moment and help you make decisions to realign your use of time with the goals you seek.[1] The four quadrants can help us understand where certain tasks fit into our lives according to our values and use them to manage time effectively and be proactive. Make seven copies of this quadrant chart and track where and how you spend your time for 1 week.

Quadrant 1 (Q-1): Urgent and important. Crises and emergencies are categorized here. All of us have encountered some of Q-1, where we must put out fires and manage emergencies, our own and the predicaments of those around us. Interestingly, spending too much time in Q-1 increases the likelihood of getting stuck in Q-1. Alice Boyes in the *Harvard Business Review* emphasizes that when someone is stuck in Q-1, they are "Too busy chasing cows to build a fence." You find yourself always managing urgent situations because you do not have time to do the necessary preventative processes to help avoid crises to begin with (https://hbr.org/2018/07/how-to-focus-on-whats-important-not-just-whats-urgent).

Quadrant 2 (Q-2): Not urgent but important. Q-2 is where effective people focus their time and energy. The discipline to prioritize tasks is key to self-management and achieving your personal mission. Q-2 includes activities that could easily be put off for their lack of apparent urgency but that will greatly benefit your life in the long term if you invest the time in them. Like pursuing your doctoral degree!

Quadrant 3 (Q-3): Urgent but not important. This is one of the more familiar of the Stephen Covey Quadrants. You are likely not aware that these situations are not even important because of the "urgency" placed on the action by someone else's implied importance. Oprah calls this the OPP-Quadrant: Other People's Priorities (https://stenovate.com/lesson-2-how-to-prioritize-like-oprah-and-eisenhower/). This might include emails, meetings that could have been communicated via email, and household chores that someone else is helping with. By spending too much

TABLE 11.1 ■ **Four-Quadrant Time Management Grid**

	Urgent	Not Urgent
Important	Important and urgent	Important and not urgent
Not important	Not important and urgent	Not important and not urgent

Reproduced from: Covey S. *The 7 Habits of Highly Effective People: Powerful Lessons in Personal Change.* Simon and Schuster; 2013.

time in Q-3 you may be letting others' goals and values guide your efforts rather than your own.

Quadrant 4 (Q-4): Neither urgent nor important. These are things you may do purely for enjoyment or out of confusion about what's truly important. Quadrants 3 and 4 are irresponsible uses of your time, and effective people tend to avoid these activities. The most common of these today would be the time vortex of social media. No one is saying that you must end all social media, but you should structure the time to maximize its value toward achieving your goal. Every time you say yes to that next Instagram feed, you are saying no to what is more important for goal achievement.

What you may find is that you spend a disproportionate amount of time on items in the other three quadrants. Effective people respond to opportunities to do what's important instead of reacting to urgent problems. When things come up, it is easier to determine what's important and what isn't once you've defined your goals and personal mission statement. Remember, pots on the back burner don't get attention. Do not fail to prioritize yourself and your doctoral education.

A wonderful anecdote from Elizabeth Gilbert, the *New York Times* best-selling author of *Eat, Pray, Love*, recalls the story when she was in a place in her life where she wanted to write a book but knew she would never have the time to take on such a monstrous goal. She lived near and often ran into one of her most favorite and personally admired authors. Ms. Gilbert had often shared her dream of becoming an author, and one evening she continued to bemoan the limited time that prevented her from taking on her dream. This respected author proceeded to ask Ms. Gilbert a few simple questions: "What was the most wonderful movie you have recently seen?" and "What magazine are you currently delving into?" Ms. Gilbert replied enthusiastically to both questions, sharing her excitement for the conversation. The respected author replied, "That movie was 4 hours of time you could have spent on your book," and "Oh, that magazine was an hour of time you could have dedicated to your book."

Now, no one is suggesting you cannot go to a movie, spend special events with family, spend time binging your favorite television show, or scrolling your favorite social media sites ever again. The point we want to drive home is that by exploring how you spend your time via categorizing each item as it aligns with your dream of earning your doctoral degree and forever transforming yourself, your goal is going to come closer. You need to identify and carve out the time it will require. Getting into school and being successful as a student will demand time away from your usual free time. And full awareness of where you are currently devoting your time is needed to engage with time management tactics and practices that will support you as you take on the stressful multifaceted circumstances that doctoral education will bring to your situation.

Moreover, attending graduate school is about something other than checking a box. You won't want to simply "phone it in." You will want to dive in, put in the effort, enjoy it, and be transformed. So, learning to manage your time is key to thriving in graduate school, just as it is key to winning at a sport, playing an instrument, or climbing Everest.

SMART GOALS

You must set goals to design your future. Jim Rohn emphasizes that goals should offer the greatest pull on you toward your future and enable you to face the future with anticipation. Goals should capture your imagination and galvanize your effort. Well-defined goals are like a magnet: they will help you to work harder, and they will pull you onward and pull you through.

Decide what you want and write it down. List your personal and professional educational goals in your journal. Track them across time starting NOW, before you apply. Tracking your goals across time allows for visibility on goal achievement and growth. It is perfectly fine (and essential) to see goals grow, stretch, and, very likely, transform through the years. Keeping track of your journey provides clarity.

Higher rates of doctoral student success are correlated to goal setting and establishing an action plan for achievement (Sorrentino, 2006; Carmel and Paul, 2015). The greatest value is not what you get upon achieving that goal but who you become upon attaining that dream. "*Set a goal to be a 'doctoral prepared nurse' for what it will make of you to achieve it!*" Set goals that will make something of you to achieve them; aim high, and "go where the pressure is on to change, develop, and grow" (Rohn, 2014). When the demands are high and doctoral transformation is in the air, the journey of who you were as a nurse and who you became as a doctorly prepared provider, researcher, leader, or faculty will be the real story.

The key to achieving and reaching any goal is clarity in the goal and its capability to be achieved. Use the "SMART" approach for goal building. SMART stands for: Specific, Motivational, Action-oriented, Relevant to your situation, and Timebound. You may also see: Specific, Measurable, Achievable, Realistic, and Timely (Box 11.1).

MENTAL CONTRASTING

Goals are pure fantasy unless you have a specific plan to achieve them.

—STEPHEN COVEY

Failure to prepare and set a plan is the main reason many of us fail to adequately move forward on a dream. We start with the goal or dream of participating in that first triathlon, and mentally we catapult ourselves to the other side of that accomplishment. These fabricated feelings of early achievement drain energy and impair

---

BOX 11.1 ■ SMART Goals

- **S**pecific: Well-defined, clear, and unambiguous; detailed and describe what you want; the more specific the goal, the clearer the goal that is set.
- **M**easurable: With specific criteria that measure your progress toward the accomplishment of the goal: I want to apply to three programs, and I want to complete a doctoral program in 5 years.
- **A**chievable: Attainable and not impossible to achieve, setting unachievable goals, it sets you up for failure.
- **R**ealistic: Within reach, realistic, and relevant to your purpose.
- **T**imely: With a clearly defined timeline, including a starting date and a target date. The purpose is to create urgency. All SMART goals have a timeline. Reinforces the seriousness of your goal. You set yourself up for driving toward achieving the goal.

https://corporatefinanceinstitute.com/resources/knowledge/other/smart-goal/

---

our ability to navigate the way forward when an obstacle occurs (Adriaanse et al., 2010; Oettingen, 2015; Hidden Brain Podcast, 2020).

To achieve goals, we must expect that there will be obstacles blocking our road to success. The ancient philosophers would advise not to think that only what we want to happen is going to happen but to anticipate everything will happen. "Premeditation malorum" is an ancient philosophy directing us to be prepared for what lies ahead, to expect certain events before they happen, that nothing should be inconceivable, unfathomable, or unforeseen (Ryan Holiday, Calm App, 2022). Preparing for the most likely obstacles on this doctoral journey increases our ability to manage more effectively and maximizes our capability to achieve the goals we have set for ourselves. This is where mental contrasting can be helpful.

Mental contrasting is a tactic whereby you consider and complement the positivity and excitement of setting the dream in motion with the clarity and consideration of what might be a barrier or stand in the way of attaining the goal. Gabriele Oettingen, author of *Rethinking Positive Thinking: Inside the New Science of Motivation*, directs us to approach dreams and goals methodically. Dreams are only the beginning of the action and do not give the action the direction to accomplish the goal.

The mental contrasting approach is Wish-Outcome-Obstacle-Plan (W-O-O-P). Think about it like this: First, what is your WISH? This should be challenging but achievable (Make it SMART). Second, consider the best OUTCOME from that. These are the positive dreams you see occurring. Oettingen stresses that keeping focused on goal attainment demands reflecting on the OBSTACLE that stands in the way. And once identified, build a PLAN in addressing this OBSTACLE. If this obstacle occurs, then the PLAN to address this OBSTACLE will be activated. W-O-O-P! (Box 11.2). Mental contrasting will be a beneficial

BOX 11.2 ■ **WOOP for Doctoral Essay**

WISH: Writing a clear and concise essay and purpose statement.
OUTCOME: Build an essay that speaks to the mission, vision, and goals of the program and demonstrates clear alignment of my professional and personal goals with the mission and vision of the program.
OBSTACLE: Time management in writing essays while navigating family demands: Little League practice, dog training, daughters' volleyball practices, etc.
PLAN: Optimize my optimal time—3 days a week, wake up 90 min before the family, and set the coffee pot early for quiet writing time.

skill throughout your doctoral journey and complement opportunity management (see Chapter 14).

BIG ROCK THEORY MOST IMPORTANT THINGS

When I am working on a book or a story, I write every morning as soon after first light as possible. There is no one to disturb you and it is cool or cold and you come to your work and warm as you write.

—ERNEST HEMINGWAY

Be purposeful about *what* you're doing and *when* it's going to happen. Ruthless prioritization is critical. If you have 20 tasks for a given day, how many of them need to be accomplished? Getting the MITs done first builds confidence to move through the day to accomplish subsequent tasks. Steven Covey offers the Big Rock Theory to better highlight the importance of MITs (Box 11.3). Spend time on the MIT (Big Rock) and not the gravel that fills up our lives, such as email, laundry, and less important activities. Let's be honest, we are not all morning people like Earnest Hemingway, and that is okay. The best practice is to put the MITs first whenever your optimal time.

Strategies to Addressing Motivation and Best Time Tracking

The following describes different tactics to put into action when managing your time.

CIRCADIAN RHYTHMS AND NATURAL EBBS AND FLOW

As you start each day, make a list and prioritize the day's actions and performance benchmarks. Set aside time for your MITs and finish them during your optimal

---

BOX 11.3 ■ Big Rock Theory

One day this expert was speaking to a group of business students and, to drive home a point, used an illustration I'm sure those students will never forget. After I share it with you, you'll never forget it either.

As this man stood in front of the group of high-powered overachievers he said, "Okay, time for a quiz." Then he pulled out a one-gallon, wide-mouthed mason jar and set it on a table in front of him. Then he produced about a dozen fist-sized rocks and carefully placed them, one at a time, into the jar.

When the jar was filled to the top and no more rocks would fit inside, he asked, "Is this jar full?" Everyone in the class said, "Yes." Then he said, "Really?" He reached under the table and pulled out a bucket of gravel. Then he dumped some gravel in and shook the jar, causing pieces of gravel to work themselves down into the spaces between the big rocks.

Then he smiled and asked the group once more, "Is the jar full?" By this time the class was onto him. "Probably not," one of them answered. "Good!" he replied. And he reached under the table and brought out a bucket of sand. He started dumping the sand in and it went into all the spaces left between the rocks and the gravel. Once more he asked the question, "Is this jar full?"

"No! the class shouted. Once again, he said, "Good!" Then he grabbed a pitcher of water and began to pour it in until the jar was filled to the brim. Then he looked up at the class and asked, "What is the point of this illustration?"

One eager beaver raised his hand and said, "The point is, no matter how full your schedule is, if you try really hard, you can always fit some more things into it!"

No, the speaker replied, "that's not the point. The truth this illustration teaches us is: If you don't put the big rocks in first, you'll never get them in at all."

What are the big rocks in your life? A project that you want to accomplish? Time with your loved ones? Your faith, your education, your finances? A cause? Teaching or mentoring others? Remember to put these "Big Rocks" in first or you'll never get them in at all.

From http://appleseeds.org/Big-Rocks_Covey.htm.

---

focus. James Clear, author of *Minimalism, Procrastination, Productivity*, explains, "If you do the most important thing first each day, then you'll always get something important done" (https://jamesclear.com/productivity-tip). During your "optimal time," willpower is elevated, and you can limit interruptions, thereby increasing the chance of completing the MITs (Kahneman, 2011). So, work within your optimal time zone.

What is this concept of "optimal time"? We all have moments in the day when we are more alert and energetic. To maximize the time you have each day, don't fight against your body's natural state. Researchers call this our circadian rhythm—a 24-hour internal clock running in the background of the brain that cycles between alertness and sleepiness. Planning to write the application essay or draft a reference letter from 9 to 11 at night may work for some, but it won't be productive for others. Whether you are a night owl or a morning person, use this time zone to your advantage. "Make sure you allocate blocks to complete the MITs during the time of day that fits your schedule" (Breus, 2021). Following a routine routine that focuses on using optimal time zones for addressing MITs sets you up for a productive day (Spall, 2021, https://rescuetime.wpengine.com/morning-routine-benjamin-spall/).

STRATEGIES TO ADDRESS PROCRASTINATION AND IMPROVE TIME MANAGEMENT

There are times we struggle to get started on important tasks, such as exploring doctoral programs or even writing a chapter on time management. Important projects bring up uncomfortable emotions such as fear and anxiety. Ignoring the work to avoid the uncomfortable feelings might improve anxiety for a short time, but it creates problems that, over the long term, will put opportunities out of reach. This coping mechanism is known as procrastination.

When you feel that pang to scan the newest items on your social media feed or get pulled into one more episode of your favorite streaming show (which can be especially difficult since the genius of these streaming services is their forced "Opt In" with the next episode automatically loading in 7...6...5 seconds), when you have a project due, notice the emotions and thoughts that are driving this action. Do your best to describe these emotions and thoughts in your journal. Ask yourself: What are the consequences if I delay? If this delay continues, what will occur? Is it worth putting off today? Write it down and face it. Create a W-O-O-P for the anticipated obstacles and forms of procrastination and have it ready to activate when the "procrastination pang" is lurking. This is the beginning of how you build a plan for lifelong personal and professional growth, as well as leadership development. The following are evidence-based strategies to guide the integration of critical thinking and analysis in order to achieve your doctoral goals.

CHUNK IT OUT

The best thing you can do is to start very small. Decide what the smallest, most doable next step is on the MIT or big project, and then list out all the next steps along with a deadline for each.

—B. CAREY, HOW WE LEARN

Burnette and Evans in *Designing Your Life, How to Build a Well-Lived, Joyful Life* (2016), encourage "reframing" the MITs into smaller projects. Let's start with the application process; it has several steps as outlined in Chapter 10. Rather than being overwhelmed by the end goal of submitting all requirements by the due date, set a daily goal of reviewing just one of the components. If the application has a 3000-word essay and this is too daunting, consider writing 500 words every night. If you can keep this up, you'll hit your goal in 6 days, leaving you plenty of time to edit and rework it. If writing even a single paragraph makes you shudder, segment out the activity with four sentences in the next hour. By coming up with doable attainable tasks that seem manageable you can minimize the fear that often leads to procrastination. We have chunked out a few components of the application process in Table 11.2.

TABLE 11.2 ■ **Reframing the Application**

MIT: Identifying Best Programs For ME	Chunk-able Actions	Considerations	Time
Program Delivery Format	How do I like to learn?	Exploring of best learning options What kind of delivery is best for me Try online webinar and course at coursera	30 min each night (1 week)
Best Program for me AACN/Nursing Centralized Application Service for Nursing Programs NCAS	AACN Website List Programs	Keep Journal/Table Explore websites; 1 program a night State/Program/Faculty/ Learning Modality	30 min every other night (4 weeks);

You might also want to list these actions:

1. Look at American Association of Colleges of Nursing website each night: 30 minutes × 14 days; journal results
2. Look and list out prospective program due dates: 30 minutes × 14 days

Continue to "Reframe" chunks of the work to successfully accomplish your MIT.

GETTING THINGS DONE: THE 80/20 PRINCIPLE

The Pareto Principle, also known as the 80/20 rule, is a timeless maxim that's all about focus. The 80/20 principle posits that 20% of what you do results in 80% of your outcomes. Focusing on the MITs results in achieving a greater output (https://www.tonyrobbins.com/productivity-performance/how-to-increase-productivity/). The Pareto Principle dispels the myth that everything matters equally. Break down that wall and prioritize the chunks, keeping in mind that MITs are your priority.

This can be challenging. There are tasks to be done daily, weekly, or monthly. This is where tracking your time can identify how you spend your time and where you might be able to recraft how you use time. I will offer some examples here, but there are others out there:

1. Dusting and cleaning. No one is suggesting that we live in squalor, but there are a number of services to support keeping your house clean.
2. Grocery shopping. Is it really essential that you spend on average 1.5 hours at the grocery store? There are services to support this process.
3. Remember, life is not 50/50. One week your partner is doing 80% because a class assignment or work demand brings your contribution to home maintance time down to 20%. The following week your partner has a new job interview and an important client for supper, and the pendulum swings from 80/20 to 30/70. And so is life.

PUSH BACK AGAINST MULTITASKING

Let's discuss multitasking. First a few questions: If you brush your teeth every day, raise your hand! Okay, just a wild guess here, but all hands are high in the air. Next, if you brush your teeth while looking through your closet for something to wear and making your bed, raise your hand higher! We have all been there, making sandwiches for lunch, orchestrating the breakfast table, talking on the phone while preparing the agenda for the afternoon meeting. Despite your best efforts, the kids get their lunches mixed up, and the meeting agenda was poorly crafted and demands even more time when you get into the office. The false allure of multitasking is well presented in this example: when you try to focus on everything at once, you end up not genuinely focusing on anything at all.

Science tells us that multitasking is a myth, divides our attention, and does not allow us to give our full attention to any of the activities we are engaging in (Bovi et al., 2011; Leland Tavakol et al., 2017). Sally Helgeson, renowned author of *How Women Rise*, explains that multitasking gives the impression that you're overly responsive to random events. She clarifies:

> *If you see someone constantly checking her phone in a meeting, you don't think,* wow, she must be important. *And you certainly don't think,* what a strong presence she exudes. *Instead, you're likely to conclude that she isn't in control of her own time or schedule and is therefore incapable of showing up for what's going on. By demonstrating over-responsiveness, she minimizes both her importance and her presence.*

—SALLY HELGESON, *HOW WOMEN RISE: BREAK THE 12 HABITS HOLDING YOU BACK FROM YOUR NEXT RAISE, PROMOTION, OR JOB*

What you are doing when multitasking is switching quickly between two tasks (if not more). You may be able to do two uncomplicated things at the same time, such as a phone conversation and walking; however, activities requiring more intellect, such as writing and painting, cannot be done at the same time. David Meyer, professor of psychology at the University of Michigan in Ann Arbor, argues that performing two complicated tasks that require the same parts of the brain does not allow us to have the capacity to do any of them well (Bovi et al., 2011). "We end up being much slower overall and can lead to worse performance than if we allow the brain to focus on just one task at a time" (Bovi et al., 2011, p. 11). Ask yourself these questions: What needs to be done? What is the MIT? Do no more than two tasks at a time.

Lucky for us, multitasking is not an incurable disease. It is the result of the bad habit of doing too much. So here are eight things you can put into action to do less better.

1. Don't start your day by looking at your phone. Experts say wait a minimum of 60 minutes before checking social media, emails, etc. You get behind immediately trying to align to someone else's schedule and time frame.

2. Prioritize your day and tackle your MITs during your Optimal Diurnal time (see Optimal Time section).
3. Be present during meetings by keeping your phone off and flipped over.
4. Set a time for distractions: A time to check email, social media.
5. Be prepared to say No (see section on Saying No).
6. Keep your work area clean. Organize your desk before you leave the office in the evening.
7. Do one task at a time. Check off each task and move on! Make your bed. Brush your teeth. *DO NOT* make your bed while brushing your teeth. One way to keep this from happening (a trap for many of us) is to brush your teeth with your nondominant hand. This slows me down every time.
8. Consider using apps to help stay focused. (See Technology Applications to Support section.)

Distractions—Staying Focused

Respond from the center of the hurricane, rather than reacting from the chaos of the storm.

—GEORGE MUMFORD

Time management is a skill to acquire and strengthen. The same 24 hours are in every day. It's crucial to prioritize tasks well and not spend too long on just one task at the expense of other MITs as well.

Today's work and home environments are chaotic at best, offering many challenges and dopamine-inducing "dings" and "pings" that call to us. Let's face it: we are going through a very chaotic time that society did not face even 30 years ago. You may find yourself completing necessary forms for your kid's daycare, answering work emails on your mobile device. Then, before you realize it, you are on Instagram or Twitter for an hour reading headline after headline about what's going on in the world. Technology offers "access to more and more gravel, burying us under a mountain of less important things" (Covey, 2013). Procrastination is easier when you have social media, shopping, and entertainment at your fingertips.

Let's revisit the time tracking addressed earlier in this chapter. The first step to better time management is to identify where you are spending your time and use this information when designing your time management strategy. In addition to the handwritten log option described earlier in the chapter, there are some exceptional time management software applications that provide tracking and align time spent with your productivity goals and metrics for more efficient working. The data from mapping and tracking your time with the Four Quadrant chart will help you select the best apps for your weaknesses.

Now it seems ironic to suggest the use of technology against technology. In the *Art of War*, Sun Tzu explains: "He who can modify his tactics in relation to his opponent and thereby succeed in winning, may be called a heaven-born captain" (p. 31). Mobile devices and computer apps offer time tracking for individual projects and provide a general analysis of how time was used throughout the day and help identify periods when you can be more productive (Productivity Apps, Table 11.3). Some apps will block distracting websites and pop up an idyllic location photograph encouraging you to take 5 minutes for yourself if you have been working ferociously for 90 minutes (Staying Focused Apps, Table 11.3). Some apps are designed to allow "surfing" for a preset time and then intermittently send an onscreen message about the amount of time that has passed. By reviewing the documented time-distracting "obstacles," you can select an app that drives the necessary re-direction and minimizes procrastination. Table 11.3 summarizes of the Best Time Management apps of 2021, updated annually (https://www.lifehack.org/articles/technology/top-15-time-management-apps-and-tools.html).

BUILDING HABITS TO HELP MINIMIZE TIME DRAIN

When the daily decisions we must make are not considered in proportion to their worth, we waste our most precious commodity: Time (Drucker, 2006). Good news is that bad time management is most often the result of poor decision-making processes and bad habits that we have developed over the years. Great news! We can build new habits for specific actions to relieve the mental strain and prevent constant crises.

For example, if every morning is a frenzy of trying to prepare for a meeting, finding the files you need, and reading last minute notes, consider the habit of cleaning your desk and printing the next day's documents before you leave the office. Cleaning up and reorganizing your desk every evening before you leave the office will help minimize the hectic start to your day. Setting habits allows for openness for the decisions that demand greater attention throughout the day. "Motivation is what gets you started. Habit is what keeps you going" (Rohn, 2014).

A second habit to establish is the "*If-then*" scenario. Let's say you want to watch another episode of your favorite streaming show, and you also need to write your application essay. Put into motion the "If-Then" rule. *If* I complete two paragraphs of the essay, *then* I will watch one episode of my favorite show. Or *if* I work on my essay for 20 minutes, *then* I will spend 5 minutes on social media.

SELF-COMPASSION

Time management is really about energy management. Your ability to generate strong, meaningful work relies on your ability to be awake, focused, and energized. To achieve excellent work and make the most of your days, you need to build a habit of self-compassion.

I have no doubt that most individuals, nurses in particular, possess the knowledge of what to do in general for self-care: lower an elevated BMI, consume less caffeine, or floss every night before you go to bed. Still, did you know that just

TABLE 11.3 ■ Best Applications for Time Management and Wellness

Strict Workflow Pomodoro Technique	Timecamp	Manic Time	Productivity Apps Todolist	The Pocket	Clockify
Pomodoro Technique times 25 min of work followed by a 5 min short break. Free browser plugin Pick one project or task to focus on. Set a timer for 25–30 min, and get to work. When the buzzer sounds, take a 2–3 min break. Repeat. After four sessions, take a longer break. Record each session with a tick or X in your journal.	Time tracking actions aimed at improving team productivity. Integrates with over 50 apps for ease of use, including Slack, Jira and Evernote.	Downloadable and runs locally Tracks time spent on a local file, or website Integrates with task-based systems, like Github or Jira. Free tier basic functionality Pro tier: a year of upgrades	Desktop and mobile Set for recurring events and tasks, Check off each task as completed Receive custom schedule of tasks at the start of each day (unless you choose not to), Enables ability to plan time effectively.	Creates a space to save articles, videos, and images found on the web or social media. instead of bookmarking everything on the internet journey. Send the image over to the app where it will be stored and saved. Option of sharing any saved media with social media platforms.	Free simple time tracker and timesheets. Provides ability to set up and manage projects and teams. Dashboards provide overview of projects as well as analytics based on use.

			Staying Focused			
Rescuetime	*Stay Focused*	*Calm App*	*LeechBlock*	*Hocus Forest*	*Focus Keeper*	*Mindful Browsing*
Time organizer app	Browser extension	Helps to explore	Web extension to	When you choose a	Helps prevents	Plugin built
Can even discon-	for productivity	and spend time	block websites	task you want to	burn out.	specifically for
nect	by blocking dis-	relaxing and	both when and	get done, set the	Times productivity	Chrome,
Lays out time spent	tracting websites	meditating.	for how long.	timer to 25 min.	sessions and di-	Interrupts long
on each app and	while trying to	Provides 2–20	A timer that	When the timer is	rects the incor-	sessions with
website in graph	work.	min guided	monitors the	up, rewarded with	porations of	beautiful pho-
Help to trim down	Block distractions	meditation	time spent on	a 5-min break (See	breaks.	tography in-
aimless surfing	either for set	sessions	certain	Pomodoro tech-	Doesn't block	stead
Goal setting avail-	times and dates	Recharge to stay	websites.	nique)	sites	Easy to setup.
able	(like 9–5, Mon-	focused on the	Blocks websites	Following four focus		type in the web-
	day through Fri-	next task.	after reaching	sessions, allows		sites to be
	day) or after		the preset time	an even longer		mindful of
	reached a limit		limit	break of about		spending too
	(e.g., no more		Redirects to differ-	20–30 min.		much time on
	than 30 min of		ent webpage,	Customizable, set		and then type
	Twitter per day).		helping to stay	the session for		in what you'd
	Simple, free, and		focused.	longer periods of		rather be
	helps keep		Password or ac-	time with longer		doing.
	productivity.		cess code op-	breaks. Either way,		Like scuba
	Aids in self-		tion, to unlock	it's habit building		diving, moun-
	discipline toward		preset websites.	for getting things		tain biking, ar-
	a more produc-			done and taking		ranging flowers
	tive life.			those well-de-		To be honest, we
				served breaks in		probably all
				between.		need to install
						this one.

Continued

TABLE 11.3 ■ Best Applications for Time Management and Wellness—cont'd

New Tools for School

Drop Box	Ever Note-Taking	Calm App (See Above)
• Organizer app to upload, save, and send files • Sync music library between computers and the cloud, so it's the same on every platform. • Ability for users to automate files • Convert an image just by dropping it in or upload your pictures right to Facebook.	• Stores important ideas, favorite movies • Capture notes with writing, recording audio, taking photos, uploading PDFs, sketching digitally • Search words/phrases, the app can look for pictures of words in images. if you snap a picture of a For Sale sign and later search for "sale," Evernote will find it. • Free or Pay Options • Paying account holders can search PDFs and uploaded documents from instances of words • Can be used for collaboration, share notes, and collectively create	• Helps meditate to focus on school • Customizable settings such as background and choice of music • Each meditation program is self-explanatory

Data from https://www.lifehack.org/articles/technology/top-15-time-management-apps-and-tools.html.

about 8% of all New Year's resolutions are met (https://www.forbes.com/sites/dandiamond/2013/01/01/just-8-of-people-achieve-their-new-years-resolutions-heres-how-they-did-it/?sh=7e83f5f0596b)? Each of us occasionally fails to achieve the goals we set for ourselves. Yet we rarely fail to reflect on our past performance and see all the things we should have and could have done differently. Then we go to war with ourselves. It is emotionally draining, and we are ridiculously self-critical (Hochli et al., 2012).

Stop knocking yourself down and start being a better friend to you. Inner critic meet inner advocate. Consider the following: If your best friend called and said that they had spent 3 hours watching this great new streaming show and didn't study like they had planned, my guess is you would reply, "That's okay friend. Don't be so hard on yourself. You got this. Let sleep refresh you and start studying again in the morning." But what do we say to ourselves? "What an ijit! I needed to study" and continue to berate yourself for the rest of the evening into the next day if not longer.

We suggest that you set SMART goals for self-care and self-compassion. Consider some of the following approaches when you start getting down on yourself:

- First, journal your journey. Science tells us that when we write down our failings, or bursts of temper it helps us let them go, so we can move on.
- Second, chunk out self-care in a manner like described earlier when completing your doctoral school application:
  - for 1 week I will schedule my sleep time in order to sleep for 6 hours for two nights.
  - today I will take two flights of stairs to the third floor and take the elevator from there.
  - call or send one email to my important supports (parents, friends, mentors, etc.) once a week for three straight weeks.
  - turn my cellphone off 30 minutes before bed on Tuesday and Thursday this week.
  - schedule a "date with my _____" (your fill in the blank: partner, kids, massage the second week of every month).

Chunk it out, set your goals in action, and when an unforeseen obstacle gets in the way, use the famous words of Ted Lasso: "Sam, do you know what the happiest animal on the planet is? A goldfish. A goldfish only has a ten-second memory. Be a goldfish!" Make use of this insight from past experiences as you set new goals but don't dwell on your failures. Consider using the award-winning Calm App for mediation, energy review, and renewal strategies. One of the most insightful and restorative components are the Master Classes, including Tara Brach and "Radical Self Compassion."

SLEEP IS ESSENTIAL

Many of us misunderstand that the more we work, the more we can get done. Prioritizing self-care is difficult, especially when choosing more work over sleep.

> **BOX 11.4 ■ Recipe for Creative Napping Ritual: The Nappa Latte**
>
> To maximize the effect of an afternoon siesta, Dr. Breus created the Coffee Power Nap: The Nappa Latte. Here is the recipe: 6 oz of drip black coffee, 3 ice cubes, drink as fast as you can, take a 25-min nap. This 25-min nap is enough to allow caffeine to block the adenosine from making you sleepy—and you wake up ready for 4 hours of creative work.
>
> From Breus M. "Tips that will put you to sleep." 2021. https://goodnewsplanet.com/renowned-expert-dr-michael-breus-with-tips-that-will-put-you-to-sleep-3-2/, CalmApp, 2022.

Getting a good night's sleep can make all the difference amid the flurry of day-to-day responsibilities. The brain is working hard during sleep, searching for hidden links and deeper significance in the day's events and getting you ready for the next day. Insufficient rest makes it harder to focus.

Restful and productive sleep requires habit building, and nighttime rituals. Nighttime rituals are as important to adults as they are to kids. Consider the following approaches to improving your sleep hygiene.

1. Select one bedtime and stick to it.
2. Stop caffeine by 2 pm (caffeine half-life is 6 to 8 hours).
3. Exercise daily but at least 4 hours before sleep.
4. Keep a journal on your bedside table.
5. Try to get get 15 minutes of sunlight every morning to naturally turn off the melatonin faucet.

Productivity is elevated through 7 to 8 hours of sleep. If that is not possible, schedule a 20- to 30-minute mid-day nap (Box 11.4) (Breus, 2021; Calm App, 2022). University of Michigan researchers have shown that napping effectively boosts productivity, perseverance, and improves decision-making. The length of the nap and the time of day can have an important influence on creativity and productivity, with the perfect nap being no longer than 20 to 25 minutes and between 1 and 3 o'clock in the afternoon (Breus, 2021; Calm App, 2022).

WEAVING "NO" BACK INTO YOUR VOCABULARY

You have heard the phrase, "If you want something to get done, give it to a busy person." Successful people have formed a reputation of being the go-to person to get requests done and done well. Successful people are easily tempted to say "yes" to the many requests for unique jobs and enthusiastically take on new opportunities because this is how they succeed (Goldsmith, 2007). The downside to success is spearheading too many projects, getting pulled in many directions, and saying yes too quickly and frequently. Successful people find themselves overloaded with a calendar of activities that eat up all their time because it's easy to oblige, wanting to please and seeking that next adrenaline rush. The shortcoming of being successful is failing to consider each request in due proportion to its worth on how it will move you toward your SMART goal. (More discussion on saying "No" in Chapter 14 under "Opportunity Management".)

WHY NO IS SO IMPORTANT

Stoic philosophy urges us to consider paying attention to each activity in due proportion to what it is worth. Marcus Aurelius directs us that we must do less to be present, focused, and creative toward achieving goals: "Don't do nothing, but do less better." With the word "no" lies the capacity to be fully present. Present for a task, for a conversation, for the moment, for an opportunity. Present for your larger purpose in the world (Holiday, Calm App, 2022).

The realm of possibilities and opportunities expands exponentially along the doctoral journey. As a doctoral student, a well-honed ability to search for meaning over efficiency in each opportunity is essential. Always ask yourself (or a mentor): "Where does this opportunity fit in relative to my goals and values?" and don't be afraid to say "No" using some of the thoughtful approaches listed here.

1. **Saying No and Mentoring Across**. "I am so happy to hear that you appreciated the presentation last year and that the student reviews were favorable. I am afraid that at this time I will not be able to offer the same attention and quality that the presentation and your students deserve. Would you be open to another colleague that I believe would be an excellent person to help you out?"

2. **Delay Tactics.** There are some delay tactics that can be used when you are currently committed to an important task and yet the request is intriguing. Use the following: "I am excited to hear about your project. Can I get back to you at the end of the day? Or week? I am very busy these next two weeks. And I need time to see how it fits into my schedule."

3. **Seek Mentoring**. Finally, if you are not sure how an opportunity could be influential toward achieving your SMART goals, reach out to your mentor (see Chapter 8). Ask for their impression of the opportunity if it is possible to decipher the likelihood that this opportunity will come again or if it is truly a unique possibility. Be willing to lean in to your mentor's overarching perspective on your current situation and the greater distant visibility of the horizon in front of you.

Summary

The best thing about the future is that it comes one day at a time.

—ABRAHAM LINCOLN

Time is our most precious commodity, and we must be prepared for twists and turns. Becoming more productive doesn't demand drastically changing your lifestyle or investing in expensive training and coaching sessions. It starts with awareness of how you are currently spending your time and then incorporating some of the many resources offered here in this chapter: establishing SMART goals that are time-limited, chunking out each activity, addressing MITs first, doing your best work during your optimal time, building habit driven strategies for stress-free decision-making, using technology to help you stay focused and minimize distractions, incorporating healthy sleep hygiene practices, and, finally, creating a habit of carefully evaluating the flurry of requests on your time so that you can say yes to your future self.

Bibliography

The 20 Fastest PhD Program in 2021. Available at: https://www.premiumschools.org/fastest-phd-programs/.

Adriaanse MA, Oettingen G, Gollwitzer PM, et al. When planning is not enough: fighting unhealthy snacking habits by mental contrasting with implementation intentions (MCII). *Eur J Soc Psychol.* 2010;40(7):1277-1293.

Amabile T., et al. *Harvard Business Review on Breakthrough Thinking*. Boston, MA: Harvard Business School Press; 1999.

Blanchard V. *Doctoral Program Completion: Grit, Goal-Setting, Social Support*. Seton Hall University Dissertations and Theses (ETDs). 2552. 2018. Available at: https://scholarship.shu.edu/dissertations/2552.

Blume C, Garbazza C, Spitschan M. Effects of light on human circadian rhythms, sleep and mood. *Somnologie*. 2019;23(3):147-156. Available at: https://doi.org/10.1007/s11818-019-00215-x.

Boss J. *5 Reasons Why Goal Setting Will Improve Your Focus*. 2017. Available at: https://www.forbes.com/sites/jeffboss/2017/01/19/5-reasons-why-goal-setting-willimprove-your-focus/#1b7c8638534a.

Bovi G, Rabuffetti M, Mazzoleni P, Ferrarin M. A multiple-task gait analysis approach: kinematic, kinetic and EMG reference data for healthy young and adult subjects. *Gait Posture*. 2011;33(1):6-13. doi:10.1016/j.gaitpost.2010.08.009.

Boyes A. *Harvard Business Review. How to Focus on What's Important, Not Just What is Urgent*. Available at: https://hbr.org/2018/07/how-to-focus-on-whats-important-not-just-whats-urgent.

Breus M. *Tips That Will Put You to Sleep*. 2021. Available at: https://goodnewsplanet.com/renowned-expert-dr-michael-breus-with-tips-that-will-put-you-to-sleep-3-2/.

Burnette B, Evans D. *Designing Your Life: How to Build a Well-Lived, Joyful Life*. New York, NY: Knopf Doubleday Publishing Group; 2016.

Burnette B, et al., Evans, D. *Designing Your Life: How to Build a Well-Lived, Joyful Life*. Penguin Randome House, LLC. New York: Penguin Random House; 2016.

Calm App. Calm; 2022. Available at: https://play.google.com/store/apps/details?id=com.calm.android&gl=US&pli=1.

Carey B. *How We Learn: The Surprising Truth About When, Where and Why It Happens*. New York: Penguin Random House; 2014.

Carmel RG, Paul MW. Mentoring and coaching in academia: reflections on a mentoring/coaching relationship. *Policy Futur Educ*. 2015;13:479-491. Available at: https://doi.org/10.1177/1478210315578562.

Chase JA, Topp R, Smith CE, et al. Time management strategies for research productivity. *West J Nurs Res*. 2013;35(2):155-176. doi:10.1177/0193945912451163.

Clear J. *The Only Productivity Tip You Will Ever Need*. 2021. Available at: https://jamesclear.com/productivity-tip.

Clear J. *Atomic Habits: An Easy and Proven Way to Build Good Habits and Break Bad Ones*. New York: Penguin Random House; 2019.

Conrad S. *The 5 year PhD: An Endangered Species*. Available at: https://figureoneblog.wordpress.com/2013/01/22/the-5-year-phd-an-endangered-species.

Corporate Finance Institute. Available at: https://corporatefinanceinstitute.com/resources/knowledge/other/smart-goal/.

Covey S. *The 7 Habits of Highly Effective People: Powerful Lessons in Personal Change*. New York, NY: Simon and Schuster; 2013.

Covey S. *The 7 Habits of Highly Effective People Personal Workbook.* New York, NY: Simon & Schuster; 2003.

Drucker P. *The Practice of Management.* Silver Spring, MD: Harper Business; 2006, 1954.

Duffy J, Moore B. *The Best Productivity Apps for 2021.* 2020. Available at: https://www.pcmag.com/news/the-best-productivity-apps.

Goldsmith M. *What Got You Here Won't Get You There: How Successful People Become Even More Successful.* New York: Random House; 2007.

Helgeson S, Goldsmith M. *How Women Rise: Breaking the 12 Habits Holding You Back from Your Next Raise, Promotion or Job.* New York, NY: Hachette Books; 2018.

Höchli B, Brügger A, Messner C. Making new year's resolutions that stick: exploring how superordinate and subordinate goals motivate goal pursuit. *Appl Psychol Health Well-Being.* 2020;12:30-52. Available at: https://doi.org/10.1111/aphw.12172.

James SM, Honn KA, Gaddameedhi S, Van Dongen HPA. Shift Work: Disrupted circadian rhythms and sleep—implications for health and well-being. *Curr Sleep Med Rep.* 2017;3(2):104-112. Available at: https://doi.org/10.1007/s40675-017-0071-6.

Kahneman D. *Thinking Fast and Slow.* New York, NY: Farrar, Straus and Giroux; 2011.

Lawrence L. *Lesson 2: How to prioritize like Oprah and Eisenhower.* 2020. Available at: https://stenovate.com/lesson-2-how-to-prioritize-like-oprah-and-eisenhower/.

Leland A, Tavakol K, Scholten J, et al. Affective and cognitive conditions are stronger predictors of success with community reintegration than gait and balance performance in veterans with mild traumatic brain injury. *Med Arch.* 2017;71(6):417-423. doi:10.5455/medarh.2017.71.417-423.

McKay J. *Time Management for Students: 10 Strategies and Tips to Maximize Your Time and Build Your Focus.* 2019. Available at: https://blog.rescuetime.com/time-management-for-students/.

Oettingen G. *Rethinking Positive Thinking: Inside the New Science of Motivation.* New York, NY: Penguin Publishing Group; 2015.

Robbins T. *How to Increase Productivity.* Available at: https://www.tonyrobbins.com/productivity-performance/how-to-increase-productivity/.

Rohn Jim. *The Jim Rohn Guide to Time Management.* Dallas, TX: SUCCESS; 2014.

Rohn J. *The Jim Rohn Guide to Goal Setting.* Dallas, TX: SUCCESS; 2014.

Sorrentino D. The seek mentoring program: an application of the goal-setting theory. *J Coll Stud Ret.* 2006;8:241-250.

Spall B. (guest author) *Is there a perfect morning routine? Here's what I learned interviewing 300+ of the most productive people.* 2018. Available at: https://rescuetime.wpengine.com/morning-routine-benjamin-spall/.

Tew A, Smith MA. *Calm* [Mobile App]. The App Store. Available at: https://www.calm.com/.

Tzu S. *The Art of War. Barnes & Noble Classics.* New York; 1994.

Waterworth S. Time management strategies in nursing practice. *J Adv Nurs.* 2003;43(5):432-440.

Weinzaepflen C, Spitschan M, eds. *Enlighten Your Clock: How Your Body Tells Time.* (C. Weinzaepflen, Illus). 2021. doi:10.17605/OSF.IO/ZQXVH.

Women at Work. Harvard Business Review. *The Essentials of being productive. How self awareness, zoning out and routines help us complete our most important work (podcast).* 2021. Available at: https://hbr.org/podcast/2021/05/the-essentials-being-productive.

CHAPTER 12

Becoming a Writer

Kim Curry, PhD, FNP-C, FAANP

I have put off going back to school for graduate study for several years now. My main concern is that I really hate writing. I feel like I am under so much pressure when I am assigned a paper that I put it off until the last minute. As a result, my papers don't turn out well and that's discouraging. I am worried about not being able to overcome this hurdle.

—Arturo, 32, Florida

Some nurses love to write and are drawn to it. For others, scholarly writing is one of the biggest stumbling blocks to success in graduate school. Writing, particularly assigned writing, can seem like a bit of a chore. Fortunately, there are a number of ways to make scholarly writing more enjoyable and less of a burden. By following some basic guidelines, writing becomes more achievable for inexperienced writers and those who have struggled with writing in the past, as well as the rest of us.

The purpose of this chapter is to:

- Review tips for writing in an academic style.
- Ensure you are organized and prepared to write.
- Help you feel better prepared to write efficiently and effectively.

Introduction

This chapter discusses scholarly and academic writing undertaken by nurses. This applies to writing that occurs in the academic program as well as other professional settings. What is scholarly writing? It is writing that focuses on evidence, knowledge, and reason. Whether done individually or in a writing team, scholarly writing is done using an academic style. This style is more formal than other types of writing. It is this style of writing that sets scholarly writing apart and creates an impression of the writer as a knowledgeable professional.

Some examples of writing that should be done in a scholarly style:

- Term papers or essays assigned in your academic program.

- Communication sent to doctoral program directors, colleagues, or other professional contacts.
- Manuscripts written for publication such as articles, monographs, or books.

WRITING SELF-ASSESSMENT

Think about where you are as a writer. Here is a quick self-assessment to think about your current skill set:

1. I wrote a few papers as an undergraduate and have not written an academic or professional paper since that time.
2. I have been a member of a writing team and have contributed to a part of a manuscript.
3. I have led writing teams and have previously published in peer-reviewed journals.
4. I currently serve as a peer reviewer or journal club member, so I'm involved in critically reading and evaluating the writing of other professionals.

You may have been able to check several of these descriptions or at least a few of them. If you stopped after the first one, don't worry. Most applicants for doctoral programs fall into this category. You can be very successful at writing just by planning, organizing, and then practicing your writing.

GETTING MOTIVATED TO WRITE

There is no doubt that fear of failure interferes with the writing plans of many of us. A lot of this fear is tied to a quest for perfection. Keep this in mind if you are just getting into (or back into) writing. Avoid the urge to expect perfection in each sentence that flows from your keyboard. Related to this is the quest for a moment of inspiration. Don't feel that you must be inspired to write. Professional writers rarely wait for inspiration. They know writing is a business and deadlines must be met, just as deadlines must be met in graduate school. Professional writers often talk about how they require themselves to write at a scheduled, regular time whether they want to or not. Even professionals talk about the struggle to stay disciplined. It's OK to let your deadline be your motivation.

ORGANIZING TO WRITE

A large part of this chapter focuses on the details and techniques of organizing, because organization relates to many components of your writing. However, there are personal components of organizing as well. These include your writing space, equipment, supplies, and competing interests. An initial step in organizing is to evaluate how to have the space and time to write without interruption and distraction. The way to achieve this varies widely from writer to writer. As you consider your doctoral program, where and when do you picture yourself writing? As you think about this, if you cannot currently envision a space or time to write, that is understandable. Most people don't have a lot of extra free time and space sitting around unaccounted for. Recognize that without acknowledging barriers they cannot be overcome. Take time to brainstorm changes you can make that fit your own needs.

The Nuts and Bolts of Writing

Let's discuss the types of papers that are written for a typical doctoral assignment, such as term papers. These papers follow a structured outline. At times, the professor will specify an outline to follow. Two types of papers are typically assigned to graduate students: review papers and research papers.

ORGANIZING A REVIEW PAPER

Most assigned papers are non-research papers, also known as review papers. These papers review and summarize information that has been previously published. They are organized in a way that allows the writer to introduce the theme of the paper, present major concepts, and then synthesize the information into a coherent whole.

Outline for a Scholarly Paper That Is Not Research-Based

- Abstract: A brief summary of the entire paper. For papers other than research papers, the abstract is often unstructured, containing no headers within the abstract.
- Introduction: Introduces the theme of the paper and provides background information.
- Purpose: Describes the goal and intent of the paper.
- Body of the paper: Each topical area typically includes a discussion of the literature the writer located and other points to be made about the subject matter.
  - Major topical area 1 and related subtopics
  - Major topical area 2 and related subtopics
  - Major topical area 3 and related subtopics
  - Etc.
- Discussion: Detailed description that describes and synthesizes the information contained in the body of the paper.
- Conclusion: The overall summary of what was learned. Includes implications for future practice, education, or research.

ORGANIZING A RESEARCH PAPER

Research (or scientific) papers are written to describe an original research study that has been completed. The organization of a research-based scholarly paper follows a somewhat different outline than a non-research paper.

Outline for a Scientific Research Paper

Abstract: The abstract of a research paper is structured and includes the same headings as the paper itself. Both the abstract and the paper are typically organized as follows:

Introduction: Background of the topic, why it is important, why there is a need for research, and a purpose, problem statements, or hypotheses.

Literature Review: Most research papers separate the literature review into a separate section that is presented before the research plan is revealed.

Methodology: The plan for research. A discussion of how the study was designed and conducted.

Results: This section is limited to a reporting of the qualitative or quantitative results based on the data collected.

Discussion/Analysis/Limitations of the Study. This section includes a broad discussion of the meaning of the findings, relates the findings back to prior literature, and addresses the research hypotheses and whether they were supported or not.

Conclusion: An overall conclusion and implications for practice, research, and/or education.

The above information summarizes the organization and outline of two main types of papers. Often professors have a preferred outline that they will provide for you to follow. If you are feeling a bit overwhelmed at this point, do not despair. The whole task may seem daunting, but it is very achievable. Writing a paper of more than a couple of pages brings to mind the old joke about how one should eat an elephant: one bite at a time. Rather than the intimidating view of the pages and pages that lie before you waiting to be filled, view one small piece of the assignment and complete only that step. Remember, you have many colleagues who have been through this and been successful. You can do it.

CONSTRUCTING A PARAGRAPH

Just like the entire paper, each paragraph needs to follow a pattern so it makes sense. Each paragraph should address one key point within a topical area. It should flow logically from the previous paragraph and serve as a bridge into the paragraph that follows it. Those who teach writing often depict each paragraph as a sandwich. The top is a sentence in which the subject of the paragraph is introduced. The "meat" is the middle of the paragraph and consists of those sentences that provide detail and discussion of the subject. The bottom is the end of the paragraph and contains a concluding sentence that briefly summarizes and provides a transition into the next paragraph.

To see an example, look at the paragraph above. The first sentence introduces the subject of constructing a paragraph. The following four sentences provide detail and explanation of the topic. The final sentence concludes the explanation and the paragraph ends. This prepares the reader to move on to the next thought.

Just as the organization of a paragraph is important, so is the length of the paragraph. Each paragraph should contain a minimum of three sentences. However, paragraphs longer than eight to ten sentences are very hard to read and understand. Avoid the urge to solve this problem by writing long sentences. Many beginning writers think that long sentences positively reflect on their knowledge, but that is not the case. Sentences should be clear, direct, and succinct. They should have a beginning, a middle, and an end, just like paragraphs. Remember to limit each paragraph to one key point. Look for natural breaks where the subject matter shifts and start a new paragraph at that point.

A FEW WORDS ABOUT WORDS

Word choice is key to sounding professional and knowledgeable in your writing. In addition to spelling and grammar, choice of words can make your writing stand out as unmistakably professional, or it can leave a less desirable impression on the reader. Word choice can also impact the impression your paper gives with regard to words that convey feelings. As a general rule, scholarly writing isn't intended to convey your personal feelings or opinions. When personal feelings are inserted, the paper is seen not as the objective analysis of a topic but as an emotional, reactive response to an issue. Such expressions are not the objective of scholarly writing. Consider carefully before putting these descriptive and technical words into your paper:

1. Crisis or disaster: These words are overused by novice writers in an effort to draw attention to the subject matter. Limit the use of these words to those instances in which a public health agency has used one of these labels to describe the problem you are writing about.
2. Fantastic, wonderful, awful, infuriating (and similar words): These are words that are used to convey emotion and feelings. If you are tempted to use these words, recheck your assignment to be sure you are being asked to provide your personal viewpoint.
3. Jargon words: We are all tempted to use our own professional jargon. Put your audience first. If your paper will be read by those practicing outside of your specialty area, the use of jargon will frustrate readers and will not be appreciated.

There is an exception to this discussion about word choice. When you are writing, there will be times when you will use quotations from other sources. The words included in the quotes should be exactly what was spoken or written by the person being quoted, even if the quote includes one of the examples above. At all other times, when you are writing your own words, you should choose carefully to ensure your paper has a professional and scholarly tone.

STAYING ON TRACK

There is a main message contained in every scholarly paper. Do you know what the message is? This seems like a very simple question for which the answer is "Of course!" However, many authors waste a lot of time and effort getting off the track of the main message and trying to get back on.

Consider this scenario: Three graduate students have been asked by their professor to collaborate on a paper on a clinical topic of their choice. If the paper is of high quality, they will have the opportunity to submit it to a journal for publication. They are very excited about this prospect. They discuss options and select the topic "herbal treatments for osteoarthritis." They also agree on the following assignments:

Author A: First author, serves as the primary author, organizes the parts into a whole paper.
Writing: Introduction, pathophysiology of osteoarthritis.
Author B: Second author, serves as the contributing author, reviews and approves the final paper.
Writing: Literature review, identification of major herbs used for arthritis care.
Author C: Third author, serves as the contributing author, reviews and approves the final paper.
Writing: Synthesis of literature review, recommendations, and conclusions.

Everyone takes a month to draft their sections of the paper, then they share the information and a draft of the full paper is created. When the group meets to review their work, they discover that they have a big problem. Author B has gotten off track and included other types of arthritis besides osteoarthritis in the literature review. Author C has also gotten off track and included other alternative treatments in addition to herbal therapy. The whole paper will have to be rewritten. Everyone is discouraged because they have spent so many hours getting to this point and now the paper must be reworked. How could this have been avoided?

Whether writing as an individual or as a group, setting parameters for a paper is key to avoid spending hours of unnecessary time writing content that cannot be used. Write down the main message, which includes the theme of the paper and the topics that will be covered within that theme. Think "what is the point of this paper?" and commit it to writing. Then write down topics that will NOT fall under the theme. Be sure to ask and answer these questions before starting to write:

1. What is the assignment?
2. What is the specific topic chosen for this paper?
3. What is the main message or theme of this paper?
4. What topical areas fall under this theme that we should include?
5. What topical areas are excluded?
6. How will we study this? What sources will we include and exclude?

In the example above, the authors could have stayed on track if they had answered the six questions. How they answer these questions is up to the authors, but the point is for everyone to commit to the same vision so they can stay on track. Here's one way the questions could have been answered:

1. The assignment is to write a paper on a clinical topic suitable for publication in a journal.
2. The topic we have agreed on is "herbal treatments for osteoarthritis."

3. The main theme of this paper will be to provide clinicians with guidance on updated research and clinical guidelines that address effective herbal treatments for osteoarthritis.

4. We will include information that addresses topical or systemic herbal therapy for osteoarthritis. We'll include herbs that have been found to be effective, and we will also mention herbs that have been found to be ineffective.

5. We will exclude any treatments that are not defined as herbal or botanical therapy, as well as treatments for other types of arthritis or any conditions other than osteoarthritis.

6. We will review research articles and national or international guidelines published within the past 5 years. Information that is more than 5 years old and that has not been published in a peer-reviewed journal will be excluded.

The authors could have answered these questions differently. For example, they could have limited their discussion to effective herbal therapy, extended the literature out to 10 years, or made any number of other choices. The point is to define the parameters of the paper so the paper they set out to write and the paper they end up with are the same paper. That only happens if you stay on track.

THE ETHICS OF SCHOLARLY WRITING

There are writing professionals, editors, and publishers who spend their careers devoting themselves to the extensive ethical issues that can occur in the field of scholarly writing. An international organization, the Committee on Publication Ethics (COPE), provides significant leadership in this area with guidelines for resolving many types of ethical dilemmas that can arise in scientific and scholarly writing (COPE, 2021).

All writers should familiarize themselves with ethical standards for research and writing. A few of the most common stumbling blocks that occur include the following:

1. Failure to protect research subjects: Lack of institutional review board (IRB) clearance and failure to follow ethical standards in research are very serious breaches of publication ethics. Any paper that addresses a research project is expected to include a statement about IRB approval for the project.

2. Falsified data: While this problem is not common in nursing science, it does exist. All writers and readers of research-based publications should be aware that data falsification occurs. This problem results in numerous retractions of research articles worldwide each year and is a very serious violation that can impact a researcher for life.

3. Not crediting one or more authors of the paper. This error can result in retraction of an article from the literature and can cause legal problems for any author who knowingly fails to acknowledge another author. It is important to note that the definition of "authorship" varies somewhat among professional journals. One of the most common guidelines for establishing authorship comes from the International Council of Medical Journal Editors (ICMJE).

According to this guideline, anyone wishing to be listed as an author must have met each of the following requirements:

A. Substantial contributions to the conception or design of the work; or the acquisition, analysis, or interpretation of data for the work; AND

B. Drafting the work or revising it critically for important intellectual content; AND

C. Final approval of the version to be published; AND

D. Agreement to be accountable for all aspects of the work in ensuring that questions related to the accuracy or integrity of any part of the work are appropriately investigated and resolved (ICMJE, 2021).

There are many times when colleagues make contributions to papers, but the contributions do not meet each of the components mentioned above. In these cases, the colleagues can be recognized through a written acknowledgement that is published as a part of the paper. However, they cannot be included on the list of authors. It is also an ethical breach to list someone as an author who did not author the paper. Be sure to follow your school's guidelines for authorship when submitting a paper written by a group.

4. Plagiarism: The American Psychological Association (APA), in its publication manual and style guide, defines plagiarism as "The act of presenting the words, ideas, or images of another as your own" (APA, 2020). In other words, plagiarism occurs when an author uses another's work without proper permission or proper attribution of the actual source of the work. Again, this is a serious violation of publication ethics standards. It is very important to follow the professional style guide required by your university and ensure that you properly credit others' work. Some instances where this needs to occur include paraphrasing the ideas of others, using direct quotes, or using a table, figure, survey, or other material developed by another author (APA, 2020).

5. Failure to properly cite sources: This is one of the most frequent errors committed by new writers. Failure to cite includes leaving an item out of your reference list, missing a citation in a text but including the reference, misspelling an author's name, and similar errors. These errors stop short of plagiarism but are still problems with attribution, or correctly crediting someone's work. Always check your work to ensure that you have properly cited all sources you have used according to the style guide required by your institution.

The nuts and bolts of writing are the keys to getting started. Organization, paragraph construction, word choice, staying on track with your message, and publication ethics are fundamental skills. They can give you the confidence to move forward knowing how to avoid basic errors and where to go for assistance.

Improving Your Writing

It is gratifying to see your skills and confidence level as a writer develop over time, and it need not require the rest of your career to grow into an excellent writer who is comfortable with the writing process. There are several practical steps you can take to enhance your skills. At the top of this list is your own reading. By taking time to critically read and evaluate the professional literature, including clinical journals, conference proceedings, textbooks, and similar publications, you will be exposed to examples of how scholarly writing is created and organized. There are also several other steps you can take to further your expertise.

WRITING AND PEER REVIEW: A SYMBIOTIC RELATIONSHIP

One of the best ways to improve your own writing is by volunteering to serve as a peer reviewer for a nursing journal with a scope that matches your area of interest and expertise. Most journals have a large panel of peer reviewers whose purpose is to review and provide feedback on the suitability of manuscripts submitted for publication. Often, journals are seeking peer reviewers who are able to provide knowledgeable feedback on a specific area of clinical practice or education. The payback for the peer reviewer is being able to read, think about, and comment on new scholarship in the reviewer's specialty area.

The purpose of peer review is to critically read, evaluate, and critique the content of a manuscript. Peer reviewers look at writing style, accuracy of content, quality of references, and many other aspects of the manuscript. In addition to critiquing the content of the manuscript being reviewed, the peer reviewer must be aware of the journal's purpose and scope and should be familiar with the types of articles that have previously been published by the journal. This awareness allows the reviewer to judge whether the manuscript fits within the journal's scope and style. Journals expect peer reviewers to be able to comment on both the specific content and the overall fit of the manuscript.

Free training is available is available for new peer reviewers (Wolters Kluwer, 2021). Those interested in serving as a peer reviewer should locate the web site of their favorite journal, find the editor's email, and send a message volunteering to serve on the reviewer panel. Regular service as a peer reviewer is both educational and inspiring. It can provide you with examples of writing styles that will improve your own work, as well as potential ideas and motivation for your own future manuscripts.

JOURNAL CLUBS

Like peer review, journal club membership can be extremely helpful to developing writers. A variety of journal clubs are available, and you should be able to find an existing local or online journal club that you'd like to join. Journal clubs meet to discuss the content of a published article as a group, and this interaction is very educational for participants. Through a journal club, you are able to assess and evaluate the publication and share differences in your perceptions of strengths and weaknesses of the paper. These different perspectives provide insight to participants about their own strengths and weaknesses as critical readers and can quickly sharpen these skills. While journal club members do not provide formal feedback on a paper that contributes to the publication outcome, they are gaining knowledge of both the subject matter and the style of scholarly writing that led to success in publication.

GETTING HELP FROM OTHERS

For a beginning scholarly writer, the importance of co-authors, friendly "unofficial" reviewers, and informal editors cannot be overstated. We have all had times that we felt a paper was right on target, only to find out that it missed key points, had gotten off track, or had some other deficiency. Of course, it's always best to find this out before submitting the paper for grading.

If you have the opportunity to write with a group, you should choose this option over an individual paper whenever possible. Even if you don't know the other members of your writing team well, the opportunity to generate and share additional ideas, discuss the direction of the paper, and develop an achievable schedule for the finished product will be beneficial to you and almost always result in a better paper. Many of us are hesitant to write with a group due to fear of missed deadlines and work left undone by one or more members. This is understandable. However, there is much to be gained from peer participants as you all support each other as developing writers, and concerns can be overcome by writing out an assignment plan first and then ensuring that everyone agrees to be held accountable.

Friendly reviewers are informal reviewers, usually colleagues, faculty, or more experienced writers, who agree to read and comment on your work prior to submission. You can often find someone who is willing to do this just by asking one or two people that you trust to give you honest feedback. Informal reviewers should be asked to check your paper for spelling and grammar errors and to comment on the quality of the content of your paper. An informal editor can serve a similar function and make comments on the overall flow, organization, and word count while making suggestions for enhancing the overall look of your paper.

WHEN YOUR GOAL IS GETTING PUBLISHED

Many graduate students rightfully want their hard work to be disseminated broadly. Having a terminal degree supports your ability to contribute to the body of knowledge of the profession (Rohan and Fullerton, 2020). While every paper won't result in a publishable manuscript, consider whether your finished paper has the makings of a potential publication.

Fortunately, nurses who are serious about becoming published have numerous opportunities. There is a wide array of journals within the field of nursing, including general publications that are intended for broad audiences and very specialized journals that cover a discrete area of practice, education, or research within nursing. It does not take years of experience as a writer to have success in publishing an article in a professional journal. It does take commitment, perseverance, and a willingness to receive and respond to feedback.

A good first step if you are considering publishing a scholarly paper is to discuss this possibility with your professor. A faculty member with experience in publishing their work can provide direction in turning the paper into a manuscript and targeting appropriate journals. Realize that all papers written for an academic program will require some significant revision to conform to a journal's style, word count restrictions, and referencing style. In the case of larger academic assignments, such as DNP project papers and particularly dissertation-length work, the revisions will be extensive, but the result will be a much broader dissemination of your findings than you would be able to achieve without publication in a professional journal (Hicks, 2015).

Once you have made the decision and located journals that may be a potential fit for your paper, it can save you a great deal of time if you query the editor of the journal to determine the level of interest in your topical area. There are times when a journal may have received a manuscript covering your topic in the recent past, or there may be page count restrictions in the journal that prevent the editors from considering your paper. It will save you time if you can identify any roadblocks before you go through the process of formal submission.

If you have identified several journals that seem to be a good fit for your work, it is fine to send a query email to more than one journal to assess interest. However, once that is done, take care to never submit your manuscript simultaneously to more than one journal. That is considered unprofessional behavior and has negative consequences for future publication attempts. Submit your manuscript to the journal of your choice, and if it is declined you may then submit it to an alternate journal.

Throughout your journey as a writer, your work will be reviewed and judged. Many beginning writers find criticism of their hard work very discouraging, and that is understandable. Try to develop the mindset that these reviews are simply feedback that helps you further develop as a writer. Believe it or not, it is true. Your ability to respond positively and meaningfully to critiques and criticisms will make all the difference in your success. Don't take feedback personally, it's just feedback. Reflect on what the reviewer is telling you that will make your paper better, make the changes, and move on.

PUT YOURSELF FIRST

Both students and academic faculty know that the time necessary to think deeply about a subject and to create original material does not fit within the busy schedule of a regular workday for most of us. That is why taking a realistic look at your calendar and budgeting your time so that you will have the time and energy to write is a critical first step. It's important to know that you are not alone in this endeavor, and you are not deficient if you cannot juggle your writing with other elements of your busy daily life. It is very frustrating to try to write with distractions and inter-ruptions. While putting yourself first is often a very difficult mindset for nurses to adopt, you are owed the time, space, peace, and quiet to write. This should be your assumption and expectation.

TIPS FOR SUCCESS

Seven Techniques to Ensure Success

1. Make time. Schedule a regular time to write and commit to not deviating from your schedule.
2. Run sprints, not marathons. Budget your time over several weeks so you stay fresh and are rested enough to do your best work.
3. Make contact. Connect with the person in charge, be it an editor, professor, or colleague. Ensure you know the guidelines to follow before starting.
4. Engage your team. If your writing assignment or manuscript is a group effort, don't start writing until the assignments are clear as well as the consequences for those who fail to follow through.
5. Follow the rules. Review all guidelines: authorship rules, research policies from your institutional review board (IRB), individual journal guidelines, and any others that may apply.
6. Make the beginning the end. Create the title and abstract after the paper is finished to ensure they accurately reflect the final product.
7. Use a second set of eyes. Scholarly writing is important. Consider having a colleague review your work before submitting it.

Top Pet Peeves of Those Who Will Be Judging Your Writing

1. Spelling and grammar errors. Multiple errors in such simple things as spelling and grammar says "sloppy work" to a teacher or editor. Solution: These basic problems are preventable by using spelling and grammar checking functions and friendly reviewers.
2. The train of thought isn't moving in the right direction. Ideas jump around. Topics are picked up and then suddenly dropped. The unavoidable impression is that the author was distracted or rushed. Solution: Be sure you allocate enough time to fully understand the assignment, organize yourself to write, and allow adequate writing time.
3. The theme is missing or buried. There must be a purpose statement that reflects the theme, content that addresses the purpose, and a conclusion that ties it all together. Solution: The old adage, "Tell them what you're going to tell them, tell them, and then tell them what you told them" is really true. Stick to the theme and review it repeatedly while writing. Don't be afraid to repeat key points.
4. Personal agendas, viewpoints, and feelings are injected into a paper that is sup-posed to be scholarly. This reflects a problem with understanding what scholarly

writing is and is not. Solution: Unless you are asked to include a segment on personal feelings or reflections, this material should not be in your paper.

Here are a few resources that can provide assistance and additional techniques for writing. There are many others available. Please see the reference list for more complete information on accessing these resources.

Comprehensive Texts About Writing for Nurses

Saver, Cynthia: Anatomy of writing for publication for nurses.
Roush, Karen: Nurse's Step-By-Step Guide to Writing a Dissertation or Scholarly Project.

Spelling, Grammar, and Style Guides

Grammarly: Spelling, grammar, and sentence construction. https://www.grammarly.com/
INANE resources for nurse authors. https://nursingeditors.com/resources/writing-for-publication/
Purdue Online Writing Lab (OWL). https://www.owl.purdue.edu/
Word processing software with integrated spelling and grammar checking functions, such as TextEdit for Apple and Microsoft Word.

Managing Citations and References

Endnote citation management tool. https://endnote.com/
Zotero reference locator and organizer. https://www.zotero.org/
Word reference manager, available in Microsoft Word.

Publication Ethics and Plagiarism

Publication ethics and plagiarism detection software
The Committee on Publication Ethics. https://publicationethics.org/
iThenticate originality and plagiarism software. https://www.ithenticate.com/
Originality software provided by your university

Summary

This chapter provides a broad overview of concepts and skills that will be used when writing at the graduate level. Writing in a scholarly style is an acquired skill. Students may also want to seek out comprehensive writing texts and style guides for more specific assistance. Writing skills are a critical component of career advancement into academia, research, and clinical leadership. Many nurses don't think of themselves as natural writers, but all nurses can write in a professional and scholarly style and can become very comfortable with this style of writing. The development of writing skills can provide nurses with opportunities for future publication and can enhance their careers as experts within their area of specialization. For some nurses, a growing enjoyment of writing can lead to a career as a nurse writer. Nurses can view the acquisition of writing skills as just one of many skills in their professional toolbox.

Bibliography

American Psychological Association (APA). *Publication Manual of the American Psychological Association.* 7th ed. American Psychological Association; 2020. Available at: https://doi.org/10.1037/0000165-000.

Clarivate. *Endnote: Accelerate Your Research.* Clarivate; 2021. Available at: http.s://endnote.com/.

Committee on Publication Ethics. *Promoting Integrity in Scholarly Research and its Publication.* COPE; 2021. Available at: https://publicationethics.org/.

Corporation for Digital Scholarship. *Zotero: Your Personal Research Assistant.* Zotero; 2021. Available at: https://www.zotero.org/.

Grammarly. *Elevate Your Writing.* Grammarly; 2021. Available at: https://www.grammarly.com/.

Hicks R. Transforming a presentation to a publication: tips for nurse practitioners. *J Am Assoc Nurse Pract.* 2015;27(9):488-496. doi:10.1002/2327-6924.12228.

International Academy of Nursing Editors (INANE). *Writing for Publication.* INANE; 2021. Available at: https://nursingeditors.com/resources/writing-for-publication/.

International Council of Medical Journal Editors (ICMJE). *Defining the Roles of Authors and Contributors.* ICMJE Recommendations; 2021. Available at: http://www.icmje.org/recommendations/browse/roles-and-responsibilities/defining-the-role-of-authors-and-contributors.html.

Purdue University College of Liberal Arts. Purdue Online Writing Lab (OWL); 2021. Available at: https://owl.purdue.edu/.

Rohan A, Fullerton J. Developing advanced practice nurse writing competencies as a corequisite for evidence-based practice. *J Am Assoc Nurse Pract.* 2020;32(10):682-688. doi:10.1097/JXX.0000000000000298.

Roush K. *Nurse's Step-By-Step Guide to Writing a Dissertation or Scholarly Project.* 2nd ed. Indianapolis, IN: Sigma Theta Tau International; 2018.

Saver C. *Anatomy of Writing for Publication for Nurses.* 4th ed. Indianapolis, IN: Sigma Theta Tau International; 2021.

Turnitin Solutions. *iThenticate Products.* iThenticate; 2021. Available at: https://www.ithenticate.com/.

Wolters Kluwer. *Peer Reviewer Training Course.* Wolters Kluwer Author Services from Editage; 2021. Available at: https://wkauthorservices.editage.com/peer-reviewer-training-course/.

CHAPTER 13

Determining Good Fit

Mary Anne Dumas, PhD, FNP-BC, GNP-BC, FAANP, FAAN, FNAP

Education is the most powerful weapon you can use to change the world.
—Nelson Mandela

Once you have determined the academic degree that best supports your career aspirations, you will want to consider several aspects of the educational programs available to earn your terminal degree.

This chapter introduces the features of the education program you will want to consider when making your decision. The objectives of this chapter are to:

1. Emphasize the importance of finding a program that is a "good Fit" for your career goals
2. Describe what is meant by program concentration
3. Discuss completion requirements and rates
4. Evaluate measures of performance across different programs of study.
5. Decode the language of tuition and financing
6. Identify opportunities that may be available to you as a student during your program of study
7. Explain instructional delivery models
8. Differentiate the various technology approaches used in program delivery
9. Understand the varied learning and student support resources available.

There are over 400 DNP programs and 150 PhD programs in the United States (AACN.org). Doctoral programs vary in the type of curriculum delivery: online, face-to-face, content focus (for example, research, practice, policy, informatics, and leadership). Each must be considered in making an informed decision. Further information is available on the American Association of Colleges of Nursing website, for example, the DNP Practice Contrast Grid (AACN, 2022).

Good Fit

Finding a "good fit" will be the focus of all your research and decision-making when choosing your program. Availability of faculty mentors whose expertise compliments

TABLE 13.1 ■ **The "Good Fit" Table**

Summary of Variables That Must Meet the "Good Fit" Criteria			
Type of Degree	**PhD**	**DNP**	**DNP to PhD**
Length of Program			
Graduation and retention rates			
Number of students admitted per academic year			
Type of admissions: Rolling/Annual			
Admission criteria and interviews			
Faculty Mentors/advisors			
Institutional resources			
Learning methodologies			
Full-time/Part-time options			
Financial considerations			
Faculty-Applicant interaction pre-admission			
Current student feedback			

your interests, academic resources, the learning methodology, full-time/part-time options, and financial considerations are all variables that determine the "good fit." Table 13.1 presents a checklist you might find useful in evaluating the "good fit" for the program you are considering.

Program Concentration

As mentioned earlier, it is essential to consider individual career goals when choosing your program. DNP programs vary in the academic areas of concentration, for example, policy, leadership, practice, informatics, education, and advanced practice. Advanced Practice Registered Nursing (APRN) includes four different roles: (1) nurse practitioner (NP), (2) Certified Registered Nurse Anesthetist (CRNA), (3) Certified Nurse Midwife (CNM), and (4) Clinical Nurse Specialist (CNS). The APRN Consensus Model provides the regulatory model for the four APRN roles. The model requires that all APRN programs include three discrete graduate-level courses: (1) pharmacology, (2) pathophysiology, and (3) physical assessment (advanced health assessment). The APRN Consensus model identified specific, "populations" for the role of the NP, which requires performing clinical hours in a clinical practicum. Nurses who choose a DNP program will want to consider the practice and scholarship of the DNP faculty.

PhD programs will vary in the area of concentration as well. It will be important to consider the program of research of the faculty members at each school. It will also be important to delve into the research methods, analytics, funding history, and scholarship generated by the PhD faculty.

Some nursing schools combine DNP and PhD students to learn in the same courses across areas of study. Another option is to pursue the combined DNP-PhD. At the time of publication, four such programs are offered (https://www.aacnnursing. org/Portals/42/LeadershipNetworks/GNAP/ 2019/PhD-DNP-Dual-Degree-Program-Presentation-GNAP-2019.pdf). These prorgrams integrate curriculum to offer both research and clinical practice experiences, and any student considering one of these programs will want to weigh the faculty qualifications and all aspects listed above.

Degree Completion Requirements

The requirements for the PhD and DNP degrees differ. The PhD is educated with the knowledgge, abilities, and analytical skills to conduct primary research and generate new knowledge. The dissertation phase of the PhD education is an intense mentored research experience with a faculty investigator or mentor (also known as the dissertation chair), usually supported by two additional committee members. The dissertation chair should have experience mentoring PhD students through their research. Ideally, the dissertation chair should have an established, funded program of research or expertise in the student's dissertation area of research. The dissertation may be qualitative or quantitative in design. Qualitative research designs use descriptive statistics and content/thematic analysis, such as grounded theory, phenomenology, or ethnography. Quantitative or experimental techniques randomize subjects and use parametric and inferential or advanced statistics such as multiple regression or mixed methods.

The DNP is educated with the knowledge, abilities, and analytical skills to bring evidence into practice to improve outcomes. The scholarly project phase of DNP education is an intense mentored experience under the guidance and direction of a qualified faculty member. The scholarly project involves desing, implementation, and evaluation of an evidence-based clinical practice innovation. The purpose of the project is to improve outcomes for individuals, populations, organizations, and communities. Expert clinical faculty and a practice mentor provide support and oversite to ensure safety and effectiveness of the quality improvement project

When considering a PhD program, some schools offer two options for the degree requirement. The first and most common option is a dissertation. This is a document comprised of five chapters (refer to Chapters 5 and 6). The second and newer option is to produce three manuscripts that disseminate your original research through peer-reviewed publications. Both options require reporting of original research conducted by the student and evidence of mastery of the content and attainment of the terminal objectives for the program of study.

Measures of Program Performance

The admissions criteria and academic requirements differ among programs and from one educational institution to another. Take time to explore program requirements (see Chapter 10). Never immediately rule out a program that identifies a minimum GPA on your transcript that is lower than the requirements on the website. Always reach out to admissions offices or faculty of the desired degree program directly to make inquiries. Email or telephone contact is acceptable to make program faculty/staff aware that you are interested in their program.

FACULTY SCHOLARSHIP, PRACTICE, AND RESEARCH

Doctoral programs that have a reputation of excellence include faculty members who demonstrate expertise and excellence in one or more areas, such as teaching, clinical practice, and/or research. Explore the program that you would like to apply to and consider the faculty members in both nursing and other departments in your area of interest. Consider these questions: Do the faculty have a national presence? Are they recognized as experts? Do they have a reputation for excellence? Do they have stature as national/international nursing leaders? Faculty serving as mentors provide opportunities and networking resources to assist your development as a successful nurse scientist, clinician, academician, and leader.

EXPECTATIONS FOR THE DURATION OF THE PROGRAM

Each program will clearly state expectations for the length of that program. This will differ based on whether students enroll full time or part time. You will want to understand these expectations and factor them into your program selection.

COMPLETION RATES

Completion rates are one measure of program performance that can help you evaluate the programs you are considering. Low completion rates for any academic program are a reason for concern. Because of the significant requirements of doctoral study, lower completion rates are not uncommon. When speaking to program faculty, it is important to investigate completion rates. When considering a DNP program, you will want to compare completion rates for any individual program with those in other DNP programs. When considering a PhD program you will want to benchmark completion rates with other PhD programs.

Coursework across programs is a very structured and guided process. In the dissertation/scholarly project phase of doctoral education, the unstructured nature of completing the dissertation or project may be difficult for some students. Students may have difficulty working individually and may feel isolated, except for their relationship with the oversight of their research/project chair and mentor.

Self-discipline and time management are required to complete the dissertation or DNP project. Setting timelines with the research chair or mentor can provide structure and guidance and enable the student to smoothly progress in a timely fashion. Failing to complete a PhD dissertation is referred to as "Going ABD (all but dissertation)."

You should be able to find the completion rates of any program you are considering listed on program websites. If these data are not available in promotional materials, do not be afraid to ask. Exploring the most common reasons for not advancing provides insight into the responsiveness of the faculty and staff and the infrastructure in place to support busy working professional students with complex and dynamic lives.

ON-TIME COMPLETION

The percent of students who complete the program of study within the expected time is another measure of program performance (Robinson & Volkert, 2018). In much the same way that you explored completion rates, you will want to understand time to completion. In other words, you will want to ask what percent of the students successfully complete the program of study within the time frame described in the curriculum plan. It is possible that some students may take longer to complete the program because of personal responsibilities. So learning about the frequency with which students require additional time and resources needed will help you understand the likelihood that you will be able to complete the program on time.

RATIO OF STUDENTS TO FACULTY

Doctoral programs do not have prescribed student-faculty ratios the way pre-licensure and clinical master's nursing education in nursing do. The faculty-student ratio for NP programs is described by the National Taskforce for the Evaluation of Nurse Practitioner Programs, 6th edition, 2022 (https://cdn.ymaws.com/www.nonpf.org/resource/resmgr/2022/ntfs_/ntfs_final.pdf). Faculty are assigned to doctoral students for guidance of the scholarly project or research dissertation. Programs often set a limit on the number of projects and dissertations a faculty member can supervise. So you will want to inquire about the number of student projects and dissertations the faculty in each program will carry. This information will inform your program selection. Please check out www.nonpf.org/resource/resmgr/ 2022/ntfs_/ntfs_final.pdf.

Program Ranking and Reputation

Some data components from the ranking structure are of interest to prospective students (graduation rates, faculty productivity, funding resources). We encourage you to investigate the reputation of every program you are considering. Graduate school rankings are generated annually and can be found in the U.S. News and World Report (https://www.usnews.com/best-graduate-schools). What are the rankings of the programs you are considering? Are any of the top ranked schools located in your area? Which factors in the rankings are most important to you?

Tuition and Debt Load

Tuition and debt load carried by graduates are two important measures you can use to consider best fit. You should consider the program costs and the debt load as a reflection of an investment in yourself and your future. Consider the words of Nelson Mandela: "Education is the great engine of personal development. It is through education that the daughter of a peasant can become a doctor, that a son of a mineworker can become the head of the mine, that a child of farm workers can become the president of a nation" (Loo, 2022). Education is an investment into your professional career and future earning.

When forcasting the cost of your education and your ability to cover your living expenses, it is important to several factors and compare them from one program to the next. You will want to consider cost per credt, total credits, assistance available from employer, assistance available from the school, and your potential to generate income while earning your degree. These factors are explained in Table 13.1.

See Table 13.2 for the most important aspects of program costs to understand and compare when evaluating your program choices.

FINANCIAL AID

When selecting a program, you will want to inquire about resources and financial support that each program will provide. There will be tremendous variability from program to program. Understanding the available support will help you evaluate the fit of the program to your particular financial need. Financial support may come from any of the following: scholarships, grants, traineeships, loans, and work-study programs. (https://www.aacnnursing.org/Students/Financial-Aid). Can the program you are interested in help you seek and find the support you need? Consider the following when speaking with the Financial Support personnel:

1. Most financial aid and scholarships from federal or other sources will only be avaialble to students who complete the FAFSA form (See #2).
2. Eligibility and need for federal funds can be documented using the Federal Student Financial Aid and the Free Application for Federal Student Aid (FAFSA). https://www.usa.gov/financial-aid#item-206091.
3. Scholarships are funds available from a variety of sources that can be applied to program expenses without obligation to pay back the funds. Scholarship awards tend to be focused on particular populations. conditions, or challenges that are of interest to the donor and contribute. In order to qualify for these

TABLE 13.2 ■ Debt Load Table

Category	Costs	Itemized Costs
Costs	*Program costs, fees, books*	• Tuition rates • Fees, books • Potential earnings as a teaching or research assistant; savings available • Income • Personal savings you can access to cover costs • Length of program
	Number of credits	• Doctoral programs vary in the number of credits required to earn the degree, and graduate credits tend to be more costly than undergraduate ones
	Employer Tuition reimbursement	• Employees are commonly expected to pay the cost of tuition and submit for reimbursement after completion of a course and earning a minimum grade of a B • You will want to research tuition benefits from your employer to understand which programs of study and which credentials will be covered
	Travel	• Commuting needs: Airfare, train, mileage, lodging, and any other related expenses as applicable
Program requirements	Time constraints and cost of living	• Conflicts with school, work, study schedules, and childcare commitments—may disrupt academic progress, lengthening the time needed to complete the degree and adding to overall expenses • Time requirement to complete the degree. If you need beyond 5 years to complete the program, you may be required to repeated some courses and incur addtitional costs.

Modified from: https://www.aacnnursing.org/Students/Financial-Aid. Retrieved March 5, 2022.

funds, your area of interest will need to closely align with the intention of the donor.

4. What federal grant programs are available through the school? This site provides information, in a table form, regarding eligibility and type of grant. https://studentaid.gov/sites/default/files/federal-grant-programs.pdf

5. Does the program offer traineeships? Advanced nursing education traineeships funded by the Department of Human Services, the Division of Nursing, support master's and doctoral degrees in nursing education, as well as some certificate programs. https://www.benefits.gov/benefit/725.

6. Experienced faculty with mature programs of research may be able to offer tuition assistance to students whose programs of study are compatible with their research expertise.

Further discussion of financial sources for educational support can be found in Chapter 9.

Teaching Assistant Opportunities

If your career aspirations include teaching, then teaching assistant (TA) opportunities will be important to you. As mentioned earlier, you will want to learn if the program you are considering can make such opporutnities available to you.

Research Assistant Opportunities

If your career aspirations are to become a researcher, then research assistant opportunities will be important to you. You will want to ask about these opportunities when exploring your PhD program of choice.

Interprofessional Opportunities

Regardless of your interests in research or practice, you will want to understand the different opportunities that would be available for interdisciplinary collaboration. You may want to explore your area of interest outside of the nursing community. For example, If your interest lies in ethics, you want to know if you will have the option to take courses or work with faculty in other university departments such as philosophy, humanities or law. Additionally, if you have an interest in a particular methodology or analytic approach, you want to know if you would have the option to choose to work with faculty or take courses in epidemiology, education, or statistics.

And though your doctoral topic may be associated with a different department within the institution, interprofessional collaboration provides a rich networking source with colleagues and can lead to even more research opportunities. Academic institutions are likely to have a Community of Scholars (COS) institutional online link, which will introduce you to the broad research interests of all faculty and researchers, further expanding your network of science experts.

Opportunities to Publish With Faculty

Dissemination is expected of doctorally prepared scholars. Opportunities to publish with faculty will support your success in this area. You will want to ask about faculty publication history and the opportunity to publsih with them. Chapter 5 offers lists of questions that you will find helfpul when speaking with faculty at the schools your are considering.

Instruction Model

There is tremendous variability in instructional models and approaches across doctoral programs (Kostas-Polston, 2018). When you are selecting your program of study, you want to consider the instructional approach or model that best meets your learning needs.

Instructional models have evolved from face to face only to online only and "blended" instruction. In order to identify the best program for you, you will want to ask several questions:

1. How is instruction delivered? Do classes meet face to face, online, synchronous or asynchronous, blended?
2. What is the schedule of classes? Run by semesters, trimesters, immersion or intensive experiences, does the program run 9 or 12 months?
3. How does the supervision and advising of your program work?
4. What support is available to you from the library, from student services, writing center, testing, information technology?
5. What resources are available to support your health and wellness?
6. What supports are in place for your project and dissertation?

Here is a quick review of the types of content delivery today's schools of nursing are offering:

- *Face-to-face learning* is a traditional model that places a premium on learning in a community. In this model students meet with faculty and peers to activitely engage with each other and the content. This experience, under the best conditions, is characterized as shared, interactive, and personalized. The traditional classroom experience has been significantly influenced and enhanced by developments in online learning. In the best case, it is very engaged, classroom environment where students come to class having reviewed the content and prepared for dynamic interaction and development of critical thinking and reflection. The focus has moved from simple presentation of content by faculty expert to mastery and competency among the group of learners.
- *Online learning* is broadly accessible and allows the student a high level of control over timing and pace. Online synchronous learning provides the student with opportunities to learn in real time with the faculty/instructor present during instruction. Class is scheduled for a specific time and day of the week. Online asynchronous learning takes place when the student chooses and proceeds at their chosen pace. Interactions between faculty and students are carefully planned and structured and largely take the form of discussion boards, voice threads, video recordings, and/or podcasts. Skills and confidence with technology and computer access are essential for success in this model.
- Blended instruction combines the best of face-to-face and online. Today, most programs use a course management system (CMS), such as Canvas, Moodle, Blackboard, Sakai, or others, to organize, store, and deliver course content and resources.
- "Executive format" refers to an organization of the learning experiences. These offerings vary from program to program. It is important to ask how

these programs are structured, what kind of support is built in, the pace at which the program proceeds, and the responsibilities of students and faculty for successful completion.

Choosing an instructional model that is a good fit with your learning style, work schedule, career trajectory, and family and personal commitments will significantly contribute to your success, progress, and completion of your doctoral study.

Time on Campus

As mentioned earlier, many schools require time on campus. Each program determines the criteria for face-to-face learning experiences, which may include lab time, simulations, interprofessional learning, teamwork, and formal presentation.

Full-Time and Part-Time Study Options

Doctoral programs may offer both full-time and part-time options. Graduate nurses often elect part-time study due to time, work, and family commitments. Attending school part time offers benefits such as home and work life flexibility and more distributed tuition costs, which may allow you to use your tuition benefits to reduce the debt load you will carry. Keep in mind that part-time students may not be eligible for certain scholarships or grants. In either full-time or part-time pursuits, solid and transparent support system communication skills are needed, as complex scheduling demands will include balancing numerous tasks and priorities. Some students employed full time in nursing may choose to voluntarily reduce their number of work hours to better enable them to complete the course demands. You will want to consider whether moving ahead briskly is to your advantage or whether studying part-time and moving a bit slower is a better fit for you.

Postdoctoral Opportunities

Postdoctoral programs (post-doc) provide independent experiences, sometimes grant funded, that enable you to pursue your research interests and publications beyond completion of your PhD. A post-doc provides newly graduated scholars with dedicated transition time to develop an independent research career, develop greater autonomy, and build networks for team science. Funding support avenues include private foundations, institutes, the National Institutes of Health, Duke University, and the U.S. Department of Veterans Affairs, which showcase some phenomenal opportunities to build your teaching and clinical research skills (https://www.registerednursing.org/post-doctoral-nursing-fellowships/). To date, most postdoctoral fellowships are only available for PhD graduates, but work is moving toward designing and delivering postdoctoral opportunities for DNP graduates.

Technology Preparation

Most graduate universities and college programs publish minimum computer hardware and software requirements (Box 13.1). Seek out the university's existing systems and how your favorite technology tools will talk with one another. If considering a doctoral program that is primarily a Windows/PC environment, yet all the technology you own is Apple-based, be sure to ask if support resources on campus offer the assistance needed to succeed in your coursework, clinical, and laboratory endeavors. (The reverse is also true!)

In general, you will be required to use technology throughout any program of study and university, and you will want university tech support to be available. Any program you are investigating should provide information about the availability of technical support to troubleshoot and repair problems when they occur suddenly and unexpectedly. Faculty and staff should be able to describe an effective process for promptly rectifying technology problems.

- For on-campus or face-to-face programs you will want to understand the availability of the technology resources, computer labs, and simulators to conduct research and perform qualitative and quantitative data analysis. Is it up to date and in good working order?
- Inquire whether purchasing a new computer/laptop is the student's responsibility. Ask whether the institution provides student discounts for purchasing new technology.

Laptops and mobile devices are helpful when moving to and from class and/or study groups. You will want to make sure your device meets the requirements. Most of the technological problems students encounter stem from using outdated software or hardware.

Most universities and colleges will strongly recommend (or require) that your system run up-to-date security software (anti-virus and anti-malware). Most modern operating systems include software that will meet these requirements, but check with the institutions you are considering before purchasing any security software.

BOX 13.1 ■ Common IT Requirements

- Modern computer (tablets and mobile devices are NOT recommended as primary device for online students)
- Manufactured within the last 2–3 years (with upgrades every 2–3 years) with the ability to reliably run the software needed
- 64-bit multi-core processor or better
- 8 GB or more of memory (RAM). *ED. Generally, more is better up to 32Gb*
- 128 GB solid-state hard drive (SSD) or 250 GB hard disk drive or larger *ED. SSDs are typically more reliable, faster, and smaller than "platter-based" hard drives. (As in, larger RAM is better.)*
- Sound card and speakers
- Headphones
- Webcam for video conferencing

Other recommended software/devices include backup software and device (usually an external drive or cloud-based service). It cannot be stressed enough how crucial a backup of important files is; you never know when your dog will push over your cup of coffee, spilling it all over your computer.

Library or Information Support

Online access to search engines, journals, e-texts, databases, and classes should be available to you as a student. Access to library services usually depends on active enrollment. It is important to know if reference librarians are avaialble to assist with literature searches for coursework and research and what types of instruction are avialble to help you become a successful scholar.

Graduate Experiences/Current Student Feedback

"Open House" information sessions are offered by practically all programs to provide you with the information about their programs and all the metrics we have described. You will want to take time to learn the answers to the questions we have provided. Often faculty and students within the program are willing to share their experiences and opinions about the program, provide information, and answer your questions. Feel free to ask the PhD or DNP program director or the admissions director to arrange for you to speak with a current student. Speaking with current students regarding the strengths and weaknesses of the curriculum/program, the availability of faculty and staff, and the innovative welcoming approaches toward building an inclusive environment for learning are all examples of lines of inquiry that will offer guidance for a successful doctoral journey (Ward-Smith, 2014). Ask questions regarding a program's flexibility and your ability to gain access to necessary resources, for example, a writing center, remedial services, and student health and wellness programs. These personal perspectives can help you evaluate the fit of the program with your particular needs and aspirations.

These personal experiences can help you appreciate how to maximize growth opportunities and prepare for potential shortfalls of program delivery.

Community Life and Community of Scholars

During doctoral study, both the DNP and PhD, your classmates and faculty become a community of great imporance to you. You and your classmates will have many shared intense experiences and will help and support each other throughout your doctoral journey and beyond. You will want to ask questions about the climate and collaborative culture in any program you are considering.

In general terms, a community of scholars is a network of individuals holding advanced degrees. The institution should list the community of scholars and their research interests. You will want to understand who are the members of this community in any program, college, or university you are considering entering. This community can contribute to your development and success.

Summary

Doctoral graduates become team players, scientific problem solvers, and expert clinical scholars. They develop new knowledge and apply evidence to improve outcomes. They develop disciplined scholarship and strong communication skills including the ability to publish, present, and persuade. Understanding the strengths of each program you consider will help you select the program that is best for you.

Bibliography

American Association of Colleges of Nursing. *DNP Practice Comparison Grid.* 2022. Available at: https://www.aacnnursing.org/Nursing-Education-Programs/DNP-Education. Retrieved April 28, 2022.

Kostas-Polston EA, Rawlett K, Miedema J, Dickins K. An integrative review of nurse practitioner education models: part three of a four-part series on critical topics identified by the 2015 nurse practitioner research agenda. *J Am Assoc Nurse Pract.* 2018;30(12):696-709.

Loo C. *Top Nine Nelson Mandela Quotes about Education.* 2022. Available at: https://borgenproject.org/nelson-mandela-quotes-about-education/.

Robinson LB, Volkert D. Support issues and nursing doctoral students' intent to leave. *Nurs Educ Perspect.* 2018;39(5):297-298.

US News and World Report. 2022. Available at: https://www.usnews.com/.

Ward-Smith P. Student nurse perception of doctoral graduate programs. *J Nurs Educ Pract.* 2014;4(5):36-41.

CHAPTER 14

Staying Motivated, Confident, and Well Focused as a Doctoral Student

Laura A. Taylor, PhD, RN, ANEF, FAAN ■
Mary F. Terhaar, PhD, RN, ANEF, FAAN

> *Wayfinding is the ancient art of figuring out where you are going when you don't actually know your destination.*
>
> —Bill Burnett

Well done! Here you are, ready to start your doctoral educational journey. We hope we have made the case that increasing the number of doctoral-prepared nurses is urgently needed, and this is where you come in. The health of our society will depend on bright, talented, and committed nurses. The world seeks nurses who develop a deep understanding of our discipline's phenomena, think outside the bounds of practice as we know it, ask new questions, bring evidence to inform care in innovative and effective ways, and form boundary-spanning partnerships. Overcoming health disparities and achieving inclusive healthcare will require people from all races, backgrounds, cultures, and gender identities.

Throughout this text, each author has provided resources and personal stories describing perseverance and creative problem-solving. They have shared evidence-based strategies and innovations you can activate to increase the likelihood of success as you embark. This next step is yours to take. You will no doubt discover some new strategies and come up with new solutions that work for you. You will likely make mistakes. Nevertheless, we have done our very best to help ensure that you will not repeat errors from which we can steer you away. So, if you make a misstep, it should be authentic and new, and you can share what you learn on this journey with others who follow you.

In Chapters 5, 6, 7, and 13, you read about the importance of knowing the right questions to ask to help determine which doctoral degree is best suited for your career goals and learning style (Smith & Delmore, 2021). In Chapters 5 and 6, you learned about the different programs of study and the demands of each. Then in Chapters 9, 10, 11, and 12, you explored how to develop a plan that addresses your finances, career commitments, family responsibilities, and personal situation as you began your doctoral educational exploration efforts (Smith & Delmore, 2021). As you read the narratives, you realize that it is a long journey, that you must want to take that journey, and that most who do begin with some trepidation, move into excitement, settle down to work, and in the end go on to do amazing and important things. As you read this chapter, we hope you realize that you are capable beyond measure, just like those who took the time to share their knowledge and experience in the narratives.

Making the Dream a Reality Will Be Challenging

Now, we do not intend to "throw shade" on the bright "can do" spirit of the future doctoral student that lies inside you. Nevertheless, as exciting as the future journey will be, we need to emphasize that becoming the next generation of nurse scientists, expert clinicians, policy drivers, educators, and leaders comes with challenges. The literature is straightforward; you will encounter speed bumps, hurdles, and thick cinder block firewalls along your doctoral journey. One can easily find statistics to reflect the statistics of completion rates in doctoral education today. The 50% dropout rate of doctoral students before attaining their degree has stagnated for 60 years (Van der Linden et al., 2018; Brill et al., 2014; GSC Graduate Student Council, 2021). Moreover, though completion rates for doctoral students in the health sciences trend a little higher, they remain concerning (Wollast et al., 2018).

These statistics are both significant, perplexing, and disheartening when considering the future of the nursing profession. Nurse leaders across practice, clinical, research, policy, and education underscore the importance of carrying today's excitement, passion, drive, and enthusiasm throughout your educational journey in order to stay on target (Vance et al., 2020). Accordingly, a need to obtain a deeper understanding of the nature of the doctoral process, the challenges enrolled students are likely to encounter, and how they relate to student well-being must be shared. In the pages ahead, we offer evidence-based approaches to mitigate some of the students' highest hurdles experienced in doctoral education: limited support and wavering motivation. Read on!

Support for Success

FACULTY SUPPORT AND ENCOURAGEMENT

The research on doctoral education has identified various harmonizing factors that contribute to a successful doctoral experience: a welcoming scholarly community, including supervisory researcher-faculty relationships, as well as fellow doctoral students, and a supportive community of family and friends (Volkert et al., 2018; Van der Linden et al., 2018; McNelis et al., 2018).

The provision of sufficient supervisory faculty and researchers for doctoral students is the foundation for developing doctoral education, yet there is a distinct challenge with our nursing faculty shortage. To increase the odds of completing studies and reducing the risk of experiencing burnout, your program of choice must provide sufficient support. Use the critical questions offered in Chapters 5, 6, 7, and 13 to explore how the program and faculty identify students at risk and how faculty strategically align success for their budding doctoral researchers by building a network/community of coauthorship and collaboration to facilitate a robust support system.

Mechanisms that foster a warm, inclusive research environment will result in a more confident and positive doctoral student community (Jeffreys, 2014, 2015). To maintain interest and passion in your concentration area, faculty mentors should promote self-directed thinking with research activities and guide self-development that aligns with your values, interests, and goals (Dreifuerst et al., 2016; McNelis et al., 2018). Passionate and highly engaged doctoral students boast greater satisfaction and increased perseverance (Volkert et al., 2018). Furthermore, the more a doctoral program can help you avoid the development of self-cynicism and exhaustion, which can be detrimental to anyone's intellectual and personal well-being, the more significant the reduction of risk of dissertation delay or dropping out altogether.

Student Support Groups and Organizations

Early career researchers share that if students learn how to support each other, it can also positively influence their progress (Vekkaila & Pyhältö, 2016; Peltonen et al., 2017; Vidak et al., 2017). Support structures embedded in the doctoral program can help you and your fellow doctoral students support each other, cope with doctoral course load curriculum demands, and learn stratagems to solve conflicts within the researcher community. These programmatic resources highlight the importance of supervisory and researcher community support as one of the most crucial assets of future doctoral education in researcher communities (Smith & Delmore, 2021; Wollast et al., 2018).

No matter the doctoral program you select (hybrid, traditional, or online), we encourage you to initiate recommendations from the literature: garnering support from peers, participating in faculty-designed and -led support mechanisms, and being active in student-led support groups. Journal clubs or dissertation/capstone/scholarly project writing groups often formalize student-driven support groups and even promote collaboration between students in PhD and DNP programs. These evidence-based strategies help mitigate barriers to completion, minimize attrition, and promote persistence (Kuchinski-Donnelly & Krouse, 2020). Table 14.1 describes four online programs/resources that are available and accessible for your doctoral journey.

TABLE 14.1 ■ Programs Available for Doctoral Support

***International Network for Doctoral Education in* Nursing** The International Network for Doctoral Education in Nursing (INDEN) is a nonprofit professional association dedicated to advancing quality doctoral nursing education globally.	https://indenglobal.org/resources
AACN Graduate Nursing Student Academy offers numerous webinars and resources for doctoral education support and networking.	https://www.aacnnursing.org/News-Information/Research-Data-Center/PhD
The Doctoral Support Team Committed to helping graduate students complete their academic programs, earn their degrees, and maintain a healthy school-work-life balance.	https://www.doctoralsupport.org/
The PhD Project Network of Support A strong support network is a crucial success factor in the journey to a PhD The encouragement and insights of other doctoral students and alums faculty members are invaluable. Only those on, or have already followed, the same path truly understands the challenges and opportunities of reaching your goal.	https://phdproject.org/network-of-support/
Online PhD Degrees is a website for those considering online programs. PhD is one of the most challenging phases anyone can choose to face in their academic life. Coping is an everyday struggle in itself. Many can attest that the road to a doctoral diploma is long and lonely. You will surely encounter struggles most fellow PhD students would understand.	https://www.online-phd-degrees.com/online-support-groups-phd-students/

Friends and Family

Friends and family support significantly impact doctoral students, and it has been noted that as family support declines, intent to leave a doctoral program rises (Vekkaila & Pyhältö, 2016). Though it is not the duty of a doctoral program to ensure well-functioning social circles, we encourage you to inquire about system supports in place to help build supportive relationships for students and their significant others/family members.

Staying Motivated

PERSISTENCE

It is impossible to remove all stressors from your future student life during doctoral studies. Obtaining a doctorate requires intensive work. Motivation is essential in doctoral study; sadly, as many as 44% will lose motivation (Council of Graduate

Schools, 2022). When you get into the heart of your research and doctoral scholarly project, a clear relationship between motivation and peer/family support seems to exist. The most successful students have a passion for the subject and enjoy the process of learning more about it, essentially becoming immersed in the topic. You are more likely to achieve your goals when maintaining a positive outlook on your future and the outcomes of the doctoral program. Those who attend graduate school because of vague expectations, under pressure, or wavering support from friends or family can struggle with an already challenging course load (Volkert et al., 2018).

There are worries that most doctoral students face. We discuss many of these earlier in the text, specifically anxiety, fear, and impostor syndrome. Let us now explore limited persistence and low confidence (Priode et al., 2020). Your ability to be persistent throughout this doctoral journey directly impacts your self-confidence and is the oxygen for more remarkable persistence. A cycle of support and motivation leads to more reasons and opportunities to stay and finish your doctoral expedition. For instance, those doctoral students who perceive themselves as members of a supportive research community are empowered to maintain motivation, which will further drive persistence in maintaining their passion for their topic. Students who maintain a passion for their area of concentration are less likely to consider dropping the program. Staying motivated, coupled with the ability to persevere, is the secret sauce to staying on to the end of this doctoral roller coaster ride (Box 14.1).

Grit

Recent work shows that nearly 67% of all doctoral students gradually develop anxiety and burnout from prolonged and extensive work-related stress (Nagy et al., 2019). The discrepancy in the student's ability to cope with and balance the stress demands of work and family with school results in an inability to keep focused on long-term goals (Baker & Pifer, 2015). Staying passionate, persistent (the quality to continue doing something even though it is difficult), and focused on long-term goals is the embodiment of "grit" (Duckworth, 2016).

When speaking of grit, what first comes to mind are stories of extreme tenacity against unlikely odds as one strives to achieve a goal that appears out of reach. For most, this includes the goal of earning a doctoral degree. Duckworth contends that

---

BOX 14.1 ■ Ways to Maintain Motivation as a Doctoral Student

See the big picture.
Celebrate successes, all successes, big or small—yours, your coworkers', and your peers'.
Focus on another passion—go back and make sure to do things you enjoy—hobbies, crafting, reading, and exercise.

grit is "the how" we nurture our perseverance and talents to confront life's everyday hurdles that "pop up" along the way. The grittiest people stay driven and focused on the task before them, even when they get bored or lose interest.

As you drive along the doctoral journey road, the data tells us this: you will get bored, lose passion, and lose motivation. It happens in some way or another to the best of us. There are parts of any career and education that are hard and annoying. School is most exciting and fun when you are leaning into your strengths and are deeply engaged and energized by what you are doing. When you feel bored or lose the drive, use the following strategies to stay focused and resist changing lanes (https://www.success.com/4-ways-to-build-grit-when-you-need-it-most/; https://www.psychologytoday.com/us/blog/here-we-are/202007/building-grit-in-pandemic; https://www.carnegiefoundation.org/blog/helping-students-succeed-by-building-grit/).

1. Focus on your why
2. Do the work in chunks
3. Build strong habits
4. See failure as a gift (more below)
5. Take a breather
6. Build a community
7. Think about times when you have needed to be gritty and use these
8. Be compassionate

Maintaining Confidence

BOOSTING CONFIDENCE THROUGH FAILURE

I have not failed; I have just discovered 10,000 ways that will not work.

—THOMAS EDISON

We all face negative thought patterns, and you will encounter them throughout your doctoral education. Take it from someone who knows: The more you try, the more you fail. Furthermore, THAT is OK! Because in doing so, you learn that failing is not fatal. And when you fail once, you are less afraid and less fearful of trying again the next time, and you are not afraid of trying harder to solve problems.

When we lack confidence, we are more likely not to move forward with an action or decision. We remain inactive mainly from the fear that we might fail—an absolute paralysis. President Truman once said that "The worse danger we face is the danger of being paralyzed by doubts and fears" (Maxwell, 2007). Rachel Hollis, best-selling author and motivational speaker, is adamant that you not be afraid to goof up the presentation and to believe in yourself to act and stare down doubt and paralysis (Hollis, 2018). A little self-confidence and simply showing up are chief components of your success and building more confidence. Hollis encourages us not to be afraid to be embarrassed. The more confident you become, the less likely you are to let your fear of failing stop you from going out and doing what you desire, like earning a doctoral degree (Burnett & Evans, 2016). Taking action gives you at least a chance. In life, as in many sports games, you miss all the shots you do not take. Moreover, people who lack confidence do not take shots. (Confidence Code: https://www.getstoryshots.com/books/designing-your-life-summary/.)

Kay and Shipman (2014) and their partners developed a quiz with resulting strategies to build your confidence: https://learnconfidencecode.com/quiz/. Take the quiz and see where you stand and build your confidence plan.

Goal Setting: Mental Contrasting and W-O-O-P It Up

Goals excite us for the future, and they challenge us to keep pushing ourselves. Earning a doctoral degree is the excitement in your professional and personal nursing exploration that we want you to embrace, but it will present challenges and obstacles. Every mentor, advisor, faculty, and fellow student you meet will be able to share an obstacle they have faced along their journey. To be successful on the other side of this doctoral educational endeavor, you must prepare for challenges; it is essential to be honest about your vulnerability and adjust your thinking to anticipate that things will be difficult.

As presented earlier, one of the fundamental obstacles in the tribulations of completing doctoral work is withering motivation. We will not sugarcoat this: studying for a doctorate is intrinsically lonely, and the workload is sizeable. On top of that, the day-to-day routine can soon become boring, and students often feel undervalued, receive little acknowledgment for their expertise, and frequently feel overwhelmed. Plus, the further you go on the doctoral journey, the more uncertain you become about the quality of your work or where you will end up when you are finished.

So be ready for what you know lies ahead, whether it be a loss of motivation or more financial challenges outside of the financial demands of paying for school (such as textbooks, supplies, or maybe even the use of vacation days for studying), or concerns about family demands. Here is a perfect place to introduce the scientifically validated work of mental contrasting by Dr. Oettingen: Mental Contrasting (https://mindfulambition.net/woop/; Oettingen et al., 2009). Mental contrasting has shown to be very effective in sustaining the energy, motivation, and persistence needed to commit to realizing the desired outcome of earning a doctoral degree.

Mental contrasting guides us to W-O-O-P it up. First, identify your **Wish** for the future (that is the entire purpose of this book), and then align the reality of your current situation with how your situation fits into this wish and its **Outcome**. Then, honestly, lay out all the likely **Obstacles**. Knowing your obstacles helps you to create a **Plan** for when they occur (and they will). Many before you have achieved this degree through thick and thin. It will be hard, and you must be sensible and honest to know that challenges lie ahead and that you need to have a plan (Table 14.2).

TABLE 14.2 ■ **Mental Contrasting Definition and Exemplar**

W—Wish	Identify your wish for the future: Describe in 3–6 words	Apply to a doctoral program
O—Outcome	The most significant benefit that will result from this Wish. Again 3–6 words here.	Submit application by Fall Due Date
O—Obstacle	Obstacles to achieving this wish. Be realistic; earning a doctorate includes time management, addressing a lack of motivation, and preparing for the loss of financial support. Be open and list as many as you can	Time management is not my strength. Use the "If then Rule: If I spend 30 min on the application, I can watch 1 episode of my favorite streaming show."
P—Plan	Make a plan to address the obstacles, not if but when they occur. Make this plan so that you are not reactive in your approach when this obstacle arises.	Carve out 30 min before the usual wake-up time and use Chapter 11 timeline to start my journey
Shout it Out! W-O-O-P W-O-O-P!		

Modified from https://mindfulambition.net/woop/.

Opportunity Management

Using this text, identified mentors, and the resources available, you will explore, select, and apply with confidence to the doctoral program that offers welcoming faculty, invites you into professional networks, and exposes you to mentors across fields of practice. As a promising, motivated, and gritty doctoral student, you will catch the eye of leaders and innovators on a daily basis. These individuals, resources, and experiences bring a vast horizon of opportunities to further your skills, accentuate your knowledge, and push you to new heights. Welcome to the world of the doctorally prepared nurse leader, educator, researcher, scientist, and clinician (https://www.ryrob.com/opportunity-management/).

What exactly do we mean by opportunity? An opportunity is an invitation or experience that is likely to have a positive effect on your future professional or personal self. Moreover, because you are demonstrating your skills, enthusiasm, and capabilities daily in pursuing your doctoral degree, believe me, people notice. You will enter the twilight zone of possibility. However, as Jim Rohn reminds us, you will be offered a lifetime of opportunities as you travel, and what you want is to choose the opportunity of a lifetime. Keep in mind that with every offer you accept or say "Yes" to you are saying "No" to something else by default. The infrastructure of doctoral education is built on opportunities. You will benefit from crafting your opportunity management system sooner rather than later.

An indispensable technique is an Opportunity Management System (OMS) for examining, evaluating, and selecting from multiple opportunities. A well-crafted decision tree process for reviewing an opportunity ensures the purpose supports the timely achievement of your goals. It allows you to maintain control of successfully achieving your essential goals efficiently (https://www.ryrob.com/opportunity-management/). An OMS will help identify the best opportunities through informed decision-making.

To build an OMS, reach out to mentors, doctoral advisors, and trusted colleagues. We suggest reaching out early and often for their guidance or wisdom. Mentors can offer insights and perspectives on how a presented opportunity will contribute to your future self in ways you may not be able to see just yet. These trusted resources can offer views on work and school demands not seen from a student's viewpoint. There may be times when exploring the opportunity with mentors and colleagues first before agreeing or declining allows for greater clarity on how the invitation will benefit your end goal and if the opportunity is genuinely beneficial at this time. Sally Helgeson (2018), author of *How Women Rise*, reminds us that not all opportunities are offered for your benefit. They are provided because you are a go-getter, and go-getters get the job done. So, who better to get things done than you? And this is one reason why reaching out to mentors and colleagues for guidance will never be a bad idea.

Saying No Can Get You to Yes

I will let go of immediately saying yes or no to requests so I can take time to think about what works for me.

—SALLY HELGESEN

Helgesen and Goldsmith guide us in realizing that to get to the next level and become a doctoral student and doctoral-prepared nurse, you must learn to carefully assess and analyze the many opportunities that will be presented (Box 14.2). Assessing each opportunity with a streamlined OMS compliments your success and maximizes growth. We understand that "No" is an unfamiliar vocabulary word. You are "all in" when it comes to taking on or performing uniquely challenging duties. "No" has always been the lackluster option in response to requests. In his book, *What Got You Here, Won't Get You There*, Goldsmith terms this can-do spirit the "Paradox of Success." Saying yes to many things got you to a place where you feel confident and successful (being accepted and enrolled as a doctoral student = very successful, in case you were wondering).

An OMS is essential to follow to best support your needs at the time of the requested opportunity. And guess what? You and "No" are about to become acquainted. Remember, saying "no" does not mean you are trapped/unappreciative/doomed to be overlooked for all great things. The mechanics of saying "no" showcase skills in being mindful of one's capabilities and emotional intelligence to direct time and talents wisely, and confidently agree to opportunities that will help you stay focused on the end goal.

BOX 14.2 ■ Specifics to Consider When Opportunity Knocks

Evaluating Opportunities

Is it...

- aligned with the above mission, values, priorities, ground rules, and marching orders?
- something you can do, ideally well, fast, and with confidence?
- an investment of time, energy, and resources in something that has a high likelihood of success and offers significant potential benefits?

Analyzing the Opportunities: The 3 Ws:

- Where do the opportunities come from?
- What are the causes and consequences of options?
- What are the uncontrollable opportunities and the level of exciting opportunities?

Tactics and Questions

- What are your career goals, and how does this opportunity help or hinder achieving these goals?
- Will you lose anything by accepting this opportunity?
- What are today's dates and times? (This will help you track how the project evolves.)
- Who is the asker?
- What is the deliverable being requested? Be specific.
- By when does it need to be accomplished?
- What resources will be required?
- Who is the source of authority on this issue, and do you have that person or group's approval?
- What are the possible benefits?
- What are the obvious and hidden costs?
- What are your non-negotiables when deciding whether to take opportunities?
- Is there anything about the offer that would need to change to become appealing?
- Will you need any support fulfilling the obligations of this opportunity?

---

https://hbr.org/2020/09/learn-when-to-say-no.

Opportunity Management https://www.inhersight.com/blog/advancement/how-to-say-no-to-professional-opportunity#.

First, prioritize delivering your response face to face. In-person is a wonderful way to highlight respect for the individual request. Second, in-person expresses confidence in the decision and appreciation for being considered. Here are phrases that let the requestor know that you are intrigued but need a little time and clarification on how and why this opportunity is a good fit. Be succinct, using the suggested responses for opportunities that come knocking.

- *I would love to understand if there are any immediate deadlines or expectations that I should be aware of that might inform my decision.*
- *I am excited to explore this opportunity, and I appreciate your enthusiasm and confidence in my abilities. Before committing, I want to make sure I have thought through a transition plan that will not result in gaps for you or the team.*
- *I want to make sure that I am setting both of us up for success, thinking through all my current responsibilities, and balancing this exciting opportunity. I want to take*

*a few days to make sure there aren't any areas where I might need additional support,
so there are no negative implications for you or the team.*

Upon thoughtful reflection with mentors and a close examination of the
opportunity, you might conclude that the invitation is more likely to pull you away
from the areas that you are most interested in or does not align with your future
goals; try this phrase:

*Thank you for thinking of me as someone who could do this job well. I am already
committed to other responsibilities and projects. I would love to do this for you at a
later time. If that is not possible, I would love to be of service somehow in the
future.*

End with confirmation that you look forward to being considered for future
opportunities that might be a better fit. Follow up with an email summary of your
conversation, and appreciate their consideration of you for getting the job done.

Conclusion

This chapter began with a discussion about the facts that indicate that achieving a
doctorate is not easy and that many try but do not succeed. Our purpose is not to
discourage anyone but to systematically identify the challenges faced along this
journey and then outline the many strategies you can implement to increase your
probability of success. As stated earlier, it is impossible to remove all these stressors
during doctoral study, yet being aware and forearmed can help you complete your
program, do so on time, and avoid costly delays and headaches!

We have identified clusters of challenges for which you can prepare. Some relate
to your personal life and responsibilities, some to logistics, others to the academic
work you undertake, and still others to your resilience and grit. By now, you will
have learned a few essential lessons.

1. <u>Nearly everyone faces self-doubt at some point on this journey.</u> These feelings
   should be understood as a caution flag. They call you to reflect, reassess,
   reevaluate, rely on mentors and friends, and then dig in and press on.
   These feelings are not indicative of your failure but may well point to your
   emotional intelligence. It is essential to listen but not linger. Winston
   Churchill is credited as saying, "When you are going through hell, keep
   going." Do not linger in self-doubt. Use it. Lean into it. Learn from it and
   move on.

2. <u>You cannot make more time</u> in the day or more days in the week. So, taking
   on the responsibilities and challenges of doctoral study will require your time,
   and you will need to carefully consider what you will actively choose to
   discontinue so you can dedicate the time you need to succeed in your studies.
   Learn to say, "NO THANK YOU!" Most of the opportunities you decline
   will be waiting for you once you are done with school.

3. Stretch goals are thrilling and fun. Be mindful and enjoy the journey.

4. Take risks. Meet new people. Embrace new things. Doctoral study is more than classroom learning; it promises to transform you in unimaginable ways. GO FOR IT and SEE IT THROUGH.

Routine change and prioritizing life's commitments require balance and creative planning. The likelihood of program completion increases when you build skills to address your persistence, grit, confidence, and optimism. Further, making sure you select a program that offers supportive structures, community-building faculty, student peer opportunities, and honest and transparent communication with significant others will lessen the chances of suffering from burnout and minimize program dropout intentions. Your inner qualities of persistence and grit, combined with an OMS, have been shown to offer the doctoral student an internal locus of control to stay focused, motivated, and driven to complete the degree.

We hope you can feel our enthusiasm for your future as a doctoral nurse. The science is precise: you will feel more empowered with every accomplishment earned on this pathway toward educational success. A strong personal desire is required to engage in learning to complete a terminal degree.

Bibliography

Baker VL, Pifer MJ. Antecedents and outcomes: theories of fit and the study of doctoral education. *Stud High Educ.* 2015;40(2):296-310. Available at: http://www.tandf.co.uk/journals.

Brill JL, Balcanoff KK, Land D, Gogarty MM, Turner F. Best practices in doctoral retention: mentoring. *High Learn Res Commun.* 2014;4(2):26-37. Available at: http://dx.doi.org/10.18870/hlrc.v2i2.66.

Burnett B, Evans D. *Designing Your Life: How to Build a Well-Lived, Joyful Life.* New York: Alfred A. Knopff; 2016.

Council of Graduate Schools. *CGS.* Available at: https://cgsnet.org/.

Dreifuerst KT, McNelis AM, Weaver MT, Broome ME, Draucker CB, Fedko AS. Exploring the pursuit of doctoral education by nurses seeking or intending to stay in faculty roles. *J Prof Nurs.* 2016;32(3):202-212. doi:10.1016/j.profnurs.2016.01.014.

Duckworth A. *Grit: The Power of Passion and Perseverance.* New York: Scribner/Simon & Schuster; 2016.

Helgeson, Sally and Goldsmith, M. How Women Rise: Break nthen12 habits Holding You back from your next raise, promotion or job. Hatchett Audio.

Hollis R. *Girl Wash Your Face. Stop Believing the Lies About Who You are So You can Become Who You Were Meant to be.* Publisher: Thomas Nelson: 2018.

Jeffreys MR. Student retention and success: optimizing outcomes through holistic competence and proactive inclusive enrichment. *Teach Learn Nurs.* 2014;9(4):164-170. doi:10.1016/j.teln.2014.05.003.

Jeffreys MR. Jeffreys' Nursing universal retention and success model: overview and action ideas for optimizing outcomes A–Z. *Nurs Educ Today.* 2015;35(3):425-443. doi:10.1016/j.nedt.2014.11.004.

Kay K, Shipman C. *The Confidence Code: The Science and Art of Self-Assurance: What Women Should Know.* Harper Business; 2014. Available at: www.harpercollins.com.

Kuchinski-Donnelly D, Krouse AM. Predictor of emotional engagement in online graduate nursing students. *Nurse Educ.* 2020;45(4):214-219. doi:10.1097/NNE.0000000000000769.

Maxwell J. *Failing Forward: Turning Mistakes into Stepping Stones for Success.* New York: Harper Collins Publishing; 2007.

McNelis AM, Dreifuerst KT, Schwindt R. Doctoral education and preparation for nursing faculty roles. *Nurse Educ.* 2018;44(4):202-206. doi:10.1097/NNE.0000000000000597.

Nagy GA, Fang CM, Hish AJ, et al. Burnout and mental health problems in biomedical doctoral students. *CBE Life Sci Edu.* 2019;18(2). Available at: https://doi.org/10.1187/cbe.18-09-0198.

Oettingen G, Mayer D, Timur Sevincer A, Stephens EJ, Pak H, Hagenah M. Mental contrasting and goal commitment: the mediating role of energization. *Personal Soc Psychol Bull.* 2009;35(5):608-622. doi:10.1177/0146167208330856.

Peltonen J, Vekkaila J, Rautio P, Haverinen K, Pyhältö K. Doctoral students' social support profiles and their relationship to burnout, drop-out intentions, and time to candidacy. *Intl J Doct Stud.* 2017;12:157-173. Available at: http://www.informingscience.org/Publications/3792.

Priode KS, Dail RB, Swanson M. Nonacademic factors that influence nontraditional nursing student retention. *Nurs Educ Perspect.* 2020;41(4):246-248. doi:10.1097/01.NEP.0000000000000577.

Sally H, Marshall G. *How Women Rise: Break the 12 Habits Holding You Back from Your Next Raise, Promotion or Job, 1st ed.* Hatchett Audio; 2018.

Smith D, Delmore B. Three key components to successfully completing a nursing doctoral program. *J Continu Educ Nurs.* 2021;38(2):76-72. doi:10.3928/00220124-20070301-01.

Van der Linden N, Devos C, Boudrenghien G, et al. Gaining insight into doctoral persistence: development and validation of Doctorate-related Need Support and Need Satisfaction short scales. *Learn Individ Diff.* 2018;65:100-111. Available at: https://doi.org/10.1016/j.lindif.2018.03.008.

Vance D, Heaton K, Antia L, et al. Alignment of a PhD program in nursing with the AACN report on the research-focused doctorate in nursing: a descriptive analysis. *J Prof Nurs.* 2020;36(6):604-610. doi:10.1016/j.profnurs.2020.08.011.

Vekkaila J, Pyhältö K. Doctoral student learning patterns: learning about active knowledge creation or passive production. *Intl J High Educ.* 2016;5(2):222-235. Available at: http://www.sciedupress.com/ijhe.

Vidak M, Tokalić R, Marušić M, Puljak L, Sapunar D. Improving completion rates of students in biomedical PhD programs: an interventional study. *BMC Med Educ.* 2017;17(1):144. Available at: https://doi.org/10.1186/s12909-017-0985-1.

Volkert D., Candela L., Bernacki M. Student motivation, stressors, and intent to leave nursing doctoral study: a national study using path analysis. *Nurse Educ Today.* 2018;61:210-215. doi:10.1016/j.nedt.2017.11.033.

Wollast R, Boudrenghien G, Van der Linden N, et al. Who are the doctoral students who drop out? Factors associated with the rate of doctoral degree completion in universities. *Intl J High Educ.* 2018;7(4):143-156. doi:10.5430/ijhe.v7n4p143.

Available at: https://www.carnegiefoundation.org/blog/helping-students-succeed-by-building-grit/.

Shared Experiences of Doctorally Prepared Nurses on the Edge of Tomorrow

CHAPTER 15

The Nurse Scientist Narrative

Krista Schroeder, PhD, RN

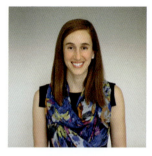

Entry to Practice

I was not a person who grew up wanting to be a nurse, yet my love of science and desire to help people led me to nursing. Once I discovered that nursing entailed applying physiology, pharmacology, and technology in a people-oriented career, I knew I found my calling. Given my interest in science, I entered practice in the most high-tech specialty of clinical nursing—the intensive care unit (ICU). I practiced as a critical care staff nurse first at Lehigh Valley Hospital and Health Network in Allentown, PA, and then at Thomas Jefferson University Hospital in Philadelphia, PA, and New York Presbyterian Hospital/Columbia University Medical Center in New York, NY. As a staff nurse in the medical intensive care (Thomas Jefferson) and critical care float pools (Lehigh Valley and New York Presbyterian), I had the opportunity to learn about cutting-edge medical technology, hone my physiological and pharmacological knowledge, and provide support to patients and families during health crises.

During my practice as a critical care nurse, I witnessed a great deal of suffering caused by non-communicable chronic diseases. I cared for patients who have had limbs amputated due to diabetes complications, experienced devastating strokes due to cardiovascular disease, and experienced pain and disability due to cancer; in addition, I was present as multiple patients were removed from life support as a result of terminal illness due to chronic non-communicable diseases. Witnessing this suffering caused me to become highly passionate about health promotion and disease prevention. I didn't want to simply make my ICU patients less sick, such as by preventing ventilator-associated pneumonia or catheter-associated urinary tract infections; I wanted my patients to not become sick in the first place.

Decision to Pursue Higher Education

My passion for health promotion and disease prevention led me to consider the next steps in my nursing career. How could I have the most impact on preventing diseases like cardiovascular disease and neurovascular accidents? Should I work as a public health nurse? Pursue a master's in nursing and become a nurse manager or clinical educator? Or maybe I should pursue a master's in public health? After much thought, discussion, and exploration, I decided I wanted to impact practice and policy at a macro level; rather than being at the bedside as the 1:1 nurse, I hoped to create knowledge about population-level health promotion. I knew that knowledge creation occurred via research, and thus I decided to pursue a PhD and become a nurse scientist.

This decision to pursue a PhD was surprising even to me! As an undergraduate nursing student, I never enjoyed my research classes. As a practicing nurse, I was on my critical care unit's evidence-based practice committee, but other than that, I was not frequently thinking about nursing research. However, after 5 years as a critical care nurse, I wanted to create knowledge to improve population health and promote well-being at a macro level, and I knew research was the way to do so.

My doctoral education began as a PhD student at Columbia University School of Nursing. At Columbia, I had the opportunity to participate in the National Institutes of Health (NIH)-funded T32 training program focused on health services research, which helped me hone skills in using data to improve health, and a Health Research Training Program internship at the New York City Department of Health and Mental Hygiene, which helped me learn about conducting research relevant to public health practice and policy. Through these experiences I realized that, in order to conduct impactful science, I needed to narrow my broad interest in health promotion to a specific area of research focus. Via communication with my doctoral dissertation advisor and engagement with a mentor's research projects and existing literature, I learned that obesity was one of the greatest threats to population health. Obesity increased the risk for and worsened almost every non-communicable chronic disease that I was passionate about preventing. Thus, I decided to focus my research on reducing obesity. For my dissertation, I conducted a mixed-methods study evaluating New York City's first school nurse-led obesity intervention.

My dissertation was conducted via my collaboration with the New York City Department of Health and Mental Hygiene; the study allowed me to conduct science in collaboration with community and school nurse partners, helped me hone research skills for working with large public health data, and provided experience quantitatively and qualitatively evaluating health promotion programs. Study findings highlighted that nurse-led obesity programs experienced challenges when occurring in settings lacking resources, community environments that hinder health, or with populations facing structural barriers and health inequities. These findings fostered my interest in using data to explore how social determinants of health impact obesity risk and obesity intervention effectiveness. I knew that postdoctoral fellowships provided opportunities for structured research training above and beyond PhD education; thus, I decided to pursue a postdoctoral fellowship that would allow me to learn more about using data-driven, population-health-focused research to reduce obesity disparities.

I completed a postdoctoral fellowship at the University of Pennsylvania School of Nursing, via an NIH T32 fellowship focused on research on vulnerable women, children, and families, and a student fellowship at the Center for Public Health Initiatives. Through the fellowships, I worked with research mentors who were experts in engaging with and centering communities' perspectives on obesity risk, conducting research to drive health equity, and approaching obesity science from an upstream framework. During my fellowship, I collaborated on research exploring how neighborhood gentrification influences access to physical activity and how neighborhood poverty impacts obesity risk. Via these research experiences, and associated coursework and training opportunities, I was able to build on my PhD skills for data-driven, population health research, and begin to build a cohesive program of research focused on how social determinants of health impact obesity risk. The postdoctoral fellowship allowed me to grow my professional network, develop increased research autonomy, and add a number of tools to my research toolbox; I consider it a key step in my doctoral education even though it occurred after my formal PhD training.

As I completed my postdoctoral fellowship, I still held my passion for preventing disease—developed as a critical care nurse—but I was also excited about using data-driven, population health research methods to do so. Because of my background as a nurse who was passionate about public health, I began my career at the Temple University College of Public Health in the Department of Nursing—an ideal place to blend my love of public health and nursing. Now, as a professor, I continue to conduct research and apply the skills I learned during my doctoral education. My day-to-day work entails doing research (data analysis), disseminating research (writing publications or giving presentations at conferences or community events), and meeting with clinical partners to discuss research results. In addition, I regularly pursue training to build on my doctoral education—even as a faculty member! For example, I have taken coursework in advanced statistical methods and geospatial analysis in order to add research skills for understanding how environments impact health. Much of my work takes place in research teams, with mentors, or in collaboration with frontline nurses. I have the wonderful opportunity to teach and mentor students, including teaching classes relevant to my research expertise and mentoring students who conduct research projects. I also engage with professional organizations and contribute to working groups inside and outside my university related to my content expertise.

Mentors

Throughout my doctoral training, I was supported by exceptional mentorship. I had formal mentorship via my NIH fellowships as well as professors who served as informal role models. There were senior scientists and new assistant professors, content-specific and methods-specific mentors, as well as mentors who provided insight about matters related to professional life more generally. Certain relationships were initiated by others—for example, I was assigned a PhD mentor; others were sought by me—for example, I would email a nurse scientist whose research interested me and ask to meet for coffee. Both types of mentoring relationships were incredibly valuable. Despite the variation in relationship structure, all presented a great opportunity to learn from another doctorally prepared nurse as well as build connections with an exceptional group of individuals.

Navigating Barriers

While my doctoral training was engaging, it was also highly challenging. When I reflect back on my PhD and postdoctoral training, I see a great deal of personal and professional growth, but also the conquering of barriers. The most notable barrier related to navigating Ivy League PhD and postdoctoral programs as a first-generation college student from a working-class family. I had never felt aware of my first-generation status when I was an undergraduate nursing student at a state university in a small town, yet I was keenly aware of being a first-generation doctoral nursing student and postdoctoral fellow at prestigious private schools in large cities. Unlike many of my peers, I had not had a close relationship with a woman who had a college degree until my own college experience. Navigating the prestigious academic settings from a social perspective felt foreign— I realized people spoke differently, carried themselves differently, and even spent their leisure time differently. None of my uncertainty was due to the nature of my colleagues—all were wonderful, and some of my dearest mentors and best friends were developed during my doctoral experiences; yet the culture did feel foreign, and I had to devote intellectual and emotional energy to learning the new norms. However, with strong family love and support, hard work, trust in myself, welcoming colleagues, and new friends, I was able to accept that I did belong in the shoes I now fill.

Another barrier to my pursuit of a doctoral education was balancing the demands of work, life, and school. I was lucky enough to have NIH-funded predoctoral and postdoctoral training, yet my time in the doctoral study was nonetheless challenging financially. I was able to work clinically for only minimal hours, given the demands of the program. Yet through careful budgeting and support from my partner, I was able to navigate the financial demands of doctoral study. In addition to finances, the time demands of the doctoral study were intense. It was taxing to work 6 days a week on my doctoral studies and then work a seventh day in the ICU, with minimal time for family and friend support. I experienced role conflict, as many of the people I cared most about, while supportive, were not familiar with the level of work required for such an endeavor and how much I needed to miss events "back home" to devote time to my studies. As a result, my fellow PhD student colleagues became key sources of support. To address the challenges I faced related to work, life, and school balance, I prioritized self-care—healthful eating, regular exercise outdoors in the fresh air, and maintaining a regular and adequate sleep schedule (no all-night study sessions). Doing so allowed me to not only survive but thrive during the challenges of doctoral study.

After PhD and postdoctoral training, and overcoming barriers related to being first-generation college student and balancing work, life, and school demands, I now have a career that I truly love and that allows me to do work about which I am highly passionate. I engage in research and pedagogy that contributes to the science of health promotion, with a focus on improving social and environmental influences on well-being. My research focuses on how social determinants of health influence obesity—one of the greatest health burdens facing the nation. My work harnesses large multi-level datasets, geospatial analysis, and advanced analytic approaches to identify family, neighborhood, and system-level obesity risk factors. I've pursued advanced training in statistics and using data-driven approaches to health—a skill set that I love using! My research is complemented by a program of pedagogy and mentorship that advances students' abilities to address upstream causes of morbidity and increases students' quantitative skills for understanding population health needs—a part of my career that I deeply enjoy. I love what I do, and the challenges related to doctoral study were completely worthwhile.

Future Goals

My overarching future goal is to grow my program of research so that I can contribute to data-driven, population-health nursing science to promote well-being. I want to continue to be a voice for nursing and obesity science to take an upstream approach to address healthcare's greatest challenges, including issues related to how social determinants of health contribute to obesity inequities. Importantly, my goal also entails taking that science, and the associated quantitative skills that I develop, and then sharing it with clinical and community partners.

Words of Wisdom

For those considering a doctorate, what should they do? My first piece of advice would be to talk with nurse scientists about their day-to-day career activities. Search for doctorally prepared nurses serving in the roles in which you are interested and ask to meet them. You can find nurse scientists as faculty at universities, but also based within non-profits or healthcare organizations. A Google search will provide you with a multitude of tips on how to ask for and engage in informational interviews. A brief Zoom or coffee meeting, to which you bring a professional presence and focused questions, can be highly helpful in informing your decision as to whether a PhD is appropriate for you and how to be successful in doctoral study. My second piece of advice would be to plan, plan, and plan some more. Pursuing a doctorate is a big step in both your career and your life—consider how will you manage the finances, how will you balance completing demands, and how you will care for yourself. You may want to journal your thoughts about the process, set goals, and talk through them with a trusted person. Current PhD students could also be a good source of advice. My last piece of advice would be to seek out resources and supports. These may come through professional organizations, such as nursing organizations, or personal networks, such as faith-based groups. The university you choose to attend may have organizations to support you, such as clubs focused on students who experience barriers in higher education or offices focused on connecting students with financial resources. Such resources are there to support you, so be sure to seek them out. After speaking with current nurse scientists, planning carefully, and seeking supports, you will be well prepared to embark on doctoral study.

Considered collectively, pursuing a PhD in nursing opens up a wide variety of avenues to impact nursing practice and policy. Given that fewer than 1% of nurses have a PhD, PhD-prepared nurses comprise a unique group. As a doctorally prepared nurse scientist, you will have opportunities to conduct engaging science focused on the topics about which you are most passionate. You may face challenges along the way, but you can overcome them with careful planning and support. We need more nurses engaged in science—join us!

CHAPTER 16

The Primary Care DNP Narrative

Mary L. Blankson, DNP, APRN, FNP-C, FAAN

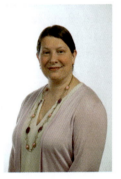

Your Initial Motivation to Become a Nurse

As a high school student who came from a family where only one person had successfully graduated college (an associate degree program for computer programming), I knew grades were important. But I didn't grow up in a family where the topic of conversation was more than just, "What do you want to be when you grow up?" There were not many conversations on how you get there, or discussions on whether the choice you made would result in a good source of income to climb out of the rural, lower-socioeconomic status in which my family had lived ever since my father passed away when I was 14. My mother was a high school graduate, who went back to school after my father passed, and got straight A's in a Certified Nursing Assistant (CNA) program so that our family still had some source of income. It was this experience (my father passing, and my mother going to school mid-life for her CNA) that made me decide the healthcare field was where I wanted to land. Secure income, secure job opportunities were the things I wanted, and maybe I could save a life for another 14-year-old who may get to hold onto their dad because of my actions/knowledge.

Your Entry to Practice

MY DECISION TO PURSUE HIGHER EDUCATION

The beginning of my story may shock people who are close to me, given that I plan everything down to the last detail. When it came to deciding that I should get my DNP, I can't even remember what prompted me to apply to my first program other than feeling it was the *right* thing to do. Whether it was because I thought it would keep me competitive with new graduates coming out of direct entry DNP programs, or that it would allow family members to call me "Doctor Nurse"—I really can't recall giving it much thought. I found myself applying to a single school, one that was near my in-laws so my husband and children could join me for the on-site weeks and spend time with their parents and grandparents. After I applied, I waited for what seemed like an eternity. I will be honest—I had never been "rejected" by any institution to which I had applied.

At the annual conference for the American Association of Nurse Practitioners, I rushed to that particular university's booth in the exposition hall. I should have received the acceptance letter the day before, but I had been out of town. So I asked the woman managing the booth if she could help me find out whether I had been accepted. She told me she would contact admissions, then meet me back at the booth during the next break in the conference.

The time came, and I rushed back excited, expecting a positive response… only to be met with hesitant eyes. She ushered me aside and lowered her voice to inform me that I had been rejected. She tried to soften the blow by reassuring me that, because the program was young, they only accepted individuals from their own state and one bordering state. No one outside those two states had been accepted. But I barely heard those details because all I could focus on was my failure to execute on my plan to get my DNP.

I shed more than a few tears that day (and the next) before trying to figure out why I was so upset. It was something more than the feeling of rejection, which had been foreign to me thus far in my career. By the end of the day, I realized that I actually did not have any good reasons to get my DNP. This degree had not factored into my calculus when I first decided to be a nurse. I was already a family nurse practitioner and primary care provider at one of the largest federally qualified health centers (FQHCs) in the country. I had been promoted to the role of medical director at two of our medical sites, supervising and supporting all providers at those sites, including the physicians. I was doing something most nurse practitioners did not (and still don't) see as possible in their typical health care culture. I was "living the dream"—practicing in a culture that valued all provider types, used provider-centric language, and allowed all of us to lead based on our skills and talents rather than on the type of provider licensure. We were all primary care providers, and we were all equally valued. That fact did not diminish our organization's physicians in any way.

Reassured by these realizations, I moved on, pushing thoughts of a terminal degree to the back of my mind. It would be 2 years before I considered a DNP again. Hindsight being 20/20, I believe this rejection was in fact the best thing that could have happened to me. There was so much I had not considered and so many new questions I had about how this degree could add to my life as a professional, not only for the organization where I was working but also for my own personal fulfillment.

The Educational Path I Chose and the Reasoning Behind That Decision

In my role at the health center, I found myself increasingly engaging in quality improvement, crafting medication management policies, and working in microsystems to solve the day-to-day problems that prevented our primary care teams from delivering the highest-quality team-based care. With these new challenges in mind, I now considered doctoral education again. I weighed whether a PhD or DNP would best serve me. After speaking with some of the PhD-prepared nurses I knew in the state where I practiced, I realized that degree would not give me the toolkit I needed in my search for practical approaches to applying evidence. The DNP met that criterion but also presented the challenge of choosing a program.

There were so many DNP programs, and they were all so very different in terms of rigor. I finally settled on a program that would ensure I learned how to complete a scholarly prosecution of the evidence, then fully design and implement a capstone project based on that evidence. The capstone was rigorous (i.e., not an education-only intervention, nor an intervention for a small population of patients or staff) and was implemented to ensure a powered study that determined whether my intervention actually solved the problem. Even though these skills were not part of my actual job description, I saw them as a job requirement. I knew they would serve me well as I continued to grow in clinical leadership roles within my organization.

I applied, and this time my application was filled with many well-thought-out and heartfelt reasons why this degree was essential for my growth as a clinical leader within primary care. My essays reflected a commitment to a new trajectory that included growth beyond my current leadership position. Not only did I need this skillset for myself and for my specific job, but I also needed it to bolster my confidence and competency as I collaborated with other organizational leaders toward achieving our performance improvement goals.

My Mentors

My experiences as a mentee have been varied. The most rewarding relationships I have had with mentors have often been the ones where I have had to hold the arms of the chair I am sitting at times when my mentor has had some feedback to give me. I have learned that a true mentor is not supposed to make you feel comfortable and supported all the time. Sometimes you will feel extremely uncomfortable, yet still you will feel supported. One of my favorite mentors once shared with me that "feedback is a gift." I believe this statement wholeheartedly, and I repeat it out loud to myself, especially when I know I am headed into a session in which I am going to receive feedback.

My best mentors do not want me to stay the same. They know I can achieve more, refine my skills more, and take on things I never would have considered as options for myself, for my career, or for the team I lead. This can, at times, leave me with butterflies in my stomach, or some amount of nervousness related to the unknown adventure I am about to undertake, because I know that I made a mistake, or because I am confronting a bad habit that has not served me well over the years. This is all part of the journey, and something that should be expected from a successful mentor mentee relationship. It is a choice to put yourself in a position where you may feel discomfort. Still, as another of my mentors always says, "this is where the magic happens." This is the type of mentor I want to be with others. The relationship is certainly not for the faint of heart, but for those truly seeking to grow and at a pace that will surprise any onlookers.

Milestones on My Path

Although I was given a virtual interview option, I traveled to my chosen university to ensure they understood how serious I was, how much I had taken into consideration as I planned for my future as an executive nursing leader. Besides fielding difficult questions mainly focused on how I was going to make room in my life for this program, I had to complete a series of writing prompts within a set time frame, most likely to show them that I had a solid foundation not just as a leader but also as a communicator and critical thinker. The experience certainly challenged me, but it also reassured me of the quality of this particular program and the transformation I would undergo should I have the privilege of attending the program.

I was delighted to be invited to join the program's seventh cohort of students on the journey of a lifetime. I still remember the in-person week that kicked off our first semester. How wonderful to be among a like-minded yet extremely diverse cohort of students. We had nurse educators, nurse practitioners in primary care, maternal/child nurses, clinical nurse specialists in oncology and the NICU, a nurse anesthetist, nurse faculty, nurse leaders, and so many others. I had plenty of experience in interprofessional education, particularly due to the team-based models of care in primary care, but this was my first real experience in intraprofessional education. We all knew what it meant to be a nurse, yet our backgrounds and experiences brought vastly different ideas to the table when we considered the many problems we were all hoping to address. Looking back, this is what I valued the most.

Some of the new friends and colleagues who gave me continuous feedback and support about my capstone had never worked a day in primary care. However, they brought with them years of working with care teams and patients, as well as their own working knowledge of the DNP skillset we were all honing. Whether we were all tucked in around a single laptop looking at data sets, or pouring over lengthy grids of journal articles rated and graded to aid in choosing an intervention to be translated, or strategically choosing a translational framework to give structure and support to our projects, we were applying our skillset over and over to build the confidence and muscle memory needed to tackle any challenge.

Challenges I Faced and Strategies I Used to Navigate Them

The skillset we were building included the development of our professional selves as leaders, consultants, experts, and so much more. We developed our presentation skills not only from a communication standpoint but also with regard to visual presentation, both of which have served me well after 8 years and nearly 100 presentations into my executive clinical role as Chief Nursing Officer. But back then, this was a fairly new role in our organization. As an FQHC, integrated primary care with medical, dental, and behavioral health services is truly our bread and butter. We care for underserved populations, and as one of the largest FQHCs (with 14 brick-and-mortar integrated health centers, and more than 200 service delivery locations throughout the state of Connecticut), we deliver care to over 100,000 unique patients every year.

I had already gained leadership experience through my role as a medical director of two of our clinical sites, but this new role was largely administrative and would change the trajectory of my career. No longer would I be changing lives one patient at a time, but I would be able to multiply my impact by changing the many team members I supported. In this way, I could help others evolve by preparing them to deliver the care that our patients needed, care that is a fundamental right rather than a difficult-to-access privilege. Instead of depending only on my own two hands and feet, I was leading 180 sets of hands and feet.

Your Future Goals

MY CURRENT FOCUS

Since becoming CNO, I have had the privilege to take on other roles including the Clinical Director of an accredited national medical assistant training school, site visitor for an accrediting agency for nurse practitioner and physician assistant residencies and fellowships, and board director of a national nursing organization. I have led grants, collaborated with research teams, supported and authored publications, created curricula, developed ladder programs, written policies, and testified before the state public health committee to advocate for the communities we serve as well as for the clinical care team members serving those communities. I firmly believe all of this is possible because of the transformation that occurred during my DNP program.

The Greatest Source of Satisfaction in My Work

I have also developed as a mentor, even as I continue to enjoy the benefits of being a mentee. This means that it is now my turn to not just walk through doors but also open doors for others. As a mentor, this means modeling the behavior I want to see multiplied in my field. It also means staying humble and teachable, as primary care continues to evolve day by day. This ensures an open culture, where people feel comfortable questioning each other and approaching relationship with a foundation of curiosity and connection, supporting the belief that feedback is truly a gift. To take full advantage of feedback, it is important to not be risk averse, for it is moments of risk that give us opportunities to identify some of the most creative and innovative solutions. These solutions benefit from the application of the DNP skillset to the evidence that informs their adaptation, the framework that translates the substance of the evidence to the specific situation and context, and the rigorous analysis that determines whether this implementation is a best practice or just a data point on the road to a best practice. In all of these contexts, the DNP skillset is invaluable.

Words of Wisdom to Nurses Considering Earning a Doctorate

Going into my DNP, I did not have an exact plan, but I was amazed to see that, as my mind transformed, my practice transformed, and the leaders of my organization noticed that evolution.

I had always thought being a nurse practitioner was the obvious growth pathway for any nurse in primary care, but in taking on the CNO role I learned that my experience as a provider made me the ideal candidate to lead the support teams that make up our care team dyads. They needed someone who could create the structure of role definitions, standing orders, continuous education, and other scaffolding needed to ensure success. Because the role of the primary care registered nurse (PC RN) is crucial to providing quality healthcare, I grew my knowledge and established myself as an expert in this area as I applied my DNP skillset iteratively to support ongoing role development.

In conclusion, here are the key takeaways:

1. Know why you need a DNP before you submit your application(s). Even if a program accepts you, the experience will not be as fruitful if you do not explore the "why" behind your decision.

2. Attend the interview in person, if you can. Even with our current videoconferencing platforms, there is just something missing from the remote interaction.

3. Just because you are a nurse practitioner does not mean you cannot take on administrative leadership or other roles. Similarly, being a nurse does not always mean becoming a nurse practitioner is your next step in growth. You have so many options.

4. Choosing a program is of the utmost importance. You do not just want to get the DNP after your name. You want to have a solid skillset that you can demonstrate over and over again. This may mean that you do not choose the least expensive program (or maybe you do). Choose based on the curriculum and evidence of the products of work created by prior graduates. Is this who you want to be? Is this the type (and quality) of work you want to create?

5. Always remember that feedback is a gift.

6. Once you acquire your skillset, use it. Every. Single. Day.

7. As you continue to rise, don't forget to give back to the next generation: open doors for people, ask them challenging questions, and be a resource.

8. Last, don't ever look back. Rise, knowing that even the sky is not the limit!

CHAPTER 17

The Entrepreneur Narrative

Taura L. Barr, PhD, RN, NC-BC

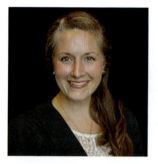

I wanted to be a biologist. My junior year of high school I went to the local college and sat in on courses. That year I had an amazing biology teacher. We had a conversation about my college plans and he shared that, aside from teaching, there weren't as many career options in biology as I hoped. However, he said that with a career like nursing, I could combine my people skills and my love of biology and have no trouble finding a job. It was my high school science teacher who helped me see that I was perfect for nursing. In fact, I had always been a nurse.

I earned my BSN at the University of Pittsburgh (Pitt). As an undergrad in my sophomore, junior, and senior year, I worked as a nurse's aide on the neurotrauma unit. I fell in love with everything about the brain. Then in my senior year I met a PhD-prepared nurse scientist who was conducting research on my unit. I met the research assistants every day and I saw how their work connected to my practice. So, I took a 10-hour-a-week work-study position as a research assistant to help collect data and measure biomarkers. It was fascinating and fun and it allowed me to feed my curiosity.

Then, I did a very simple research study of my own under the direction of this nurse scientist. As a senior nursing student, I submitted a poster, and it was accepted to the Society of Critical Care Medicine conference. I loved everything about research: being able to ask questions, study and learn new things, develop and home in on my science skills. It was the coolest thing, and I couldn't believe I could do this as a nurse. I was given an opportunity to present at a scientific conference about research that mattered to my patients. I was hooked. I came from a very poor family. And here I was at a fancy and expensive hotel presenting my research and swimming in this beautiful pool. I was smitten. Why wouldn't I want to do this with my life?

Up until then, I had wanted to be a nurse practitioner. But research just kind of fell into my lap. My mentor encouraged me to take the chance and submit for the National Institute for Nursing Research Graduate Partnership Program (GPP)

Predoctoral Fellowship. She said I probably wouldn't get it. But it was good practice, so I gave it a try. And I got it! Here is how it went.

As a BSN, I continued to work in the neuro ICU. One day I got a call on the unit and learned that GPP faculty liked my application and wanted me to join their program. I completed my course work at Pitt while continuing to practice in my ICU. Then, after my course work was complete, my husband and I and our two tiny kids moved to Bethesda to work on my dissertation research at the NIH campus.

Entry to Practice

In the neuro ICU, I fell in love with the brain and the immune system. Why would many young people, often of the same age, same gender, with the same injuries, and who seemed so similar have such different outcomes? I started wondering why some people recovered, and others succumbed to complications. This led me to study genetics and genomics, and I began to ask some very basic questions: Are some people just better able to handle the trauma? Are some more vulnerable? Is there a predisposition to poor outcomes? How does the immune system affect genetic expression?

Over time I began to study neuroimmunology, to better understand the interaction between the nervous system and the immune system and how this interaction can lead to different outcomes following brain trauma. In the unit, we would have family meetings, and families would ask, *"What happens next?"* Many times we could not give them an answer, except to watch and wait. I wanted to be able to answer those questions and give those families more information. That desire fueled my research program, which was a combination of genetics, genomics, immunology, and brain recovery.

Your Decision to Pursue Higher Education

As I look back, I was very influenced by my mentors. Originally, my goal was to become an NP. I didn't know this other option, becoming a scientist, existed. I didn't see myself as a person who could pursue such a path. My faculty mentors led me, and I followed their lead. Early in my career I was very busy, very motivated, and very young. The downside to this scenario is that, to this day, I regret not getting an NP degree. I did all my course work and wanted to continue to my clinicals before moving to my post doc. But things kept moving and I was doing great. So, I kept on this path.

Mentors

My first mentor was a nurse researcher, and she always stayed with me. Then I was dual-mentored by an MD-PhD and a neuro-geneticist at NIH. Those experiences and those mentors propelled me in my career. They were helpful, generous, boosted my confidence, and helped me navigate the barriers along the way. I still keep in contact with them.

Barriers Faced and Strategies Used to Navigate Them

My GREs were terrible. I am not a good test taker. But I had the GPP award, and I entered my BSN-PHD program on provisional status. I had to perform and get good grades, so I worked overtime making sure that happened. At the same time, I was continuing to work as a full-time ICU nurse, had one small child and was breastfeeding a new baby, and was pressing myself very hard. When we moved, we had no family with us, my husband decided to stay at home with the kids, I worked weekend alternative to pay the bills, and that is how we made things work. It was incredibly hard for 6 years, but we did it.

You don't know what you are capable of doing until you don't have a choice. My doctoral study is a blur and I don't remember much, except that I ran full steam ahead. If I had choices, I might have slowed down a bit and enjoyed the process. But finances were a barrier. I worked full time to make ends meet, and my husband, who was in construction, quit his job, and really changed everything around to help me achieve this goal and raise our family as we wanted to do.

For us, relocating presented an additional challenge. We had no family in the area to help with the kids. We really didn't know much about childcare in the area or schools. These things were stressful. We felt disconnected and unfamiliar with resources and people around us. But we found a way to make it work for our family. And we got through because we knew this moment in time was only temporary and would set us up for the rest of our lives. So we pushed through.

Milestones

Because it was so tough, I moved briskly through my coursework and then did the same through my dissertation. I was running on a hamster wheel and took all of those bad working habits with me when I took my first faculty appointment. Then, in the 12th week of my 4th pregnancy, I had a pulmonary embolism followed by lots of complications including a probable MI. After delivering our beautiful baby boy, I had to go through cardiac rehab just to walk up my stairs. It was painful, but necessary, because it allowed me to see how my behaviors and patterns of overworking had contributed to this illness and pain. I had been making good progress toward tenure and overnight all of that came to a screeching halt.

My Current Focus

It was then I knew I needed to make a change. This experience helped me see that I could take my research program and build a neuroimmunology company to better diagnose and treat head injury and contribute to the way we recover stroke and head injured patients. I say that out of my biggest setback came my greatest success, and hence Valtari Bio was born. Valtari Bio is a neuroimmunology company focused on bringing products to market to improve the diagnosis, treatment, and recovery from stroke and head injury. We bring science back to the bedside to improve outcomes. We have conducted clinical trials (Cincinnati & Austin), have a partnership with big pharma, and we are on a path to FDA approval in the next 3 to 5 years. This work directly connects to my early motivation to answer difficult questions and improve outcomes for neurotrauma patients, and that passion is what has gotten me through the toughest moments of my career.

At the same time I launched Valtari Bio, I launched a second company, Deep Roots Healing. The goal with Deep Roots has been from day one to help people engage in self-care and understand and practice holistic healing. As I told my story in the scientific community, many people began to reach out for guidance. The logical next step was to build a wellness coaching company, and then that extended into consultation to help other entrepreneurs and innovators who wished to begin their own businesses while honoring their own health and healing.

Believe it or not, I am still figuring out where exactly I fit. I love science and academe, but neither perfectly supports my goals. So, I am moving ahead with a focus on my own aspirations, my health, my values, and my family.

Your Future Goals

We probably have 3 to 5 more years of work left in Valtari Bio. If we do these clinical trials well, I believe our partner will buy us out or at least help us get through FDA approvals. This has always been our goal and each year we get closer.

I plan to work as Scientific Founder in Valtari Bio for the next 5 years, while keeping my foot in the door of academia. Right now, I take no salary in Valtari because investments in diagnostics have virtually dried up unless you're doing something COVID-19 related. I really want this company to survive and thrive, so it has been a hard decision, but worth it. Eventually, I would love to bring all of this full circle, integrating my work in brain trauma, immunology, genomics, and holistic healing. I do not know if this will grow in academia or as another business enterprise. I will find my way.

The Greatest Source of Satisfaction You Find in Your Work

For me, the greatest source of satisfaction has always been from working with patients who share their stories of survival, healing, and hope for a better future. This is why I do this work, to create a better future, and every study leads us closer to changing practice. I truly believe we are blessed to be a blessing. So when I get to use my gifts in ways that bring others healing and hope, that is tremendously satisfying.

Any Words of Wisdom to Nurses Considering Earning a Doctorate

1. Ask for what you want. The worst that can happen is you don't get it. But you could, and it could change your life.
2. Be sure to take time to look up and see where you are going. Take your blinders off every once in a while just to make sure you are still on the right path.
3. Make sure you are on your own path, not a path that others have chosen for you. Stop and reflect, don't just run ahead.
4. The biggest lesson I have learned is that you have got to create a sustainable career. It is not about work life balance. It is about integration.
5. You cannot drain yourself. You must make sure that every day you are continuously filling your bucket.
6. Create a daily schedule that allows you to fuel your soul at the same time you are fueling your career.
7. Eliminate the language of "I need to take a mental health day." You must take care of your mental health every day.
8. If you are in that place where you have no time for family and friends, you need to take a step back, set boundaries, say "Yes" to what matters and "No" to those things that don't.

Along the way, there were lots of women who had families and careers and they told me, "You can do this, you can keep having babies, raise your family, and build your career without having to sacrifice anything." I began to believe it. Unfortunately, that led to my burnout. It created a situation where I began to question, "Am I good enough, why can't I seem to keep it all together?" We need to support women to create situations that are right for them. Understand that there are times in your life you will need to adjust your plans. And that's ok! You go through seasons, and sometimes you need to spend more energy on family than your career. We can't make women feel bad for doing that. We all make choices to meet our own goals, needs, and values.

We may choose to:

- Go part time.
- Take leave.
- Take a completely different job.
- Remember, there are seasons in your life. Ask where you are and what you need to let go of.

To close, let me tell you a story. I was working with my children, changing out the clothes for the seasons. We were putting items into totes and carrying them down to the basement. I gave my son a tote and asked him to take it to the basement.

He told me, "Mom, this is too heavy for me."

I remember that I responded, "You can do it. It's not that bad."

And so he tried. And again he said, "This is just too heavy for me."

That is when I realized he needed to decide for himself what he could carry. I should not decide that for him. That is an important lesson we all need to remember. We need to be responsible to decide what we can carry and what we want to carry. And we need to respect other people's choices for themselves as well. Know what you can do (and carry). Then carry that, and do not accept extra loads from others just because you've done it. We are all uniquely designed to carry different things.

CHAPTER 18

The Postdoc Narrative

Shanina C. Knighton, PhD, RN, CIC

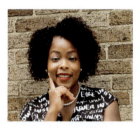

Without a family road map and as a first generation to finish high school and college, I had no idea that my passion and drive for nursing would also lead me to becoming the first person in my family to get a PhD and become a scientist.

Becoming a Nurse

I will never forget the day I knew that my calling was to become a nurse. It was 4 months after graduating from Baldwin-Wallace College, the day that I gave birth to my firstborn son. As with any new mom, there were a million things running through my mind. Will I make the right choices? Will I be able to give my child things I did not have? In all the chaos going through my mind, I found calmness and peace when a nursing student and nurse came in to care for me and my baby. It was the most genuine love that a stranger could give. When I left the hospital with my baby 3 days later, I knew I would not continue with sports medicine and that I would become a nurse.

Many of us do not know where life will take us, and in nursing there are so many endless possibilities. However, after working in nursing for 3 years, I "kind of" knew where my nursing career was headed simply because I knew everything I did not want to do. I knew I wanted to improve healthcare in some capacity. After having worked through pandemics, caring for my Grandma Ruth, and visiting my bonus mom and sixth grade teacher Ms. Anita, I was constantly seeing the same reoccurring theme of patients not cleaning their hands. When I went to visit Grandma Ruth, who had a stroke, I would watch her meticulously use her right hand to pick dirt from under the fingernails of her left hand, which had been affected by the stroke. During one of our hospice visits together I observed Anita's food sitting on her table. I asked her why she had not eaten when I clearly saw it was past mealtime, and she said, "My food got cold, because no one had time to come help me clean my hands so that I could eat." By that time, I had strategically mastered not getting H1N1 or giving it to my husband, small child, or unborn child through meticulous infection prevention techniques. I remember wearing my personal protective gear, swabbing patients' nasopharyngeal cavities, cleaning my hands, and ensuring I did not take anything into the room or take anything out. However, patients would often be so sick and weak that they would cough in their hands and sometimes without covering their mouths. I could not help but be paranoid that I would contract their illness while trying to help them get better. I would also observe how patients interacted with the hospital environment as if everything were as clean and safe as at home. And with my years of experience at this point of my career, I was pretty confident that this was the case.

Know Your "Why?"

I remember going to the Frances Payne Bolton School of Nursing open house event and speaking with faculty. I recall saying, "Respectfully, I don't want to become a nurse practitioner; I want to study germs on patients' hands and find ways for to clean them." Awaiting a response and expecting to hear about a Public Health/Master's in Nursing Program, I was shocked instead when a faculty member with the warmest eyes looked at me and said, "Well, let me tell you about our PhD program." I remember my stomach turning, becoming anxious and confused as if she was talking to the wrong person about a PhD. I mustered up a little confidence to say, "OK." After learning about admissions requirements, and speaking with faculty and students about their personal experiences, I became amazingly confident that I could work toward a PhD! I remember studying for my graduate entrance exam, crafting my essays, seeking out recommendation letters, and planning how I would need to adjust my life come my first semester of my PhD program. I knew that I wanted a career studying what I was driven to study, whether that was in academia or a clinical setting, and that I would have to position myself to work in these settings.

I immediately did a few strategic things, and I encourage you to do the same:

- Search the school's website thoroughly.
- Speak with the Director of Financial Aid and ask if he/she/they know of any funding opprtunities available for which you can apply.
- Speak with faculty who may have similar interests as yours and ask, "Do you have funding available for students to participate in your research?" Express interest if they do and FOLLOW UP!
- Speak with faculty who may have similar interests as yours; you may want to ask them to be your dissertation chair.

I Just Got Accepted! Now What?

I can still remember how amazing it felt to start an intimidating, scary, yet revitalizing journey. I just knew that this was something I wanted for myself. I needed to prove to myself and some of the people in my world that I could do this. Still, when the journey of my doctoral program began, I did not have everything figured out.

I knew that I wanted to study germs on patients' hands and ways for them to be more involved in infection prevention, and I knew that I would have to work harder than my peers. Why Shanina? Many may assume that I am thinking about being a Black woman as the reason; however, it is more complicated than that. I am the first in my family to finish high school, and I attended Cleveland Public Schools, where the graduation rate was less than 20%. I did well in undergraduate school—doing well enough to get by but was also learning what I could while working two jobs to help my parents back at home. I knew that when it came to learning, I was dedicated to it but oftentimes could not be fully submerged because I had adult responsibilities a lot earlier than what I had hoped.

I remember going into my theory class on the first day and doubt starting to creep in. Like you, I set upon this daunting goal for myself knowing full well that it would be like no other challenge I had set previously. I was a full-time employee, a part-time adjunct professor, a wife, and a mother of two small children. The goal sounded great to me, and I was confident. However, once it was upon me to begin, I wondered just how in the world I would finish the task I had before me.

It started with three classes and continued for several years. I worked as a research assistant for my research practicum hours during the day and worked the night shift while caring for my husband and children. I took one research course and then two more to start developing my own research and decided upon the potential data and sources I would need to complete my dissertation. I designed small pilot studies to learn more about the process. I worked with my mentors and chair on their studies to gain hands-on experience. After that last class, and with the experience I had gained, the dissertation process began. Then, it became possible to put my timeline into action! This is when I established a set timeline for when I wanted to complete my doctoral degree. I committed to complete my dissertation in 1 to 2 years, and I did it!

Now, I Am a Nurse Scientist!

I remember like yesterday the exhilarating experience of my dissertation defense, and then it hit me: "Graduation is right around the corner, what's next?" In all actuality, from the moment that I began my program, my PhD advisor and mentor asked me a question regularly that I began to ask of myself: "Shanina, what are your goals for this year… for the next 3 to 5 years… and where do you see yourself in 10 years?" I learned very early on to make an individual career plan and monitor my own success.

The first time I answered her question, I responded that I would be an independent researcher in an academic institution or in a clinical setting. She praised my courageous answer and then brought me back to reality by asking, "Shanina, do you seriously think you will be prepared to write a federally funded grant and execute it if you receive funding?" With a puzzling stare and no answer, I asked an important question, *"What should I do following graduation so that I am successful in academia?"* She answered, "a post-doc."

After you've spent years doing doctoral study, working as a research assistant, and learning constructs, theories, and statistical methods, the last thing you want to hear is that you need more training after your terminal degree. Still, if you become a nurse scientist who commits to a career in research, you likely will not go directly into a faculty role, but instead obtain extra training in the form of postdoctoral studies, a postdoctoral fellowship, a "post-doc."

Acquiring Professional Skills and Advance Research Skills

A postdoctoral fellowship experience has been acknowledged as a critical stepping-stone to provide opportunities for PhD-prepared graduates, including nurses, to acquire professional and/or advanced research skills needed for a productive research career. According to the National Postdoctoral Association (2014), a post-doctoral scholar is "an individual holding a doctoral degree who is engaged in a temporary period of mentored research and/or scholarly training for the purpose of acquiring the professional skills needed to pursue a career path of their choosing." Compared to 20 to 30 years ago, there are now more postdoctoral opportunities across all fields, including nursing (Kelsky, 2015).

The application to your post-doc fellowship is the faculty's first objective en-counter with you. A strategic, calculated approach is essential because the docu-ment you present will serve as evidence of what you value and what you have achieved. It reflects your attention to detail, quality of your logic, and your passion.

Schools of nursing receive hundreds of applications every year—far more than the number of spaces available for admissions and certainly more than there are faculty to support. The faculty and staff who are charged with making admissions decisions seek to find applicants who are a good fit for their program and are likely to be successful. Reviewers do not want to eliminate people: They want to find the very best. Your challenge is to present an application that gives those reviewers confidence that you will be successful and that you are just the person that they will be proud to claim as an alumnus.

The main goal of a postdoctoral fellowship is to develop your professional and academic skills under the mentorship of an experienced researcher. The skills and experience you gain as a post-doc can be key to future applications to tenure-track faculty positions. A post-doc fellowship may also be beneficial to government agencies, nonprofit research organizations, research-focused corporations, healthcare centers, or other scientific/research-driven organizations, although it is not strictly required. As you complete your post-doc, you can expect:

- time to publish your dissertation
- limited teaching or administrative responsibilities, freeing you to publish and pursue further research
- opportunities to complete requirements for specialty licensure (psychology for example)
- opportunities to receive additional training or mentoring
- time, training, and opportunity to write a grant

- time to send in multiple strategic job applications
- time to think through what you want to do with your career.

Some post-docs are renewable, allowing you to be productive and receive mentoring while you search for the perfect career opportunity.

Words of Wisdom

The words from the president of my college resonated with me as I prepared for my final defense, and they stay with me when I face challenges today. She advised, "Don't think of it as a defense; think of it as a discussion." Simple yet very profound. She continued (by the time you get to your defense), "Remember, you are the expert in this area; you've done all the research; you are merely sharing it with the members of your committee and anyone who participates." And finally, I remember her sharing this: "If your dreams don't scare you, they're too small. I dream big, and I eat nothing for breakfast."

I encourage you to dream big and to join those who eat nothing for breakfast.

Bibliography

American Association of Colleges of Nursing. 2021. Available at: https://www.aacnnursing.org/Students.

American Association of Colleges of Nursing. *The Research-Focused Doctoral Program in Nursing: Pathways to Excellence.* November, 2010. Available at: https://www.aacnnursing.org/Portals/42/Publications/PhD Position.pdf.

American Association of Colleges of Nursing. Enrollment and graduations in baccalaureate and graduate programs in nursing. 2019a. 2019–2020. Available at: https://www.aacnnursing.org/News-Information/Research-Data-Center/PhD.

Benderly BL. GREs don't predict grad school success. What does? Taken for Granted Column. 2017. doi:10.1126/science.caredit.a1700046.

Burnett B, Evans D. *Designing Your Life: How to Build a Well-Lived, Joyful Life.* New York, NY: Knopf; 2016.

Farrington R. *5 Mistakes That Could Get Your Graduate Application Rejected.* Forbes Advisor; 2019. Available at: https://www.forbes.com/sites/robertfarrington/2019/08/29/why-your-college-application-was-rejected/?sh=2383a668513f.

Gonzalez Y, Finnell DS. Promoting and supporting a Doctor of Nursing Practice Program of Scholarship. *J Nurs Educ.* 2020;59(9):526-530. doi:10.3928/01484834-20200817-10.

Hoover E. *Georgia's Public Universities will Reinstate ACT/SAT Requirement.* Chronical of Higher Education; May 25, 2021. Available at: https://www.chronicle.com/article/georgias-public-universities-will-reinstate-act-sat-requirement.

How to Look Good on Video Calls/Zoom Face Time Skype. Bloggers Secrets. How to Look Good on Video Calls. Available at: https://www.youtube.com/watch?v=ACNGhPKnmok.

Jones KD, Baggs JG, Jones MR. Selecting US research-intensive doctoral programs in nursing: pragmatic questions for potential applicants. *J Prof Nurs.* 2018;34(4):296-299. Available at: https://doi.org/10.1016/j.profnurs.2017.11.005.

Russell-Pinson L, Harris ML. Anguish and anxiety, stress and strain: attending to writers' stress in the dissertation process. *J Second Lang Writ.* 2019;43:63-71. doi:10.1016/j.jslw.2017.11.005.

Stanfil AG, Aycock D, Dionne-Odom JN, Rosa WE. Strategies and resources for increasing the PhD pipeline and producing independent nurse scientists. *J Nurs Scholarsh.* 2019;51(6):717-726. doi:10.1111/jnu.12524.

Taylor LA, Terhaar MF. Mitigating barriers to doctoral education for nurses. *Nurs Educ Perspect.* 2018;39(5):285-290. doi:10.1097/01.NEP.0000000000000386.

Weiner OD. How should we be selecting our graduate students? *Mol Biol Cell.* 2013;25:429-430.

CHAPTER 19

The Academic Narratives

Latina M. Brooks, PhD, CNP, FAANP ■
Amy Bieda, APRN, PCPNP-BC, NNP-BC

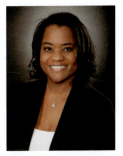

Latina M. Brooks, PhD, CNP, FAANP

Initial Motivation to Become a Nurse

I knew from an early age that I wanted to work in healthcare. When I was 3 years old, my family was involved in a severe motor vehicle accident that permanently disabled my mother. As a result of her injuries and subsequent rehabilitation, I spent quite a bit of time in healthcare facilities, both inpatient and outpatient. As I grew up, I became more and more interested in the people who were taking care of my mother. The older I got, the more questions I had and would ask regarding her care. I took it upon myself from a very early age to make sure she was getting good care. I think this translated into who I would ultimately become as a nurse, educator, and administrator. I have always been curious, and I have always been a caregiver.

I was considered the "smart kid" in my neighborhood. If you were smart and did well in school, your family and friends automatically would tell you that you should be a "doctor," and of course they were referring to becoming a physician. Being a physician was considered the ultimate success. So, of course, being the obedient child that I was, I bought into it, and I was going to be a doctor! True to form, a few days after graduation from high school, I was invited to start pre-med courses early during the summer term at a small private liberal arts college in Atlanta. Everything was going well. I loved my courses and my friends. I even planned who I would room with during the regular academic year and the sorority I would pledge. Life was good and going according to plan. I finished the summer session successfully and came home to visit before the start of the Fall term and everything changed. My mother became very ill, and I decided I could not go back to Atlanta; I had to stay close. So, I changed my plans. I had applied to a university in the city where I grew up when in high school, just to see if I could get in. I had been accepted and was already attending my first-choice school. However, because the Fall term had not started when my mother became ill, I was able to accept admission to the local university and start classes there at the beginning of the academic year.

Despite the change in location, the plan remained the same. I started as a pre-med student whose actual major was still undecided. When planning to become a "doctor" was the goal, you could major in anything you wanted! The local university was research-intensive, and my first work-study job was in general pediatrics. They were writing a major grant, and I was able to participate in the process. I loved it!

My next work-study job was in the AIDS clinical trial unit, where they were doing the early research on antivirals and the early work related to pregnant women with HIV. I absolutely loved working there and stayed for the duration of my undergraduate experience. I fell in love with research during this time. I worked with "doctors" most of whom were PhD-prepared and medical doctors. I also worked with the research nurses on the team who had more direct contact with the patients, which I enjoyed. So, I had two loves at this point: patient care and research. It was explained to me at the time that to be formally educated to do clinical trials and intervention research, you needed to obtain a PhD. I discovered that you could get a PhD in nursing but not in medicine. I still wanted to be involved in direct patient care, but I also saw myself fully engaged in clinical research. I had not explored nursing much before this. However, as I did, I discovered the possibilities a career in nursing would afford me and ultimately started in the School of Nursing and received my BSN.

Entry to Practice

My first regular position as a registered nurse (RN) was in major medical center on the surgical transplant team. On this specialized surgical unit, we provided postoperative care for solid organ transplant patients, which included patients who underwent kidney, liver, and pancreas transplants. This was a phenomenal experience. These patients were direct admissions to our floor, so they did not go to the ICU first. We were specifically trained to take care of critically ill surgical patients and were set up somewhat like an ICU, including our patient-to-nurse ratios. This was a great experience even though it could be very sad at times. As nurses, we developed close relationships with these patients. Not only did we provide their day-to-day care, but we also were responsible for educating our patients on their new reality of an array of antirejection meds, taken at specific times with specific parameters that the patients would have to follow for the rest of their lives. As a result, we had daily teaching sessions with our patients. Additionally, when a transplant patient needed to be hospitalized for any reason after their transplant, they would return to our floor. That meant we saw the same patients for very long periods of time. The relationships we as nurses developed with our patients were the most gratifying aspects of our job. It was also one of the hardest parts because we inevitably lost patients we had taken care of for months, and in some cases, years.

My experience working on the transplant unit was one of the best experiences of my career as an RN. I learned a lot and saw how the care provided by nurses truly makes a difference in people's lives. I had other experiences working as an RN, but those were more moonlighting. I covered shifts on subacute units in skilled nursing facilities. As a PRN nurse, there is less continuity of care, and most patients did not stay on the unit very long. With these experiences I could certainly see the impact of nursing firsthand.

Decision to Pursue Higher Education

The other aspect of my work as an RN on the transplant unit was staying current with the literature. This was a must because there were a lot of developments occurring with solid organ transplantation at the time, especially related to liver transplantation. This part of the job resonated with me because of my interest in research and confirmed my desire to pursue a master's degree and become an advanced practice nurse.

Soon after I started a master of science program in nursing (MSN) to become a family nurse practitioner. Toward the end of my nurse practitioner program, I had the opportunity to travel abroad for several months and work on a research project with pregnant women. This reignited my desire to pursue a research career. Prior to this international inexperience, I was not necessarily planning to continue directly on to the PhD; however, the dean wanted to meet with me upon my return to the United States to discuss my application for the PhD. She felt I had the aptitude for research. So, I decided to start my doctoral studies as soon as possible and was paired with the person who would become my PhD advisor and mentor.

Mentors

I did not really have true mentors until I started my PhD program. I did not know anyone who was an advanced practice nurse, nor did I know anyone who had earned a PhD. I knew people who would support and advise me as much as they could, including my mother, but I pretty much navigated my educational path alone for a while. This was unfortunate. However, I found my way. Once in my doctoral program, my mentors included the associate dean for research and two other nursing faculty members. I worked as a research assistant for the associate dean for research, and she and other faculty members helped me navigate through my doctoral program. One faculty member would recruit me back to my alma mater years later to take on a leadership role. During my postdoctoral fellowship, my mentor was a physiologist, and I worked on several of his clinical and bench research projects and published with him.

Milestones on My Path

There were many milestones on my journey.

- I was selected to do research internationally with a World Health Organization Collaborating Center.
- I had the opportunity to work as a research assistant and project manager and publish with my mentors.
- My PhD dissertation work was funded by a competitive National Research Service Award from the National Institutes of Health.
- I received funding for my postdoctoral training from the National Institutes of Health.
- I have been able to practice as an advanced practice nurse for over 20 years and work with minority and underserved populations, including serving women with developmental and cognitive disabilities that other providers did not want to see.
- While in full-time practice, I also was able to serve as principal investigator on several clinical trials.

I believe my greatest milestone is that I fulfilled the dreams of my family and friends. I became a "doctor," just not the physician kind. At the same time, I fulfilled my own dreams. I have to become Dr. Brooks, but more importantly, I have been able to remain engaged in each of my passions throughout my nursing career, including clinical practice, research, academics, and administrative leadership. I am not done yet!

Barriers I Faced and the Strategies I Used to Navigate Them

One of my biggest barriers was not having true mentors early in my education. However, I did as much research as I could about different nursing roles and educational programs and was able to successfully navigate through my educational programs and early career.

Early on in my practice and research career, there were not many people to look to for mentorship in nursing. There were not many people that I knew who were advanced practice nurses (APRN) with a PhD, much less doing a formal postdoctoral fellowship. I looked to medicine to navigate my way through these varied roles. Most of the PhD-prepared people I knew in nursing were full-time academics and/or researchers, not clinicians. Once I finished my postdoctoral fellowship, I had to choose between a full-time tenure-track academic appointment and going into full-time practice. There were not many avenues for a PhD-prepared nurse practitioner to integrate both the research and clinical worlds during that time. For many reasons both professionally and personally, I chose to stay in full-time clinical practice after the completion of my postdoctoral training. In an effort to continue with some aspects of research, I was able to take on a role conducting research on the industry side for pharmaceutical and device companies in the practice setting. So, not my own program of research pathway as I once dreamt, but our clinical research team did impactful work that has become integrated into clinical practice over time.

My Current Focus

My current focus is graduate nursing education. I work primarily in APRN education, program development, and administration. I am currently the director of an MSN program with several APRN program tracks. I also direct a Doctor of Nursing Practice (DNP) program with several program tracks while still finding time to practice clinically 1 day a week.

My Future Goals

My future goals: I would love to be the dean of academic programs/affairs someday. I look forward to working with other countries to develop advanced practice curricula and promote the role of APRNs globally. I will continue to practice on a part-time basis, as I am a people's person, a natural caregiver at heart, and always staying connected to the patient. I would love to volunteer with medical missions to assist in those areas where healthcare is not readily available. I think medical missions will be my retirement work!

The Greatest Source of Satisfaction in My Work

The greatest source of satisfaction in my work comes from caring for people in their time of need and making a small difference in their lives. People are central to being a nurse, and for me the patient and their outcomes are at the core of everything that I do.

I also find great satisfaction in educating future advanced practice nurses and nurse leaders. I enjoy engaging with students and imparting knowledge and lessons learned over my career. It is very satisfying to know that our patients and our profession are in good hands with the next generation of nurses, and I get to be a part of the development.

Words of Wisdom for Nurses Considering Earning a Doctorate

Know why you are pursuing a doctorate. Ask yourself how a doctorate will support what you want to accomplish in your career in the short and long terms. Determine what you want your career to look like.

I ask my advisees and those who I mentor these simple questions: "What do you want to be when you grow up?" and "What are you passionate about?" I believe you must start with your passion and what you see yourself doing for the long term. Starting with your passion and where you see yourself in your career will direct your educational pursuits. Knowing your why, your passion, and your focus will help you decide whether a clinical doctorate or an academic/research doctorate is more appropriate.

The beauty of nursing, in my opinion, is that there are so many opportunities that will become available as nurses progress through their careers. Whether in clinical practice, academics, research, administration, health policy, or elsewhere, opportunities for nurses exist in all sectors. Earning a doctoral degree in nursing is an important path to taking advantage of the many opportunities that exist for the nurses of today and tomorrow.

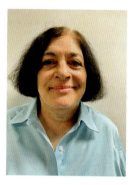

Amy Bieda, APRN, PCPNP-BC, NNP-BC

Your Initial Motivation to Become a Nurse

I had no intentions of going into nursing. I was a product of private school, so I had two choices back in the early 1970s as a female: be a teacher or a nurse. At the time, I certainly didn't want to be a teacher. Medical school for women was just in its infancy. My parents always told me if I wanted to go to college, I was going to have to pay for it myself. After investigating multiple programs, I entered a 2-year associate degree in nursing (ADN) program at a community college.

Things didn't get off to a stellar start. As directed, I attended the beginning skills labs for vital signs using glass thermometers with mercury and making of beds before fitted sheets. Then, on the first day of clinical, we had to go into the patient's room, introduce ourselves, and take their vital signs. Except I had a major problem. When I went into my patient's room, I realized she was dead. Understand that this first clinical experience was before most patients were placed on monitors in the hospital. My instructor didn't believe me. That is until she went into the room.

Nursing school improved after that, but I always thought something was missing. At the end of the program, the ADN program director called me into her office and told me that the ADN degree was just the first step in my professional career and that I needed to continue my education in nursing. Her decision to discuss this with me has remained in my head all my professional life.

Entry to Practice

I graduated when nursing jobs were scarce. I wasn't adventurous and ready to move out of state. I always loved children, especially toddlers, and wanted to go into pediatrics. I didn't want to take care of adults, but I needed to work, so I took a job in a skilled nursing facility. After orientation, I was the RN on the evening shift and had one licensed practical nurse (LPN) and one aide to take care of 60 patients. During those 6 months, I learned the following three things: (1) how to pass meds efficiently; (2) how to take care of decubitus ulcers; and (3) how to perform postmortem care.

I finally got a job in a local community hospital on their general pediatrics floor because I hounded the Human Resource department weekly. This pediatrics unit was a 40-bed unit with a General Pediatrics and Pediatric Burn Unit. Interacting with children of all ages with different diagnoses was an incredible learning opportunity. After my shift, I would go home and read about child development or review a pediatric disease of a patient that I had cared for that day. After 1 year in general peds, I started covering the pediatric intensive care unit (PICU) for the charge nurse at lunch. This was a whole new world of nursing that was compelling for me. The patient's acuity was relatively high, but the opportunity to increase my knowledge base was immense. I transferred to the PICU as soon as there was an opening. The day charge nurse was an excellent teacher and mentor. She taught me so much about PICU nursing and prioritizing. We discussed new ideas and therapies.

Rapid changes were occurring in nursing during this time. Kardex (not electronic records) were the norm. The new Nurse Practice Act allowed nurses to diagnose (nursing diagnosis). Compensation and working conditions for nurses also improved. Hospital equipment was becoming disposable. IV bottles were no longer made of glass, and single-use, disposable needles and syringes became available. I heard Marie Manthey speak in 1975 about primary nursing and thought it was the most brilliant idea.

The hospital decided that PICU nurses needed to learn how to insert IVs in pediatric patients. We learned by spending shifts with a member of the adult IV team who placed IVs in adults. Not my forte, but the ability to master a new skill and learn more about medications and their side effects was an opportunity that I could not turn down. All these new experiences and knowledge helped me change my perception of what nurses were capable of.

Decision to Pursue Higher Education

I always planned to continue my education, but it took several years for me to go back because of other life choices and responsibilities. I moved to Texas in 1981 and took a job at a regional medical center. I was hired for their PICU, which was behind schedule for construction and expansion, and I was asked to go to the Neonatal Intensive Care Unit (NICU) until the PICU was completed.

Here, I found my niche. I loved taking care of premature infants and their families, but more importantly, two events occurred. First, I could not learn fast enough about the pathophysiology of premature infants. I was a sponge. Second, and most importantly, I had two physician mentors who answered my millions of questions, gave me articles on current treatment modalities, and taught me skills like x-ray interpretation, intubation, arterial blood gas drawing, and line placements. This NICU was high tech. Everything was computerized, including nursing notes. We practiced primary nursing at its best. During this time, I had the opportunity to become a nurse on the transport team, which was composed of an NICU RN and a respiratory therapist. The team went by ambulance and fixed-wing aircraft, but mostly flew via helicopter. The first time I applied, I did not make the team. I was upset, but that experience just made me more determined. I did make it the second time the team had openings and enjoyed my 4 years of transport along with working in the NICU.

Then, I decided it was time to return to school. I started taking prerequisites at a local community college, including premed inorganic and organic chemistry, biochemistry, and basic statistics. After completion, I attended an accelerated RN-to-BSN program at the University of Texas at Arlington. The junior year and the senior year were one semester each. I thought, "How bad could it be?" It was a tough program, but we had dedicated faculty, and education was the primary goal. I had a wonderful advisor and mentor, and when we met, we discussed nursing and the importance of lifelong learning. She encouraged me to continue my education after I completed this program. I set a new goal and decided to become a pediatric nurse practitioner. This time, it was not enough that I found an excellent school; I wanted to be at a school that was affiliated with a major academic medical center.

I was recruited by University Hospitals of Cleveland in 1988. I worked in their NICU and went back to school 6 months after moving. I completed my MSN and became certified as a pediatric nurse practitioner. The department chair of neonatology heard I was job hunting and asked me to stay and practice as a nurse practitioner (NP) in the NICU. This was before Ohio state laws required you to have certification in the specialty area where you were working. I had an excellent orientation with five incredible practitioners and an array of world-renowned physicians. Then, I went back to school and got a post-master's certificate as a neonatal nurse practitioner (NNP). I worked crazy hours on weekends, holidays, and nights. That is the nature of the beast for an NNP. My favorite shift was the Friday, 16-hour nights. I think it was the autonomy of taking care of critically ill patients, prioritizing, attending deliveries, and making decisions based on specialized knowledge and skills I had learned in basic nursing—thinking critically, being observant, and staying calm. My responsibilities also included teaching residents how to perform a spinal tap, draw blood, or simply answer a question. There was great interprofessional teamwork on this unit. I enjoyed rounds because every discipline contributed to the care of each infant. It was a golden opportunity to present what you did know, learn from others, and realize what you didn't know.

In 2002, a professor from Case Western Reserve University, Dr. Donna Dowling, asked me to be on a grant she and a colleague had written to start an NNP program. A requirement of the grant was to have an NNP on the faculty. I resisted at first because I was not interested in stepping back into an academic environment. I enjoyed working in the private sector. Dr. Dowling was persistent—extremely persistent. After giving it a great deal of thought, I agreed.

At first, I sat in on classes taught by other faculty and then I started giving talks. Dr. Dowling critiqued my lectures and was instrumental in helping with teaching strategies. I knew the content and enjoyed gathering current information. However, presenting information to students in a manner that they would understand, retain, and enjoy took an incredible amount of work. It took several years to refine the course work and keep it current.

During this time, I was very intrigued with the DNP versus PhD. I listened to faculty in both camps. Frankly, I never considered either, and then I had my first evaluation as a part-time faculty member. It was terrifying. I sat before four full-time faculty members, including Dr. Dowling, who discussed my teaching evaluations, and at the end of the discussion one of the members asked if I was going to pursue my DNP. The academic dean slammed her hand down on the table and said, "Amy is going to get her PhD." I nodded up and down like a bobble-head doll. Dr. Dowling smiled.

I took my first two courses as a nonmatriculated, or special, student to determine if this is what I really wanted, and more importantly if I could do it. The program was rigorous to say the least. The first course I took was nursing theory, which is truly a foundational course for a PhD. Then I took epistemology, the study of knowledge. That was when I had my "ah-hah!" realization: a true "Where have you been all my life?" moment. I realized that epistemology was what I had been missing in all my years of practice and education. I was completely hooked. I applied, got accepted, and enrolled into the PhD program. Although it took me 5 years to receive my degree, while taking care of elderly parents, it was worth every minute.

How do you survive doctoral studies?

- First, you must believe in yourself. You can be your own worst enemy when things don't go as planned. Don't beat yourself up. Keep moving forward.
- Second, you must be organized and understand time management. I was working full-time and moonlighting at another hospital, plus going to school and teaching, through my doctoral program. I had wonderful nurse practitioner colleagues who looked out for me and understood my insane schedule.
- Third, make sure your family understands what your life will be like. You will have to sacrifice time with family and friends. So what if you can't go to your second cousin Judy's third wedding? Family members understand—but only to

a point. For the next 3 to 5 years, your *life* will revolve around pursuing a PhD. It is all encompassing.

- Fourth, develop a network of fellow PhD students. Whether it is to study together, bounce off research ideas, or just to commiserate, these relationships are extremely important, and you will likely make lifelong friends in the process.
- Fifth, jump through the hoops. Every doctoral program will have things you have to do, don't want to do, or care less about doing.
- Find a good mentor/advisor in your area of research. This is extremely important and may take some investigation. Don't be afraid to reach out to scientists who are not at your university. They love to hear from doctoral students who are interested in their research.
- Meet with your advisor/mentor on a regular basis. This is crucial to keeping you focused.
- Meet your deadlines for course work! It is a reflection on you as a student working on a terminal degree. Not meeting deadlines can increase your stress level exponentially.
- You must let some things go—what are a few more dust bunnies when you have a presentation to give or an abstract due?
- Most importantly, take time for yourself. Meditation, yoga, walking, exercise, reading a book (besides structural equation modeling), going to a movie.

Doctoral work is not for the faint of heart. It requires discipline, motivation, perseverance, and a thick skin.

Will you ever think that you are completely losing it? Yes, you will.

Is it worth the time and energy? Absolutely, it is worth it all.

CHAPTER 20

The Nurse Informatician Narratives

Katherine Dudding, PhD, RN, RN-NIC, CNE ◼
Kathleen McGrow, DNP, MS, RN, PMP

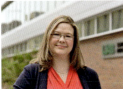

Katherine Dudding, PhD, RN, RN-NIC, CNE

Motivation to Become a Nurse

During my formative high school years, my family moved to Panama; this experience impacted my life in a way I never imagined and became my motivation to become a nurse. I attended a high school that enabled me to take advantage of incredible classes, in particular science classes. This is where science opened my eyes to the endless opportunities to which I could apply myself. I immersed myself in the sciences: biology, chemistry, anatomy, and physiology under the teaching guidance of a husband-and-wife teaching team. In my anatomy and physiology class, I realized that perhaps I could merge my curiosity for the sciences with helping others. I couldn't think of a better occupation than to become a nurse. My twin sister, Chrissy, decided to join me in this journey to pursue the nursing profession, which made it even better.

Entry to Practice

I attended East Carolina University, earning my Bachelor of Science in Nursing. During a nursing school lecture, a nurse from the local Neonatal Intensive Care Unit (NICU) visited us. I recall this being a pivotal moment in my life. Seeing these helpless neonates cared for by these exceptional nurses really touched me. I was just in awe of their compassion. At that point, I knew I had to take care of this vulnerable population. So, I began my nursing career at the Neonatal Intermediate Unit at Pitt Memorial Hospital in Greenville, North Carolina.

Decision to Pursue Higher Education

After 18 years as a neonatal and pediatric nurse, holding various roles as a nurse, including linical lead, and nurse educator, I was ready for the next challenge. I knew I enjoyed sharing my knowledge and clinical experiences with novice nurses.

Additionally, I thought the current best-evidence practice, specifically related to technology, within the NICU could have been better and could have improved neonatal outcomes and family experiences during hospitalization. This is when I realized that I wanted to make a broader impact on the actual *science* of nursing.

One day, I was discussing the possibility of pursuing an advanced degree with a clinical instructor from a local college. She told me she knew someone I needed to meet and asked for my email. Honestly, I didn't think anything would come of this meeting. However, 3 days later, I received an email introduction to a person who would become my mentor. I scheduled a meeting shortly after our email exchange to discuss options for furthering my nursing education.

Educational Path and the Reasoning Behind That Decision

It was never my intent to pursue a doctorate, but doing so aligned with my career goals and aspirations to develop a new technology to improve outcomes for neonates. Ultimately, I decided to pursue a Doctor of Philosophy in Nursing with a focus on Informatics at the University of Arizona.

In the summer of 2015, my mentor began an innovative model where students further in their doctorate studies (PhD and DNP) would assist her mentees with course navigation and questions. I recall an email explaining this model to us all and asking for suggestions of people to be a part of this community of scholars. Several of us emailed suggestions. I had the honor of recommending the selected name for our group, "The Carrington Cats."

I mention this group because a doctorate program can be highly challenging. The support I received from my colleagues was undeniably the best experience of my academic program. We supported each other through challenging times (e.g., comprehensive exams, dissertation defenses) and celebrated our successes (e.g., graduation, conference presentations). We created a community of lifetime friendships and a network of colleagues across the United States unintentionally. Though we all have gone on to our respective new roles and careers, we remain receptive even now to assisting a fellow Carrington Cat in need. I would not be where I am today without this community of scholars.

My goal as a doctoral student was to achieve a solid academic foundation in informatics. My PhD program was online, and my program of study required a minor degree. Since I was a local to the area, I could broaden my horizons outside of the College of Nursing and take advantage of earning my minor degree coursework in person. Naturally, my program of study evolved to include methods to facilitate my interest in informatics and technology. We decided that I would take courses in cognitive science, specifically in artificial intelligence (AI) and machine learning, to inform my studies and future research. This path guided me to amazing mentors and the formation of my future dissertation committee.

Mentors

As you can see so far, this journey was not accomplished in a silo. I had several mentors who guided me through my doctoral program. My dissertation committee chair was my primary mentor. My committee guided my thinking as well as selection and application of the theoretical framework for my research, my understanding of cognitive science concepts, and my foundational knowledge of AI and machine learning. Without the mentorship of my committee, there is no doubt I would not have successfully defended my dissertation.

Unofficially, I had mentors who guided me through my nursing career. I keep in close contact with my undergraduate instructor at East Carolina University, who guided my early professional nursing career. I also have a practice mentor and role model who has guided and supported me throughout my nursing career. Additionally, I would like to acknowledge the impact of the Carrington Cats and their role in guiding me throughout my PhD program and beyond. Peer mentors are so very important to our success.

Milestones on My Path

Though earning a doctorate can be challenging, it is also extremely rewarding. The milestones I reached while earning my PhD are not unique. They are a process. The first milestone was getting accepted into a program. Admission to my program involved a robust application process and interview before being invited to enroll and attend the University of Arizona for my doctorate. The next major milestone was earning my PhD candidacy. This involved a comprehensive examination testing knowledge of coursework content. It included both a written and an oral component. After successfully passing the comprehensive exams, I officially became a PhD candidate and moved on to the dissertation phase of the program.

The next milestone was defending my dissertation. For my dissertation, I completed a research study. I documented the project, which included background, literature review, theoretical underpinnings for research, research study and design methods, results, and discussion of research findings. Then, I presented my findings in a public forum, answered questions from the audience, and defended my work and the findings to my faculty and the public. Once I successfully defended my dissertation, I officially became Dr. Dudding. In my humble opinion, academia has no greater honor than the first time you are called a doctor by your dissertation chair. In my case, my mentor called me "Dr. Dudding" after 3.5 years of work.

My most recent major milestone was obtaining a position as an assistant professor. After several applications, telephone interviews, and site visits, I was offered this position at the University of Alabama at Birmingham. Currently, I am teaching in the MSN Informatics Program and conducting my research.

Barriers and Strategies to Earning My Doctorate Degree

The most significant barrier to earning my doctorate degree was financial. I faced several obstacles in paying for my schooling and living expenses as a full-time student. I had to get creative, but it was doable. I applied for and was awarded the Nursing Faculty Loan Program (NFLP) to use throughout my studies. I was able to cover some of my expenses by working as a research assistant for a couple of faculty members. This assisted me in paying for schooling, and at the same time I gained experience as part of a research team. This was how I managed the situation, and many other opportunities exist for scholarships and funding. This was a challenging time financially, but it was well worth it.

Current Research Focus

My current research focus is merging both my areas of expertise—neonates and informatics. Specifically, my research focuses on increasing our understanding of neonates with pain. I study neonate-to-nurse communication of pain for quicker detection of pain and pain relief to improve outcomes for neonates using technology-based interventions.

Future Goals

My future goals are to continue to disseminate research findings through publications, presentations, and grant submissions. Funded grants will enable me to make the most impact on the neonatal population and improve outcomes. I will continue as an independent nurse scientist through my research, teaching, and service. Overall, I hope, in some small way, to grow the body of knowledge in research and impact the nursing profession.

Greatest Source of Satisfaction in My Work

So far, my most significant source of satisfaction in my work is the finding the "why," the meaning of my work. Why I do what I do makes a difference and improves outcomes for neonates who are experiencing painful events. Gaining the educational skills to conduct research has been challenging and rewarding at the same time. I am always learning something new, which keeps me on my toes. My other source of satisfaction is the interactions with future nurses, nurse informaticists, and nurse scientists. I enjoy mentoring students with the same mentoring philosophy I learned from my mentor and the Carrington Cats. Moreover, I have a great sense of satisfaction knowing my work today has the potential to impact the future of nurses.

Words of Wisdom to Nurses Considering a Doctorate Degree

Words of wisdom for earning a doctorate degree: I would never say it is easy, but it is doable if you want to achieve this goal. Here are a couple of tips I have found to be helpful.

1. *Be organized.* This will assist you with determining what and when assignments are due. I always kept a yellow legal pad to add to my "to-do list." Other organizers were never quite big enough for my evolving list.

2. *Manage your time well.* If you can accomplish #1, you are already halfway there in terms of time management. I admit this can be challenging, especially if you tend to procrastinate. It is a process of becoming proficient with time management.

3. *Earning a doctorate degree is an exercise of persistence.* During your course work, you will have days where you want to give up—don't, you can do anything you set your mind to, and it all will be worth it in the end.

4. *Mentors, mentors, mentors…* They will be instrumental in obtaining your academic dreams. You will have many mentors, both official and unofficially, guiding your path to success in earning your doctorate degree. Not to sound cliché, but it truly takes a village.

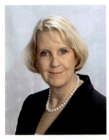

Kathleen McGrow, DNP, MS, RN, PMP

I receive a multitude of requests for speaking on podcasts, panels, and fireside chats to offer thoughts about leadership. Recently, I participated on a panel with a physician on the topic of workforce burden and burnout. The panel had an interesting start. Prior to the session, the facilitator inquired how the physician would prefer to be addressed, as "Dr. Groves" or as "Robert." The physician replied to introduce them as "Dr. Groves, as I believe that increases my credibility in speaking to the subject; moving forward, please address me by my first name." The facilitator proceeded to begin the session. I politely stopped her and requested her to do the same for me, to address me as "Dr. McGrow during the intro and then use my first name throughout the session." I have to mention this occasion, as I have found many times people do not consider a nurse as having a doctoral education. I almost did not speak up, but I am extremely glad I did. It was arduous work earning my doctorate, and I should be recognized as having my degree. Let me tell you a little about how I arrived at my current professional phase.

My Initial Motivation to Become a Nurse

My initial motivation to become a nurse was nurtured by my mother. She did not have the opportunity to go to college and worked as a nursing assistant for many years. I remember her saying she wished she had gone to nursing school so she could help people more. During high school I volunteered in a Baltimore hospital, and while I enjoyed it, I was still a little uncertain that nursing was the profession for me. My hesitancy impacted my selection of nursing schools, as I chose a 2-year AAS degree to obtain early clinical experience. My thought was that I needed to get exposure to clinical care to ensure I was on the correct career path.

Entry to Practice

My entry into practice was at a time when it was much more difficult to obtain a job when I graduated than upon entry into my nursing program. Hospitals required experience, and as a new graduate, obviously, I had none. After many interviews, I was hired to work in a medical-surgical oncology unit at an urban hospital on a permanent evening shift. I was 1 of 100 registered nurses (RN) hired at the same time. The hospital had just made the decision to change from a majority of licensed practical nurse (LPN) staffing to mainly RN staffing. This was quite the situation to walk into as a new graduate RN. I was the shift charge nurse for LPNs with over 25 years of experience. Our unit followed the team nursing integrated care model, and we cared for 40 patients with 2 RNs, 2 LPNs, and 3 nurse technicians. Some of my best knowledge was obtained from the expert LPNs who took me under their watchful eyes and helped me learn patient care skills.

Once I got the hang of patient care, I knew I wanted to take care of the sickest of the sick patients, and obtaining a BSN was important to my career path for critical care. I was in the first AAS-to-accalaureate Nursing (BSN) program at the University of Maryland's accelerated 18-month program. As a native of Baltimore, I was aware of the renowned R. Adams Cowley Shock Trauma Center and during my BSN program had the opportunity to do clinical time in the multitrauma step-down unit. I set the goal to one day return as a staff member, but first I needed to obtain critical care experience. My first critical care position was in a medical ICU where I was fortunate to work with a pulmonologist who spent time teaching about disease pathology at the cellular level.

I leveraged my experience and became a travel nurse. I worked in a variety of critical care areas across the United States. Travel nursing gave me the opportunity to live somewhere new every few months and really learn about the area. It was a fantastic experience, and upon my return home I was able to start as a travel nurse at The Johns Hopkins Hospital in the surgical ICU. I immediately looked for a position at the shock trauma center. I was informed by my hiring manager that I was the first nurse to ever be hired directly into the trauma resuscitation unit (TRU) from outside the University of Maryland system. It took time but was worth the effort. I was working in the care area that I thought I would be in for the rest of my career. I truly relished getting a call on the red bat phone, running to the helipad, off-loading critically injured patients, and whisking them into the unit where we would be able to address their life- or limb-threatening injuries. Pure adrenalin. In a good way!

Then a life event occurred that made me reassess and develop a new plan. That event was an injury I sustained while off-loading the helicopter. The patient was a critically injured 16-year-old motor vehicle crash victim. Intubated, his face was so bloody that I had one hand securing his endotracheal tube and the other was squeezing the ambu bag. In the rush to the helipad bunker my knee was hit by the stretcher and my left patella dislocated. At the time, I was not aware of the sustained impact of my injury. While in recovery, I assisted the information technology department on a trauma patient data study where I searched for codified data in paper medical records; it was tedious manual labor. I learned coding was rife with errors and the manual work required double and triple checks. I truly missed my unit and doing hands-on bedside nursing and patient care.

Upon returning to the bedside and realizing my injury would have a lasting impact, I reevaluated my next career step. Then another patient had a tremendous effect on my career, an 18-year-old female car driver status post motor vehicle crash with rollover. In the rollover her left arm flew out of the window and her hand was crushed. She was going to the operating room for wound washout, complete amputation of the left thumb, and hand salvage procedure. Time was of the essence; using the computer terminal at the nurses' station, I was searching for her lab results, as she had significant blood loss.

At the time, nurses had limited access to information via the computer. We could mainly access admission demographics and laboratory results. There was no computer mouse, so I typed in the string command "2.3.1" for hematology results and then "2.3.2" for chemistry results. It seemed to take forever to load, and I asked my coworker, "Why can't I see all the labs on the screen at the same time?" Her reply, "Because some engineers in the basement built this <expletive> and they never asked us what we wanted." She said it in a very casual, matter-of-fact manner, but this statement brought up a lot of questions for me. Who were these engineers? Why did they not talk to us, the nurses, and learn what we needed and wanted? Why were they in the basement? These questions started many thought processes.

As I continued working in the TRU, I saw the increasing use of computers and technology for patient care. I believe as nurses we need to make an impact on the information systems in which we work. Nurses need to own our workflows. Nurses should communicate our needs for the information systems we are using. Nurses should collaborate directly with the engineers and programmers that work on the information systems we use. It is our professional responsibility to ensure we have input to make healthcare better for both clinicians and patients.

Decision to Pursue Higher Education

One benefit of working at Shock Trauma was the location. It was located directly across the street from the University of Maryland School of Nursing. In searching for programs for advanced education there were a few options, but the one that seemed most intriguing was the master's in nursing informatics that was within walking distance and just across Lombard Street. My informatics path was chosen as I saw a need for nurses to engage with the technology they were increasingly using, as well as the proximity of a school with a nursing informatics program.

During my master's program I accepted the opportunity to precept with a project manager who was deploying clinical information systems. Electronic medical records (EMR) were becoming mainstream and offered options for employment as a nurse informaticist. I thought working for a vendor corporation would allow me the opportunity to understand information technology development and deployment.

Mentors

My career path has been guided by standout mentors. My first corporate manager helped me learn how to apply organizational theory to the complex adaptive system of a large for-profit organization. I had much to learn, as previously I had only worked at nonprofit health systems. At this organization I was required to be certified as a Lean Six Sigma Green Belt within 6 months of employment. My mentor, a Lean Six Sigma Blackbelt, was a former navy F-16 pilot; he had zero tolerance for error, and he understood there was a similar need in healthcare. When discussing technology regarding patient care, quality, and safety, his analogy involved an incident when he looked out his cockpit and saw oil steaming down the side of his jet. This was a zero-tolerance issue, and I still remember his story, as it was impactful to me when thinking about how information systems for patient care cannot fail.

One last mentor of note was my director at Microsoft. He stated, "If you ever want to be the Chief Nursing Information Officer at Microsoft, you must have your doctoral degree." More importantly, he continued by saying, "and I will support you in returning to school." His encouragement and my investigation into degree options were the catalysts to my returning for my DNP. It was a difficult path, but attending a hybrid program was very beneficial.

Milestones

My career path has taken twists, turns, setbacks, and breakthroughs. I have learned that change is constant and overcoming obstacles many times leads to a better path. It is essential to stay positive and embrace opportunities as they arise. My choice to take the nursing informatics path was a huge milestone. As a nurse informaticist I use my unique skills and knowledge to translate and disseminate information obtained through clinical practice and apply scientific processes through critical thinking, analysis, and application of standards necessary to develop health information technology solutions. My nursing and analytical skills are complemented by information literacy, management, and leadership competencies. I also have the ability to understand systems analysis and design, heuristics, and human factors interaction. I leverage people, process, and technology to translate my nurse knowledge and skills to solve health information technology problems. Obtaining my doctoral degree is another milestone and contributes that to my credibility as a thought leader. My manager was correct, as in my position of CNIO at Microsoft I deeply engage with leaders across healthcare organizations, and my doctoral degree is recognized as an asset.

Barriers

I have encountered barriers including both personal (such as illness and losing a family member) and professional (such as being part of a reduction in force, the dreaded "RIF"). All these events were traumatic but in different ways. As someone who prides myself in always offering my best, being let go from an organization was a huge ego blow. I learned no employee is ever "indispensable." I developed a skill set in the art of seeking a new job. In the end I landed in a much better position, so it all worked out for the best. Something that appears to be the worst situation ever can end up providing the best outcome. My path was convoluted; I tried to meet new challenges as an opportunity to reframe my priorities and develop a strategy for success. Making connections, building a solid, trusted network, and identifying knowledge development requirements are essential to continuing to advance one's career path and achieving success.

Current Focus

In my current position as CNIO at Microsoft, I focus on working with organizations to embrace innovative technologies to enhance clinical, operational, and financial performance. I am an expert on how technologies can best be deployed to address digital transformation imperatives including workforce crisis, consumer engagement, provider enablement, using analytics for population health, and using cognitive computing to support a learning health system. I am recognized as a thought leader on data, Artificial Intelligence (AI), and the workforce crisis. I have published articles including how AI transforms clinical data into wisdom and how the rapid evolution of AI will transform healthcare delivery more broadly.

My Goals

In the future, I would like to continue to grow as a leader. My goals include learning about data and AI in healthcare, which will be key to healthcare transformation, and broadening my efforts on understanding the healthcare workforce crisis and identifying where technology can improve providers' workflows and experiences through innovative solutions that improve the patient experience. In addition,

I would like to expand my network and leadership skill set through service on a board of directors.

Greatest Satisfaction

I find the greatest satisfaction in working with organizations on digital transformation through identification of problems and discovery of solutions. Mentoring and cultivating future leaders who desire to advance their practice of clinical informatics is also personally rewarding.

Words of Wisdom

For those considering obtaining their doctoral education, I advise them to cultivate a high-performance mindset. A high-performance mindset includes the ability to be resilient, optimistic, and focused on goals in the quest for excellence. I encourage you to bring a desire to grow, learn, and do things better than ever before. Trust and believe in yourself and set goals that align to your values.

In reflection, my doctoral degree is a key asset as I have increased my knowledge of healthcare informatics. I am considered a trusted source of innovative ideas and opinions as I have assisted in developing and delivering successful healthcare information technology solutions. In the beginning of my narrative, I spoke of the panel where I was participating with a physician who clearly articulated the use of "doctor" upon introduction as serving as a sign of credibility for his presence on the panel. This was a firm reminder that earning a doctoral degree brings a level of credibility, but it is our responsibility to develop and strengthen our credibility and elevate our practice expertise to be considered thought leaders and influencers.

CHAPTER 21

The Population Health Nurse Narratives

Laura Sinko, PhD, MSHP, RN, CCTS-I ▪
Nancy Rudner, DrPH, MPH, MSN, APRN

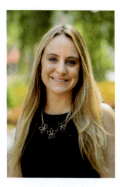

Laura Sinko, PhD, MSHP, RN, CCTS-I

Entry to Practice

There is no greater feeling than seeing the true person under the exterior they present to others—to hold space for them to authentically bring forward their fears, joy, questions, sorrow, and hope. That vulnerability is the most beautiful thing in the world to me. In my opinion, it is what makes us most human. Being able to witness and create space for vulnerability is why I decided to become a nurse. It is truly a privilege every day to be trusted with an individual's health and be a resource for education, support, emotional processing, and decision-making during one of the most challenging times in a person's life. As a patient in our healthcare system, it is easy to feel completely out of control, particularly when struggling with something that impacts how you want to live your daily life. As a nurse, I take it as my responsibility to give some of that control back—providing choice, informed decision-making, and amplifying a patient's perspective to the rest of the healthcare team. Being a nurse is so much more than I could have imagined. As a nurse, you are a caretaker, an advocate, a confidant, a medical professional, a scientist, a teacher, a resource provider, and even a counselor at times. Being able to serve in all of those many roles—to figure out creative approaches that center prevention and healing—is one of the many reasons I am so glad I decided to become a nurse.

As a nursing student, I had many great clinical rotations. I learned what areas brought me joy and purpose and what areas did not suit me. Looking back, the common thread between the patients I resonated with and provided the best care for centered around mental health. In my medical-surgical rotation, it was the patient who was recovering from a Tylenol overdose. In my pediatric rotation, it was the child we found bruises on due to physical abuse and neglect. In my neonatal intensive care unit (ICU) rotation, it was the baby going through neonatal abstinence syndrome and supporting the mother as she grappled with guilt and the fear of losing her child. When I got to my inpatient psychiatric rotation, I realized I finally found my home.

The discovery of my love for mental health brought me to my first clinical job as an inpatient child and adolescent psychiatric nurse. There, I created groups and individual activities about shame, identity, vulnerability, symptom management, emotion regulation, substance use, and grief. I was also able to work with families and caregivers to support and build their capacity as we transitioned youth back into their homes. It was through this job that I realized that most of the patients I was working with were not "ill" in the traditional sense, but instead were growing up with a set of circumstances that would cause any child to experience feelings of hopelessness, disconnect, or fear. This recognition helped me realize my true passion: trauma healing. I knew there had to be a better way to support these patients holistically, to help them reach their healing goals, including, the alleviation of their mental health symptoms and more.

Decision to Pursue Higher Education

I started my doctoral education in a less traditional way than most. I was given the opportunity to apply to the University of Michigan's PhD program as an undergraduate through the Hillman Scholars Program in Nursing Innovation, a BSN-to-PhD program that creates nursing change agents by introducing nurses to doctoral study early in their careers. I remember the feeling when I heard the statistic that less than 1% of nurses have their PhDs and that by joining this program I could revolutionize the art and science of nursing while also bringing my valuable clinical experience to solve real-world problems. It motivated me to get out there and dream big, to try to find solutions to many of the issues that bothered me throughout my clinical training within healthcare systems.

While my path may have appeared "straight" from the outside, finding my niche was hardly something that came naturally to me. I found that many different areas enchanted me and that I struggled to find focus. As others in my program progressed, I felt stagnant. I started to get down on myself and felt like a total impostor. What was I thinking, believing that I could pursue something as difficult and prestigious as a PhD? This feeling of inadequacy created constant roadblocks as I struggled to find the mentorship I needed to thrive. Four research mentors later, I found myself halfway through my first year of the PhD program, completely lost, falling behind, and feeling hopeless that I would ever even make it to graduation.

Mentors

But then, something truly amazing happened. A researcher at my school, Dr. Denise Saint Arnault, came to one of my classes and started talking about her work on help-seeking and recovery after gender-based violence. The concepts she brought forward (e.g., the idea that those who experience trauma are not "ill" or "broken," the focus on survivor strengths rather than deficits, the theory that experiences of trauma are cultural and do not occur in a vacuum) resonated with everything I was feeling during my clinical practice but just couldn't put into words. After class, I found myself at her office's doorstep to casually inquire if she needed any help in her research lab while desperately trying to hide the fact that I needed someone to take me under their wing. Without asking many questions, she fully embraced me as a critical part of her research team, helping me discover my true passions. She was incredibly generous with her time and resources while providing opportunities for me to network and travel internationally, write numerous first-author publications, manage her growing lab and projects, and find my voice as I began to take control of my craft and realize that I did have what it took to succeed. I discovered my passion reignited and felt willing and motivated to do everything I needed to make this woman proud, a mentor who believed in me when I had nothing to show for myself.

Within weeks of working together, Dr. Saint Arnault invited me to go overseas with her to attend an international research meeting in Lisbon, Portugal. There, I met her colleagues from around the world who respected and admired her. I was amazed at how she carried herself throughout the meeting, respecting everyone's ideas but always keeping the well-being of the women we were researching (survivors of gender-based violence) at the forefront of the conversation. Months later, we presented our work in Dublin, Ireland, and I had my first experience discussing research orally at a conference. In Dublin, no less! I was nervous, but Dr. Saint Arnault's confidence in me was grounding. Through that experience I was able to get over my fear of speaking in front of large crowds, and my feelings of being an imposter slowly disappeared.

As I continued my research training, I passed my preliminary exam with flying colors. As a result, I was able to work on a dissertation I was proud of, seeking ways to better understand the nature of healing after campus sexual violence. Dr. Saint Arnault encouraged me to be creative in my approach. I gathered quantitative surveys, narratives, and photo-elicitation data to holistically understand a process that can be difficult to describe with words alone. During my dissertation I continued my international work and got on-the-ground experience interning at my university's rape crisis center. This was something that some people discouraged, but Dr. Saint Arnault knew I needed to truly understand my phenomena of interest. At the end of my experience I was able to conduct a nontraditional dissertation defense. I wrote three papers, orally defended my findings, and created a campus-wide healing exhibition that displayed the photographs and narratives I gathered throughout my project. This helped me recognize the importance of creatively translating my work to be helpful and relatable to the people I am trying to serve.

Navigating Barriers

It is incredible to reflect on my journey and recognize that I had all the tools I needed within me to succeed; I just needed to find the right people to help me discover them. My PhD from Michigan brought me to Philadelphia, where I pursued an interdisciplinary postdoctoral fellowship at the University of Pennsylvania focused on health policy and health equity. During that time I worked as a sexual assault nurse examiner, where I focused on learning the impact and healing journeys of individuals who have experienced violence or abuse. Fast forward to the present, and I achieved my dream of being an assistant professor at a competitive research-intensive university: Temple University College of Public Health.

Future Goals

As I look toward the future, I have a clear mission: to create a more supportive healing world for survivors of trauma and abuse by holistically exploring pathways to recovery, and exposing, challenging, and eliminating social, cultural, and structural underpinnings that promote violence and inhibit healing. I have this mission statement written on the bulletin board in my office and will use it to be my North Star as I choose what projects I want to involve myself in as I progress in my career. I have many goals. I want to be a teacher and mentor who can inspire those who feel lost to discover and pursue solutions to the problems that keep them up at night. I want to be a high-impact researcher others can look to guide them in making policy decisions that positively impact survivor well-being. I want to transform the culture of academia from within to create a more healing-centered and trauma-informed entity where people feel that their lived experiences and differences in identity are valued. I want to help survivors recognize that healing is possible, and that their stories and well-being matter.

I find great satisfaction in the work that I do. As a nurse with a PhD, I wear many hats and can tailor my time to focus on making a dent in the issues that I care about. Every day looks a little bit different, which keeps me feeling fresh and motivated. I have space to create, problem-solve, and innovate. I can think critically about our healthcare system and patient care to solve real-world problems impacting public health. I also have the freedom to maintain a small clinical practice as a sexual assault nurse examiner, keeping my work grounded in the needs of those I serve. My research connects me with like-minded leaders across the country, allowing me to learn from their expertise and contribute to a larger mission. It also connects me with highly passionate and motivated students whose energy keeps me afloat and hopeful for a brighter future.

Most importantly, my work has given me the privilege to listen and learn from countless survivor stories and healing journeys. Witnessing their courage, strength, and vulnerability has given me hope that healing after trauma and abuse is possible, never losing sight that it is not easy. It is a privilege to amplify these stories and see others respond to them and feel less alone in their situations. It has also helped me with my own healing through witnessing and learning from the lived experiences of others both similar and different to myself.

Words of Wisdom

If you are a nurse thinking about getting a PhD, do it! If you had told me in high school or even when I started my undergraduate nursing degree that I would have a PhD by 25 years old, I would have never believed you. I was not the valedictorian of my class. I was not a 4.0 student. But I had the motivation and vision to recognize that the world needs more nurses conducting good science and that the voices and experiences of our patients need to be amplified to create actual change for the well-being of all. Of course, only you know what makes the most sense for you, but we need more people like you teaching, conducting science, and working to improve healthcare policy. If you decide this may be the right path for you, here are 10 tips.

1. **Mentorship is key.** Sometimes it takes a while to find the appropriate mentor to meet your content, methods, and professional development needs. Shop around and do not underestimate the importance of a personality and work style match. It may not be realistic for one mentor to meet all your needs. Create a mentorship team and be a mentor to others. It takes a village.

2. **You may feel like an impostor. You are not.** I learned that everyone feels like an impostor at some point in their career, even at the highest levels of leadership. Embrace the uncertainty. Just because you don't know everything doesn't mean you don't know anything.

3. **Find a topic that ignites a fire in your belly to keep you going when things get complicated.** People say your doctoral dissertation does not need to be your life's work. That is true, but it is also essential to find something that can keep you going despite setbacks that may occur. Whether you are doing quantitative or qualitative research, get to know your population. Hear their stories. Humanize the work you are doing. It will go a long way.

4. **Do not feel the need to work on an island.** Depending on where you land for your training, academia can feel like a hypercompetitive environment. Find your people. Don't try to get through it alone. Team science is the way of the future. You do not need to know everything to lead a project; you just need to know what you don't know and find people to fill those gaps.

5. **You are more than your CV.** It is easy to lose yourself in pursuit of your goals. Remember that your well-being and your life outside of work and school matter. Your personality, what makes you you, is what makes you unique and will set you apart from others. Many people will have publications, grants, and conference presentations, but none of them are you. What sets you apart?

6. **Stick to your mission.** If you choose to pursue a PhD, it can feel like drinking from a firehose once you hit your stride. Learning to say no to opportunities is difficult but necessary (and something I continually struggle with). Defining your mission and focusing your efforts in that direction can help you realize what opportunities are worth taking and what opportunities you may want to pass along to others.

7. **Don't be afraid to innovate and disrupt.** Do not underestimate the power of creativity and the courage to take a different approach or path. Some people are fearful of change. That doesn't mean you have to be. To truly improve population health, we need to be willing to make bold moves and come to terms with the fact that many of our ways of doing things are not working.

8. **Find colleagues with whom you can be authentic.** If you pursue a PhD, you may find that people who do not have experience in the academic-research world may not understand what you are going through. Trying to find people who "get it"—someone in your cohort, a teacher, a mentor, a mentee. I have found it extremely helpful to talk candidly with people who understand me and understand the pond we are swimming in. They can help you when things get hard and can be a sounding board when you need to make tough decisions. Don't forget to return the favor as well.

9. **Mentorship is the gift that keeps on giving.** No matter what stage you are at in your career, you can always be a mentor or mentee. Working with my mentees has brought me the most fulfillment in my academic career so far. It has also furthered my career in a big way. Amplify your mentee's work. Be generous with the opportunities you present them. When they succeed, you also succeed. Publish with them. Present with them. Help them find their niche within your work. This doubles what you can do with a set of data and your impact on your population of interest.

10. **Commit to a lifetime of learning.** No matter what stage you are at in your career, never stop learning. Learn from the communities you are trying to impact. Learn from your students. Learn from your colleagues and mentors. Learn from the successes and mistakes of others. The beauty of this profession is that there are always opportunities to learn and grow. Please take advantage of them.

Pursuing a nursing PhD was an adventure full of highs, lows, and a whole lot of learning along the way. I owe my success to the mentors who believed in me: the ones who challenged me to be the best version of myself. I also owe my success to the schools and funders that recognized my potential and invested in me. Without them I would not be where I am today. There is so much you can do with a nursing PhD. You can work in academia, government, a healthcare setting, a nonprofit organization, or even a large corporation. The sky is the limit. Create your own path. Take what you need and leave the rest. Know that you have all the tools you need to succeed inside of you. I believe in you. Now get out there and change the world for the better.

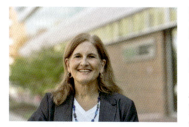

Nancy Rudner, DrPH, MPH, MSN, APRN

Motivation

As part of my bachelor's degree in history, I studied and traveled through South America. I witnessed the "social determinants of health" in their starkest form and explored the historical roots of our world order. I wanted to be a positive force in the world. Education and health care are society's two most important services. A friend working on a PhD told me about the potential of the nurse practitioner role. When I returned to the States, I graduated, worked a few years as an adult education teacher, and then enrolled in an accelerated program to become a registered nurse and nurse practitioner. The program was intense and challenging, demanding endless hours of studying. A steely focus on my goal to master the skills and work in the community with the underserved while simultaneously embracing the academic challenge kept me going.

I had clinical rotations throughout New York City, including a chronic disease long-term care facility on Welfare Island, a women's prison, a community health center, and a variety of hospital experiences. Together, these clinicals exposed me to many conditions in worlds so different from mine. A summer internship at the National Institute of Cancer was enough inpatient nursing experience to convince me that I wanted to work in the community and focus on preventive care. I love the wide range of experiences and options in nursing.

Entry Into Practice

A community health center in an impoverished neighborhood in Hartford, Connecticut became my preceptorship site and, later, my employer. To address the multiple needs of the families of the community, the health center model offered numerous resources: social workers, community health workers, specialty services, and dental care. My preceptor and mentor, Doc, taught me clinical care and how to identify and build on the assets in the community. He pushed all of us to look at the big factors influencing health, embrace diversity, and never blame the victims of inequalities.

One spring day, instead of the usual staff meeting, Doc took the clinic team for a walk in the neighborhood, helping us see the conditions affecting our patients every day. In my line of nursing, I treat many children with asthma and extract too many cockroaches from little ears, especially among children from one housing complex. To compel the landlord to clean up the roach problem, The Legal Aid Society asked me to give testimony in court. I was part of collective legal action that could prevent the problems instead of treating the consequences in each affected child. I went to court on behalf of my patients; I told the court how the housing conditions affected the children. We won, and the landlord was compelled to clean up the problem. We got to the source of the problem instead of just treating the ear invasions and roach-related asthma. **This was prevention**, changing the living conditions that negatively impact health. This was **nursing advocacy and population health nursing**. It made a difference.

Decision to Pursue Higher Education

Ready for more education and broader skills, I took the opportunity to earn a Master's in Public Health (MPH) at the University of North Carolina (UNC). With its strong commitment and connections to local and national public health, UNC is among the best in the country. I was in my element from day one with interesting colleagues and compelling courses. Public health opened a whole new world to me, building on my nursing background.

I took courses that focused on the care of populations, impacting aggregates instead of one-on-one care: epidemiology, environmental health, biostatistics, health policy, program development, and evaluation. In the community health center, I could see 25 patients in a day and 25 more with the same problems the next day. Public health helped me see the potential and gave me the skills to impact hundreds or thousands of people at a time, get ahead of the problems, work on the prevention side of the health equation, and design new ways of treating old problems.

The biggest challenge was that the nation entered a deep recession when I completed the MPH and public health jobs were scarce. I worked a combination of clinical jobs and population health projects while pursing my public health passion. I have written state and national reports on the need for expanded maternity services and co-developed a practice manual for preventive care and a guide for diabetes care for Hispanic patients. I have facilitated state task forces on adolescent pregnancy. Later, I wrote successful grant applications and developed services for human immunodeficiency virus (HIV) programs, extended comprehensive services for women with substance misuse problems, and community development resources.

Going for the Doctorate

I moved to an area with fewer resources and opportunities. I realized then that I needed more skills and a broader skill set. I went back to school to get a DrPH-doctorate in public health- with a scholarship as a Pew Scholar in Health Policy. One of the early distance-accessible programs, the program drew public health and health policy practitioners from across the country. We met on campus one long weekend a month for two years. Our cohort of 12 bonded and pushed forward, refining our skills in policy analysis, economics, program evaluation, research design, and other population-based areas. My dissertation looked at service delivery factors associated with higher rates of childhood immunizations.

Milestones in My Population Health Path

While completing my doctorate, I had the opportunity to work with a visionary leader who had learned community development skills in Latin America. Together, we developed new models of care delivery, revamping some drug misuse treatment programs to serve as community development centers. I wrote a proposal and received national funding to develop a community health worker program. The work was grueling, forging new roads in areas resistant to change. Once the program was well developed and had a proven success record, I facilitated transferring control of the program to the community it serves. One of the greatest satisfactions in my career has been to see this program sustained. Twenty years later, the women trained in the community health program still serve the community.

After the transfer of the program, I had the chance to develop an employee health program for the global headquarters of a large corporation, infusing it with a strong prevention focus. This combined my nurse practitioner expertise with population health skills. I was paired with a wonderful occupational health nurse practitioner who loved new ideas. Again, a visionary leader in the executive team paved the way, giving us free reign to develop the program. Together we developed service delivery models for employee programs for weight loss, workplace ergonomics, mental health counseling, clinical preventive care, and health coaching. We tracked our outcomes and demonstrated significant health improvements and other health outcomes. We worked with executives, warehouse laborers, clerical staff, buyers traveling internationally, and everyone else in the company. We had fun doing it. It matters who you work with. While my partner was quite unhealthy and died young, he understood and believed in the benefit of prevention.

Once that model was established, it was time for a new challenge. My next move was to be director of population health for a large health plan. I was charged with utilizing population health skills and nursing expertise to improve the health of over 100,000 "members" of the program. I analyzed the data to identify gaps in care and improve needs. I developed patient, provider, and system interventions to improve chronic disease management, preventive care utilization, and community resources. We improved diabetes care, increased mammogram rates, and raised childhood immunization rates. This was quintessential population health! We defined the population with specific, measurable baseline and outcome data, clear opportunities for improvement, and applied evidence-based strategies.

Another population health innovation I implemented was a frontline worker employee health strategy to provide ongoing health coaching and education to low literacy employees, primarily manual laborers. We have a medical-industrial system with high-tech care that does not help patients manage their chronic health issues. Further, our health system does not reach low-literacy and low-income workers very well with the employees. It took quite a while for me to establish the needed trust. Once that was achieved, employees made great strides in managing chronic conditions with a nurse guiding employees to better health each week at the workplace.

Disaster nursing is another area I deployed my population health skills. After hurricanes struck the Caribbean, I worked with response organizations to provide basic nursing care and problem-solving for population-based post-disaster issues. I volunteered to provide care to refugees at the southern border, ensuring they could recover from the journey and detention safely and continue on their journey to reunite with family. My population health skills helped me put their needs in context and help establish systems to facilitate care.

As part of my commitment to public health, I wrote and published on my innovations and findings. If it was an innovation worth doing, it was worth writing about to disseminate the information as we move forward collectively.

Now I have great satisfaction teaching the next generation of nurse leaders. It is so satisfying to see the population health nursing goals achieved and to help others develop the skills for health care innovations to change the paradigm of health and healthcare.

Satisfaction

As you can see, the opportunities are wide open for creating avenues to better address the health of large populations. Sometimes it takes a visionary employer or organization; sometimes, it takes a creative grant application.

Our nursing skills, combined with advanced practice expertise in population health, position us well to lead change in health care and develop new policies and models of care to build healthier populations. The *Future of Nursing 2020–2030* maps out our great potential.

Enablers, Barriers, and Obstacles

Throughout my journey obstacles were multiple. Employers without vision blocked creative options or were threatened by out-of-box thinking. One outstanding leader advised me, "If you are good, you become a target; if you are not good enough to be a target, why bother?" I encountered nurses who bemoaned change or failed to see the strengths in the communities they were supposed to "help." I encountered visionaries who took risks and were committed to making meaningful population-based change. I encountered problems in need of solutions I had the skills to solve.

While working on my doctorate and developing impactful programs, I found it nearly impossible to balance work and home life with two young children and caring for ailing parents. It may not have been possible without the tremendous help from a supportive and equal partner in my personal life.

Considerations Regarding Earning a Doctorate

Aim for the highest quality school possible if you are considering a doctorate. Avoid getting done quick schemes with large cohorts and too easy processes. Look for a program with vision and faculty who are leaders eager to teach. Challenge yourself to learn in new ways. So much is changing in health care and in nursing. You can be the change. Together, we can make a healthier world.

CHAPTER 22

The Policy Expert Narrative

Khalilah McCants, DNP, MSN, RN-BC

I ascribe to the adage "Life is really simple, but we insist on making it complicated."
—Confucius

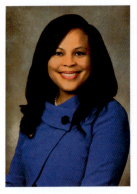

I always knew I would enter a profession that would serve others, but I didn't know in which role. My first undergraduate degree was in political science. It was work that appealed to me deeply, and I had the tremendous opportunity to work for a member of the United States Congress and the U.S. Attorney's Office. I aspired to a career in service, and this experience taught me about service, policy, collaboration, and communication. But my mind's eye searched for a job where my efforts would make more of an immediate and direct impact on individuals' lives.

I returned to school in search of a career more fulfilling. I began my work in healthcare as a research coordinator and dose manager of radioactive isotopes. In that capacity I worked with patients enrolled in clinical trials who were undergoing positron emission tomography (PET) scans. After working with several patients with Lyme disease and cardiovascular disorders, I realized nursing would be the natural progression; therefore, I applied to nursing school. What helped me see that was a female physician who steered me away from applying to medical school by advising me that if I wanted to have time for family, becoming a physician would not be a good fit for me. In hindsight, I realize that her advice may have been projection because I know several female physicians who successfully manage family and work as physicians, even though it is a delicate balance.

Entry Into Practice

After passing the nursing certification exam, I established a solid foundation for my nursing career by working at the bedside in the Medical-Surgical unit. As a medical-surgical nurse, I was confronted with a variety of diagnoses. This was ideal because it helped me increase my knowledge base in clinical nursing and sharpen my judgment. While working on this unit, I found I enjoyed the procedures. It was gratifying to remove staples after a wound healed, manage dressings, place intravenous fluid line (IV)s, manage drains, and delegate/train patient care technicians. I also enjoyed the variety of conditions and diagnoses I encountered, and I liked developing unique plans of nursing care to address many different needs and challenges of my assigned patients. My growing ability to successfully care for individuals with various illnesses required me to assess my patients thoroughly and determine abnormalities without delay. You see, hesitation can contribute to poor outcomes. And I worked diligently to avoid those. Still, even when I was thorough and timely in recognizing a negative shift in a patient's clinical picture, I, like any nurse, could not execute corrective action alone. I learned that a team approach is imperative for delivering quality patient care, and communication and coordination among team members are essential to achieving optimal patient outcomes.

EARLY EXPERIENCES AT THE BEDSIDE

Despite my hard work and care, not all of my patient outcomes were optimal. Case in point: I worked the day shift on a 45-bed Med-Surg Telemetry unit with highly complex patients. As a new bedside nurse who had just completed orientation, I was beginning to discover a routine where I felt comfortable applying nursing theory to my practice. My morning routine was obtaining hand-off reports, reviewing labs, anthropometrics, and orders, and performing my morning assessments. Here is where I met the patient, Ms. B.

The morning I met Ms. B, I received the report. I also self-acknowledged my feeling of sadness that my grandmother had been diagnosed with, and later succumbed to, complications of the same disease that afflicted Ms. B. This was a first for me. As such, I also self-acknowledged that I was still new to the clinical aspect of nursing; therefore, absorbing as much information as possible from the veteran night nurses and my more experienced colleagues was imperative to assist in my success as an entry-level nurse. However, at the time, I did not realize I could confide in my colleagues about that. A platform for reflection had not been developed yet at my facility.

During my review of Ms. B's vitals, I noticed a decline in her blood pressure throughout the night. I considered the significance of the patient's gradual decline and immediately contacted the treating physician. I explained that Ms. B had been recently admitted with a history of lupus and was currently receiving IgG therapy. I reported my concern about Ms. B's blood pressure to the treating physician. The vital signs taken at 11 p.m. and then again at 3 a.m. showed a downward trend. The physician sounded dubious. She concluded that the patient care technician likely had not used the equipment to correctly measure the patient's blood pressure.

I was bewildered by this response. Typically, a physician orders fluids when the blood pressure values decline. I also thought it was unusual that the physician did not visit the unit to assess the patient face to face. I immediately reported this interaction and my concern to my nursing director. This delay in care may have contributed to the development of a rare condition, idiopathic thrombocytopenic purpura (ITP) or other sequelae, and the patient passed away shortly after transferring to the intensive care unit (ICU).

Identifying a deviation from the standard status or process is an attribute I would hone throughout my career. For instance, when I worked as a Senior Quality Registered Nurse (SQRN), I noticed variances in how healthcare providers were documenting and billing services to the insurance company. The ramifications of the providers' erroneous documentation resulted in reimbursement delays and other associated penalties. To address this documentation challenge I developed a solution to educate the enrolled providers on more appropriate documentation and billing. As a result, the plan ranked top 3% nationally among 340,000 colleagues worldwide, 85,000 of whom are nurses and physicians.

Another instance of recognizing variances in the healthcare system was when I worked for the Medicaid program. My responsibilities included the review of procedures and medications that physicians had requested to be covered by Medicaid. I would research these medications and policies, make recommendations to approve or decline them based on my findings, and present a financial analysis. I became aware of the considerable practice variability and observed that evidence did not always inform care or improve outcomes. I began to understand that I needed to make the system work better. That became my motto: *make the health care system work well for everyone.*

The Decision to Pursue Higher Education

Early in my career, I observed that healthcare delivery was too often compromised by lack of access to quality care, low health literacy, difficulty navigating the healthcare system, a breakdown in interprofessional empathy, or other barriers (Adamson, 2018). I wanted to be better prepared and better able to address these problems. For example, I provided case management services for one patient who shared that a thorough history and documentation regarding the interaction of a significant dietary change and the onset of the patient's chief complaint was lacking. This detail was overlooked either from inexperience or lack of time on the provider's part, which are barriers that could be remedied after conducting a root cause analysis. As a principal investigator once told me, healthcare providers should know that saying "I don't know" is the best answer, and the statement "let me research that and get back to you" shows concern and empathy.

My decision to pursue advanced education was based on a deep desire to marry my passion for policy and my commitment to improving access to and quality of healthcare. I returned to school to earn a Master's in Nursing with a concentration in Health Systems Management and continued graduate study to earn my doctorate in nursing practice (DNP). Currently, I am completing a nurse practitioner certificate program at the University of Massachusetts in Boston in Adult-Gerontology.

My doctoral education allowed me to develop, influence, and execute policies that could favorably impact our healthcare system in the United States, improve patient satisfaction, and achieve a broad range of better outcomes by reducing barriers and strengthening facilitators. Further, I believed that earning my DNP would help me develop a more scholarly, collaborative, and rigorous approach to problem-solving and evaluation of outcomes. Such critical analysis and thoughtful, evidence-based recommendations would strengthen my impact on health policy and the health of society. I wanted to learn how to effectively interact with stakeholders and become a more credible and persuasive influencer on behalf of those in need of healthcare and those who endeavor to provide it.

Mentors

I have benefited from mentorship from many remarkable nurses and experts in the policy arena. I remember attending the American Academy of Nursing (AAN), where I presented my DNP project and learned from a living legend that we cannot brave this nursing journey *alone*. We all need help. I can attest to that. Numerous experts have been instrumental in my growth and development throughout the years. I attribute my success as an advocate to my parents, who taught me to be a courageous, determined, and proactive self-advocate, and support those less fortunate. My mother would always say, "Respect the janitor and the chief executive officer in the same manner." She taught me to be reticent. My father taught me how to be resilient. Once, he was mugged coming home late from work. He fought the assailant and managed to drive himself to the hospital to treat a deep gash under his eye. The scar remains, roughly 35 years later. My father did not allow that crime against him to derail him in any way. My father continued to be the best provider, father, husband, and lawyer he could be.

My husband (not faculty, but former military), my dean, and a cluster of faculty from the Graduate School of Nursing and School of Medicine at the Uniformed Services University of the Health Sciences (USUHS) have helped shape my career as a civilian in a military enterprise. These individuals embraced me and introduced me to many exciting opportunities. Through it all, I have gained valuable insight and experience that have catalyzed my ascent to new heights in the military and as an assistant professor.

My strengths as a writer have developed over the years through practice. I write a lot: I used to write speeches and summarize bills for the Congresswoman I worked with early in my career, and now I journal and write manuscripts. One of the reasons I returned to school to obtain my graduate degree was to fortify my emotional intelligence in a way that allowed me to message stakeholders and colleagues effectively. There are several faculty at my alma mater, the University of Virginia, who contributed to my achieving my goal. Their assignments and feedback were invaluable and provided sound guidance that helped improve my literary skills, among other competency-driven skills.

Milestones

I am a goal-oriented individual. Meeting my milestones is important to me, including attaining undergraduate and graduate degrees, and obtaining specialty certifications. At present, I plan to complete certifications as a nurse practitioner, in simulation, as a nurse education, and in wound care. It is most important to know that reaching milestones takes time. I have been working to achieve my goals one by one for over 20 years now and I expect to continue to set new goals for the next 20.

While the process was sprinkled with challenges along the way, I developed the skill set and strength to trust the process and manage the challenges. For example, I have improved my soft skills and emotional intelligence. I learned how to lean in to meet a common goal shared by many partners. Case in point: In my current role as an assistant professor at USUHS, I was selected to lead an interprofessional education (IPE) collaboration between a core course within the Graduate School of Nursing (Global Perspectives Seminar in a Complex Healthcare System) and the School of Medicine (Leadership in Health Systems). As a result of careful listening and discourse between both schools, I ensured that my messaging addressed both schools' objectives and responded to the interests of both groups of students. As a result, we are entering the second year of the IPE partnership and have achieved a 70% student approval rating from more than 200 graduate students.

Overcoming Obstacles

As nurses, we carry many responsibilities simultaneously. We are daughters and sisters, wives and mothers. We are often working full time while we are earning our graduate degrees. We balance so many challenges. My life is no different.

1. I am a mother of three young children and a supportive, loving, and attentive wife. I work hard to be a good wife, mother, nurse, and faculty member. It is a challenge. In the process, I have learned a few important lessons:
   a. Prioritizing is essential, owing to managing life's delicate balance.
   b. Competing priorities should be revisited daily.
   c. Honesty and working to exceed expectations are my work ethic.
   d. Aligning with policies and procedures ensures predictability and standardization.
   e. Kindness conquers all.
2. I understand that the best way to achieve equity and access to care for everyone is to build more effective health care teams that are inclusive and respectful.

3. I have found it particularly challenging to complete my practicum and clinical hours while carrying out other responsibilities. I have learned a few important lessons here:

   a. The key is to find preceptors whose schedules are compatible with your own.
   b. Your primary employer will need to take priority.
   c. Anything outside of work hours can be arranged according to your schedule.
   d. Communication is key. Leaning in is critical. Once details are agreed upon, one can navigate clinical and practicum successfully.
   e. Being vulnerable and feeling intimidated does not mean you are weak. As people of color, we are told and, most times, forced to be and act strong. Leaning in occasionally makes space for more knowledge, wisdom, and vigor.

My Current Work

My current focus is teaching students how to work effectively with colleagues from many disciplines to achieve the best outcomes for those in our care. Together, we examine clinical scenarios from our disciplines' perspectives and explore strategies to be successful together. I intend to advance to Associate Professor, knowing that much work will be required to earn this goal. I continue to provide the most up-to-date knowledge for my students.

I recently was a member of a team that led the conduct of a root cause analysis based on a scenario addressing patient admissions where participants had to consider patient experience, provider preference, and hospital expenses. This was the first cycle of this particular interdisciplinary immersion experience. I was excited to play a role in this complex and transformational student-driven directed-learning near-peer teaching experience.

Also important to me is my work with my nonprofit group, Pine Cone, Inc. (PCI). (www.pineconeinc501c3.org), which educates the community on health promotion and disease reduction. This organization seeks to improve access to breast health education and empower the target population with dietary and cognitive information that will encourage a sense of autonomy over their outcome. I hope to continue to expand the work and impact of this nonprofit to provide wellness case management services to vulnerable populations.

Greatest Source of Satisfaction

Congresswoman Shelia Jackson Lee is my mentor and North Star. I am most proud of several accomplishments that align with the lessons I have learned from her.

- I am proud to serve as an assistant professor at the USUHS, where I prepare members of our tri-services for their unique clinically oriented roles serving in the Army, Air Force, Navy, and Public Health Service.

- My 72 students were invited to join me on a visit to Capitol Hill and watch from the Galleries. This day was one of the most significant sources of satisfaction because it underscored the importance of relationships.
- I am a proud member of Alpha Kappa Alpha Incorporated (AKA), the same sorority of which the congresswoman is a member.
- I graduated from historically black colleges and universities (HBCU).
- I cultivate strong and impactful relationships.
- My most excellent satisfaction is providing students with relevant policy-related opportunities.
- I work at the top of my license, utilizing all my knowledge and skill.
- I stretch students academically.

For nurses considering earning a doctorate, lead with compassion. You may encounter barriers to advancing in your practice. Therefore, it is your responsibility as a leader to develop strategies to overcome obstacles. Maintaining relationships is equally important to your development. Practice forgiveness, stay encouraged, and ensure the policies justify the actions.

Bibliography

Adamson K, Loomis C, Cadell S, et al. Interprofessional empathy: a four-stage model for a new understanding of teamwork. *J Interprof Care*. 2018;32(6):752-761. doi:10.1080/13561820.2018.1511523.

Arnold ER. As a new nurse myself, how can I become a mentor to new nurse colleagues? *Clin J Oncol Nurs*. 2018;22(1):120. doi:10.1188/18.CJON.120.

Hou C, Moffat KA, Gangji AS, et al. Circulating heparin-like anticoagulants: case report and review of literature. *Transfusion*. 2021;61(3):968-973. doi:10.1111/trf.16236.

Millstein JH. My mentor. *Fam Med*. 2019;51(9):779-780. doi:10.22454/FamMed.2019.588459.

CHAPTER 23

The Nurse on the Board Narrative

Cheryl Lynn Fattibene, DNP, MSN, MPH, FNP-BC

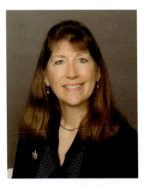

The seed was planted for my nursing career in a small village in Senegal, West Africa, when I joined the Peace Corps as a volunteer after finishing college. I had just graduated with a Bachelor of Arts in French after spending a year abroad. My roomate and I lived in Rouen (just outside of Paris) with a French couple who welcomed us for our "Junior Year abroad."

During that time, I learned more than any classroom could have taught me about the history of Europe and World War II (both host "parents" had lived through the war as teenagers and recounted many stories about that time to us) as well as trying to assimilate into French culture. Being outside of the United States helped me grow and learn more about myself than ever before.

It was clear after graduation that I would face a mountain of student debt, and job prospects were poor unless I wanted to become a French teacher (a path I didn't want to pursue). One day while walking around campus in my senior year, I saw a sign stapled on a post about a talk being given by a Peace Corps volunteer that evening. I decided to go. That evening changed my life.

I quickly applied for Peace Corps after graduation but discovered that getting in was not as simple as I thought it would be. There was paperwork to submit, verification of education, most importantly references from people who believed I would be a good fit, as well as extensive psychological testing and question-naires. Once that was done. I waited to be contacted regarding placement. My only request was to go to a French-speaking country, as my fluency was evident after living for a year with people who spoke no English. The first offer was for Rwanda, East Africa, which I turned down along with Togo (in the South Pacific), as neither were French speaking and I figured that was my best asset as a Peace Corps volunteer. The months stretched into almost a year. My last and final offer was Senegal, West Africa, a Francophone country, which for me seemed like a perfect fit.

The rest, as they say, is history. I was sent to a village of 800 people in the northern part of the county, which was a desert. The program I was in (Animation Rurale, i.e., education for rural development) charged the volunteers with "finding out what the villagers wanted and helping them achieve their goals." This proved to be an elusive task because what the village wanted was to build community latrines and deepen their communal well. These goals were well beyond anything I could actually do for them with limited resources. While disappointed, they figured they should at least take care of me for the 2 years I would be living with them.

During that time, villagers began coming to my tin hut to get medical advice for a variety of illnesses and conditions. The only doctors they had known were white. The word in their native language of Woloof was "*tubob*," which means both white person and doctor. The villagers believed that the reason I came to their remote village was to offer medical help. The Peace Corps had issued us a book entitled, *Where There Is No Doctor*, which became dogeared with use over time as I encountered vitamin A deficiency blindness, malnutrition, dehydration due to diarrheal illness, and festering wounds that would not heal due to lack of soap and water.

Each morning I would open my door and find villagers lined up for a "consultation." I was fascinated by the medical role I had assumed as well as the lack of basic knowledge about rehydration for sick children and the use of soap and water for open wounds (soap was used for washing clothing, not people). While living in the village, we experienced an outbreak of measles. I was able to give basic care with limited resources and I watched helplessly as many young children in the village died. This experience had a profound effect on me. As we went through our first rainy season, I realized how prevalent malaria was (I myself got malaria twice and fully understood the danger and risk for death without treatment). I was able to contact local authorities and reopen a dispensary that had been closed for 2 years so we could distribute antimalarial drugs to the villagers. This program was very successful. We achieved the lowest death rate from malaria for this village in many years.

Entry to Practice

Four years later, I found myself back in the U.S. with a mission and a drive to find out how I could continue the work I had done in that small village by pursuing a healthcare profession of some sort. I knew then that I wanted to pursue a degree in public health but was encouraged by another volunteer to pursue a clinical degree as well.

I decided to interview people in healthcare and ask them all the same question: "*If you had to do things over again, would you pick the same profession you are in now and why?*" My list included nurses, doctors, physical therapists, occupational therapists, and others. On the advice of my family doctor, he suggested I talk to some of his colleagues who were nurse practitioners (NP) working in a nearby alternative "wellness" program. Of everyone I interviewed, only the NPs said unequivocally, *"Yes, I would choose the same profession again."* I had my answer and discovered the world of NPs. I made the decision then to pursue a career in both public health and nursing, and have never once looked back. Nor would I have done it any differently. Serendipity is an extraordinary thing.

Pursuit of Higher Education

I am the first and only one of my siblings to pursue higher education. When I told my parents of my interest in going to graduate school after returning from the Peace Corps, they wished me good luck and offered no financial help. It was a "sink or swim" situation, and I decided to swim. To help pay my tuition, I created a window-washing business (We Do Windows) that helped me finance my schooling. There were only three programs across the U.S. that offered a dual-degree program in both nursing and public health for non-nurses at the time: Mass General Hospital, Pace University, and Yale University. Yale was the closest, so I applied and was accepted there. The 4-year dual-degree program had me matriculating in Yale's schools of nursing and medicine at the same time alongside medical students and physician assistants. While this was an extraordinary challenge, I was motivated by my experience in the Peace Corps to learn more about healthcare and somehow make my mark in the combined fields of public health and nursing.

After finishing school, I got married and moved with my spouse to Pennsylvania where he had been transferred. I left family and friends and started my new career in a new place not knowing anyone. I was a National Health Service Corps (NHSC) recipient, which helped me pay back my student loans, and I found a placement in a small clinic in a homeless shelter in Trenton, New Jersey. It was there that my nursing career really began. I was given a small clinic to run and five staff to oversee. The clientele were homeless men, many of whom were Vietnam veterans living on the streets.

Mentors

Knowing that my time with NHSC would end in a few years, I sought out connections through the Pennsylvania chapter of a local NP group in Philadelphia and started going to their monthly meetings. Here I met my first mentor, who was part of this group. She was a family nurse practitioner (FNP) like me. I was so impressed with her that I asked if she would hire me once my NHSC stint was over. At first, she said "no" because she did not have an opening for me in her new clinic. So, I offered to do "house calls" in the community where she hoped to open a clinic within the next year if she could find the funding. For a year, I went door to door in a very poor and underserved community in East Falls, Philadelphia. Essentially, I conducted a "needs assessment" during that time, which helped identify the medical needs in that community, which I used to secure Housing and Urban

Development (HUD) funding to build a primary care clinic there. It was a great success, and my mentor and I went on to work together for 11 years in that community to meet the needs of its residents.

Milestones

Leaving that practice was a milestone in my career. I realized that I was unable to grow professionally in that position for a variety of reasons. While it was difficult to say goodbye to my patients, my professional growth depended on my ability to make changes in my work trajectory.

That is when I decided to pursue managerial roles that would allow me to grow both personally and professionally. I chose a completely different type of facility in which to work: long-term care for adults with disabilities. This job enabled me to be part of an executive team that both ran the facility and cared for its patients over the long term.

Here, I was able to play a strategic role for both patients and families as I guided them through medical coverage issues, care plans, and the long term with their loved ones. We provided 24/7 nursing care for our patients. I would "round" with my staff on all shifts to get a better sense of the challenges and needs they encountered. This proved to be invaluable when faced with a temporary nursing exodus due to the introduction of a computerized medical record system, which required all caregivers to use computers for documentation, many for the first time. I understood then that "walking in someone else's shoes" in any field (but particularly in nursing) as a servant leader is an essential part of nursing leadership.

As I moved through my career to "for profit health" care entities (Rothman Institute, CVS), I began to better understand the "business" of healthcare in a way I never did before. This was a time with a steep learning trajectory. As has been my practice. I sought out mentorship from NPs I admired, which was invaluable. I maintained my commitment to servant leadership and learned even more about the business of healthcare, the importance of nursing leadership, and the impact of the "shadow you cast" as a leader. I learned that the higher up you go in any organization, the more people will scrutinize who you are, what you do, and how you treat others. I learned to appreciate that we can all chose the shadow we cast in nursing.

This was another milestone in my career. I realized that leadership carries immense responsibility not only to oneself but to those you work with each day. It was during this time that the idea to pursue a doctorate came to my awareness. Many of my colleagues were back in school pursuing their DNP degrees. After 30 years as an NP, I knew it was the next step I should and would take. I wanted to educate new nurses about the amazing profession of nursing and the role of the Advanced Practice Registered Nurse (APRN). I wanted APRNs to understand the many ways nurses could make their mark on our healthcare system for the better.

Current Focus

Over the past 5 to 7 years, I have made it my mission to push myself professionally to reach new goals and expand my understanding and influence. I have become much more aware of movements that are holding NPs back, at the state level and nationally. Working as the Chief Nurse Practitioner Officer for a nonprofit in Philadelphia opened up a new global perspective for me, one that reconnected me with my early years in the Peace Corps and the root of my motivation to enter nursing.

Future Goals

My passion now is to give back to my profession by serving as a book editor (*Transition to Practice: A Practical Guide for NPs*), sitting on numerous community and national boards that promote health and wellness (as only a nurse can), running for local office, and working with immigrants in the detention camps at our southern border.

Helping others has always been my passion. I am so very grateful to have found this path for my life's work, as it has given me great joy, as well as a sense of purpose. Working again with students gives me hope for the future of nursing both in the U.S. and abroad. The roles of nurses across the globe are changing, and countries look to the U.S. with our advanced model for the nursing profession. We can and should add to the body of knowledge that supports and improves care for communities around the globe.

Words of Wisdom

To those of you considering a doctorate in nursing, please join the growing group of committed and dedicated nurses who have chosen this path. Nursing is and always has been a work in progress. This new chapter for our profession will elevate and expand the breadth and scope of our influence throughout the healthcare industry in the U.S. and help us shine as a beacon of hope in countries that aspire to realize the promise of nursing. To achieve the bright future to which you aspire, be sure you find mentors to guide you and be sure to mentor others for professional success. In this way we will help nursing thrive and grow for generations to come.

CHAPTER 24

The Leader Narrative

Bethany Hall-Long, PhD, RNC, FAAN

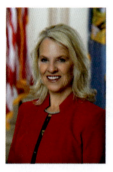

As the 26th Lieutenant Governor of Delaware, a former Delaware House and Senate member, and a Professor of Nursing and Urban Affairs with the Biden Institute at the University of Delaware, I hope my story inspires students or nurses to consider public policy and politics as an integral focus of nursing practice, research, and education. Ultimately, nurses need to "enter the ring" and run for local, state, or national political office, and perhaps my story can serve as an example of possible career options for fellow nurses.

Politics and policymaking are tools that have allowed me to sponsor over a thousand pieces of legislation and multiple proclamations with the ability to cultivate the next nursing and health workforce along with innovative research and education models. Ultimately, students and faculty must "be at the policymaking tables because if they are not, they are often on the menu." Nursing students can begin to apply research, evidenced-based practice, and clinical stories to policymakers to make significant changes for health care access, scope of practice, care delivery, systems coordination, workforce development, and so much more.

Nurses easily transition the critical bedside skills that ensure the health and safety of families to the policymaking sector. Nurses are adept at applying critical thinking, effective communication, discretion, and upholding rules and regulations. These nursing skills apply to elected office or policymaking. They have assisted me since day one, when I first ran for office due to my desire to help homeless, mentally ill veterans. As Lieutenant Governor, I serve all of Delaware's patients and communities' best interests. In turn, as Chair of the National Lt. Governors Association, I have been honored to collaborate with other lieutenant governors and policymakers across the nation on physical and mental health, education, economic, justice reform, climate change, and more. I am not a former legislator who happened to be a nurse I am a nurse who entered the political arena to deliver results and to reform health policy. I am a nurse first and a politician second. In fact, during the COVID-19 pandemic, I administered over 4000 vaccines in the arms of Delawareans up and down the state. In short, being a nurse legislator has greatly enhanced my effectiveness in state government and public policy as well as being able to apply scholarship and faculty in the classroom or clinical setting.

Initial Motivation to Becoming a Nurse

My motivation to become a nurse was simple: my desire to help people and communities in need. Having been a child in a household with both parents and a brother with cancer and disabilities, I grew up knowing there is a need for a healthcare system that works for all. At the age of 13, I started candy striping at an area hospital, and when I graduated high school, I was accepted into an accelerated medical school but changed my mind and followed my heart and chose the number one Gallup poll trusted profession—nursing. A career in nursing has given me the broadest, most flexible experience: direct patient care, research, education, and administration. Nursing was, without a doubt, the correct decision. I have had wonderful opportunities in my nursing career: I was a hospital floor nurse manager, practiced in-home care and public health, provided clinical care, and worked for three decades as a Professor in Nursing at the University of Delaware (UD) and George Mason University. Most importantly, I have been able to apply nursing skills to a career in elected office for 20 years.

I was raised on a farm with a grandmother who had an eighth-grade education. As the oldest daughter among eight children, she was tasked with working long hours in a field behind a mule. She later tragically became a young widow. Thus, she always said the most important thing a woman could have was an education and to never depend on anyone else for success. Her advice motivated me to become a first-generation college graduate. My grandmother was an early mentor, who inspired me to become a nurse and was a source of support during those days of nonstop classes and exams. She always said that a career in nursing was a lifetime profession of helping others, and she was right. My grandmother encouraged me to complete my PhD in Nursing and Health Care Administration. My passion for helping those in need is as strong as ever as the Lt. Governor of Delaware.

Decision to Pursue Higher Education

My personal higher education journey began with a Bachelor of Science in Nursing (BSN) degree from Thomas Jefferson University in 1986. I worked in America's first hospital, Pennsylvania Hospital in Philadelphia. There, I practiced in maternal health and was a certified childbirth educator. My husband was in the military and transferred to a base in South Carolina. This is when I first discovered how essential nurses are in policymaking spheres. I was working with mentally ill homeless veterans and minority communities without access to health services at the time, and I witnessed the necessity for nurses to be advocates for their patients. Therefore, it is key for nurses to be at the policy table to give these invisible, forgotten communities a voice.

I continued on to complete my Master of Science in Nursing (MSN), focused as a Clinical Nurse Specialist in Community Health Nursing at the Medical University in South Carolina. My interest in politics began while working with underserved residents at the same time I was completing my master's degree. A surprise to many is how I got assigned to "nurses in politics" for a yearlong assignment and focus on my issues class in the MSN program. I was late to class, and all other various topics were assigned, and I really wanted to cover the homeless, but instead I got the one topic nobody wanted - nurses in politics and policymaking. It was a life-changing, eye-opening assignment that became my career and changed my life. Therefore, words of wisdom were applied here: "*Always see the glass as half full versus half empty.*" For the next year, I worked at a couple of hospital units in maternal child transitional nursery in childbirth education.

When I entered the doctoral program in Nursing and Health Care Administration at George Mason University, I was the youngest applicant at the age of 25. I had the minimum 3 years of clinical experience, but there were days where I clearly was the youngest, carrying a backpack versus my classmates with a briefcase. During my educational experience in the doctoral program, I literally picked up the phone and created internships with the U.S. Secretary of Department of Health and Human Services (DHHS), Secretary's Commission on Nursing, and a Senate Fellow for Senators Cochran's and Kennedy's offices and worked with Dr. Hazel Johnson-Brown, who was my PhD advisor at George Mason University. She encouraged me to become involved politically so nurses can be at the table, not on the menu. Dr. Johnson-Brown was the leader of the Army Nurse Corps and the first Black female general in the Army. Her legacy continues to inspire me.

I became involved with my local city government, the League of Women Voters, and a federal health clinic. My work allowed me to be in the field and keep in touch with people on the ground. I went on to volunteer with nonprofit and civic organizations, and joined professional associations.

To complete my studies, I was appreciative of getting Nurse Training Act (Title VIII) funds, and as a student I taught in the undergraduate and graduate nursing lab. It was during this time that I discovered my passion for teaching. Little did I know that I would not go directly back into clinical for policy, but that I would spend a few years teaching in the classroom before taking a leap of faith to run for office

As Lieutenant Governor, my political priorities remain the same: to improve the lives of many citizens who lack life's necessary resources by crafting, sponsoring, and implementing policies that target at-risk groups. Wearing my public health nurse "hat," I have an interest in improving the services available to vulnerable populations such as the homeless, teen moms, people with substance use disorder (SUD), the mentally ill, and those with diabetes.

My Greatest Source of Satisfaction

The greatest satisfaction that I find in my work as a professor of nursing is linking scholarship, education, and clinical practice into policy changes that impact the state's overall health and healthcare workforce. For example, in the case of chronic disease management, I link students and community health workers with at-risk vulnerable clients and yield research that shows significant insurance costs savings and improved health outcomes. I am a practicing Full Professor with a scholarship portfolio of over $50 million in grants/research, and I teach undergraduate and graduate didactic and clinical courses, including leading students during the COVID surge. I am very proud to be the first faculty member of the School of Nursing at UD to receive the UD Excellence in Teaching Award. I also oversee the DE Medical Reserve Corps of over 2000 Delaware volunteers. My focus is inspiring more nurses to work in public health and policymaking while making a positive impact on Delawareans' lives. What I enjoy most about being a nurse is helping others in need, especially people with SUD, the homeless population, and veterans suffering with post-traumatic stress disorder (PTSD) and suicidal ideation.

As Lieutenant Governor, I am most fulfilled when I help pass bills relating to healthcare in Delaware. One of my greatest achievements is being the Chair of the Behavioral Health Consortium (BHC), to address mental health and SUD as legislated in 2017. The BHC is a collaboration of stakeholders including patients, families, providers, advocates, and government agencies. The goal is to improve the resources and structures of the statewide "cradle to grave" mental health and SUD system to reduce overdose fatalities and advance health outcomes through prevention, education, treatment, and community support. Bringing people together and building consensus has been essential in my policymaking role. Consensus building is a skill nurses possess and is critical to create an equitable healthcare system. But any goals or accomplishments will come with adversity and challenges. Nothing will change until we raise awareness of the opioid crisis and develop successful strategies and policies to prevent and effectively treat SUD.

My Current Focus

My current focus as Lieutenant Governor is cost and access to health care, behavioral health, business/job creation, education reform/early education, women's health, chronic care and quality of life, and disaster preparedness. The cost of healthcare is an important factor in determining when and how frequently people access healthcare. The rising costs of going to the nurse practitioner (NP) or a medical doctor (MD) for care and medications can have a negative impact on those struggling to make ends meet. More importantly, it can lead to detrimental health outcomes when an elderly patient skips an expensive but critical medication or avoids seeking treatment because they can't afford to see a provider. I also oversee the Lt. Governor's Challenge for physical and mental health. I focus on places where individuals work, play, and pray. I believe that frequent and preventative healthcare, nutrition, and lifestyle management are essential to preventing disease and minimizing the effects of illness.

I am committed to improving Delaware's response to disaster management and preparation. It's hard to predict the next natural disaster, or even a global pandemic, but there is much we can do as healthcare providers, governmental officials, and citizens to improve our response to potential threats and to address the critical workforce. Policy-making is key here. Mitigating the impact of a natural disaster by assuring hospitals and healthcare providers have the training, resources, and experience to respond timely and effectively is one of my main priorities as Lieutenant Governor. During the COVID-19 pandemic, I co-chaired the DE Pandemic Resurgence Advisory Committee. I was hands-on as a nursing faculty member with doctorate and undergraduate students doing COVID testing, vaccines, and mental health follow-ups.

Telehealth (TH) is a solution to improve access to healthcare, and fortunately we had TH available in Delaware before COVID. I was a prime sponsor of Delaware's law for telehealth after a nurse lobbied me on behalf of a patient who had a move-ment disorder and could not travel to his doctor's offices. I worked with nurses, students, and other health leaders to help pass the bill and overcome resistance from the insurance industry. Little did we know that this piece of legislation would play a critical role during the COVID pandemic.

I also look toward the future of our profession. I believe that as mentors and role models, it is incumbent upon all of us to share our knowledge, skills, and abilities. Mentoring the next generation of nurses is essential to building a highly professional workforce best prepared to assure the highest quality of care and care delivery.

I was the only healthcare professional and nurse in the Delaware General Assembly during my legislative years. During this time I was the prime sponsor of important health bills and participated on task forces such as the necessary code changes for the state's Health Exchange as a result of the federal Affordable Care Act (www.health-care.gov), the Governor's Cancer Council, and the Health Fund Advisory (Master Tobacco Settlement Committee). I have worked on numerous licensure/scope-of-practice, public health, and environmental policies. These policy issues have included occupational health, substance abuse prevention and treatment, cancer, minority health, early childhood education, prescription assistance, and end-of-life care deci-sions. I found that having a nursing background is extremely valuable in influencing a wide variety of policy issues.

I have sponsored and cosponsored a range of legislation as a member of the house and senate Health, Education, Transportation, Veterans Affairs, Agriculture, Natural Resources and the Environment, Homeland Security, Community and County Affairs, and Insurance committees. Chronic illness is a major issue for Delaware, as it is for the nation. I sponsored legislation to establish a blue-ribbon task force to analyze the problem of chronic illness and develop policy recommen-dations. The task force identified strategies including disease standards of care for health professions, improved communication between insurers and providers, out-reach to the at-risk communities, and the use of disease management approach with Medicaid patients and among the business community.

I was the prime sponsor of a variety of cancer screening, treatment, and education bills. This group has completed a comprehensive assessment and is now tackling high cancer mortality rates. I am pleased to say that the cancer incidence and rates have dropped since the creation of this body. The state has implemented the consortium's many recommendations, including establishing a free treatment program for cancer patients who lack insurance, adding statewide caseworkers, and creating screening programs.

Treating serious disease doesn't always require a prescription. I spoke up and supported alternative therapies, such as art and music therapy, and encouraged health insurance pay for these effective treatment options. As the wife of a veteran, I am most aware that many who served unfortunately have high suicide rates triggered by PTSD from their combat experiences, and benefit from these alternative therapies.

I am working on some exciting initiatives and projects that aim to improve the health, education, and safety of Delaware. For example, I lead the Veterans PTSD Challenge and the Lt. Governors Challenge for Physical and Mental Health, and I co-chaired the Healthy Lifestyles Committee. In addition, I chair the Early Childhood Learning Taskforce. These programs are designed to engage clientele to address problems that have been frequently overlooked and undertreated. Beyond healthcare initiatives, I am engaged in programs to make Delaware a safer community, with an emphasis on a compassionate approach to the incarcerated transitioning back into society, presiding over the Board of Pardons.

Many of these initiatives address problems that are not unique to Delaware. As a small state, we have the opportunity to engage with our communities, local institutions, schools, and healthcare facilities. This positions us to react effectively at the individual level. As the previous Chair of the Lt. Governors Association, and current Democratic Chair of the Lt. Governors Association, I see how nurses and nursing students shape solutions that impact the 50 states as well as territories, and showcase best practices that improve safe, healthy living by promoting effective policies that boost responsiveness to our greatest challenges from opioid abuse, mental and behavioral health, and at-risk youths.

Words of Wisdom

What have I learned as a legislator that can help other nurses who are seeking to influence policy? You must communicate in emails, phone calls, letters, etc., if you want to make a change. We have two ears and one mouth; use them wisely and in proportion. It is important that you are prepared when meeting with elected officials. Have a one-page fact sheet to leave behind, and be prepared to summarize your issue and offer potential solutions and courses of action in less than 5 minutes.

Getting involved in politics was my path and could be yours, too. As you take the journey of your nursing education at all levels, remember that there are many other ways you can make a change in your community outside of politics. Participating in professional associations, being involved in a taskforce, or exercising your expertise and voice about important issues do make a difference.

Life as an elected official has been better than I could have imagined. Though it has taken some time away from my family and scholarship, it has been worthwhile. I encourage other nurses to consider how they might serve the public, including running for elected office. The fact is that out of all professions, nurses have the best skill set to run for office. We're problem solvers, accustomed to hearing both sides. That's politics. It's about a tug-of-war over resources. According to a 2022 Gallup poll, nurses are ranked the most trustworthy occupation for the 20th straight year. The public needs elected government officials that they can trust, especially considering how polarizing the political climate is right now.

Belonging to professional organizations, attending hearings, getting to know your elected officials, and writing letters/emails to share your ideas and problems are all ways to connect with your local government. Nurses need to communicate with policymakers at the local, state, and national levels. Professional organizations and the academic settings have relationships with government affairs teams in a legislative committee or regulatory hearing. If nurses don't speak up on health care issues, who will? Physicians? Hospital associations? Insurers? If nurses don't speak up, legislators will only hear from other groups. Increasing your influence by working with a group or a coalition is an extremely effective strategy. Learn from your failures and get back up when knocked down. Remember, your attitude will determine your altitude. I hope that you consider the impact you will have in the nursing profession if you decide to get involved in the world of politics and policymaking.

CHAPTER 25

The Advocate Narrative

Lydia D. Rotondo, DNP, RN, CNS, FNAP

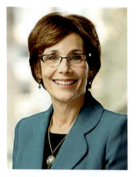

Initial Motivation to Become a Nurse

A love of science, a strong desire to make an impact, and motivation to be part of a team have served me well over a four-decade nursing career. They were not necessarily at the forefront of my mind when I entered college. My nursing education at a Jesuit university brought rich, challenging, and wide-ranging coursework in philosophy, theology, and social as well as hard sciences, all of which expanded my worldview and inspired me to pursue a life of significance in service to others. A career in nursing has provided myriad opportunities to achieve this goal.

There were no healthcare professionals in my family. I did not have any healthcare volunteer experience or receive any direction from a high school guidance counselor about pursuing nursing. In a somewhat unorthodox way of selecting an area of study, I chose the university I wanted to attend first, and then decided to apply to the nursing school within that university because of my interest in human biology. Once I matriculated, however, I quickly realized that my undergraduate experience was preparing me for a career that would offer diverse opportunities for contribution not only as a clinician but also as a leader, advocate, scholar, and educator. Engaging in bioethics debates in class, attending the Department of Health and Human Services hearings on Capitol Hill, and developing my nursing professional identity through the lens of Dorothea Orem's self-care theory that guided the nursing curriculum expanded my understanding of nursing's importance and reach. By the end of my freshman year, I was excited that I had fortuitously chosen a career that would provide a lifelong opportunity for growth and contribution.

Entry to Practice

I entered practice as a new graduate working in a surgical intensive care unit. At the time, nurse residencies or transition to practice programs did not exist. In such a high-stakes and intimidating setting, my early months as a registered nurse were simultaneously terrifying and exhilarating. I was a sponge seeking out every resource I could find to expand my knowledge and hone my skills. I was fortunate to have three exceptional staff nurse mentors who guided my development and modeled excellence. They were expert clinicians, strong communicators, staunch patient advocates, and wonderful teachers. Their impressive knowledge of pathophysiology and the therapeutic management of critical illness, combined with their commanding confidence in delivering patient-centered care was inspiring. Their examples set a standard of nursing excellence that I have spent my career emulating and ignited my desire for lifelong learning.

Decision to Pursue Higher Education

I have always believed that education provides a pathway for self-discovery and future opportunity. After working for 3 years as a staff nurse in a surgical intensive care unit at a university-affiliated medical center in Washington, DC, I moved to Philadelphia, where I practiced in cardiac surgical critical care and pursued a master's degree in advanced nursing practice. Two decades later, having had diverse professional experiences in leadership and practice roles as a master's prepared nurse, I realized that additional education would better prepare me for the increasing complexity of the healthcare environment and potentially offer new professional possibilities. I decided to pursue a terminal degree in nursing practice to achieve the highest level of education within my discipline in order to maximize my professional contributions at a very exciting time in nursing.

Educational Path and the Reasoning Behind That Decision

In the early 1980s, there were limited options for graduate study in critical care nursing practice. The acute care nurse practitioner role had not yet emerged, and clinical nurse specialist (CNS) programs in adult health did not offer a critical care specialization. Fortunately, the graduate school I attended started a critical care CNS program the year I applied, and I was fortunate to be in the second graduating cohort. With CNS coursework in advanced pathophysiology, pharmacology, and clinical management of critical illness, I began to more closely collaborate with colleagues from many disciplines to improve care delivery within complex health systems and to support the professional development of other critical care nurses.

Two decades later, I was working in a thoracic and vascular surgery practice developing clinical management programs for a variety of populations and participating in translational research. I realized that I would benefit from additional education to help me adapt randomized controlled studies to our practice populations as well as evaluate and disseminate the outcomes of our innovative clinical work. Initially, I explored PhD education, having never heard of the Doctor of Nursing Practice (DNP) degree. During a PhD program open house, one of the attendees asked about the DNP, which piqued my interest. Soon thereafter, I looked into the DNP curriculum and I realized that pursuing the practice doctorate would best advance my professional goals. I looked forward to applying my education to my advanced nursing practice as a member of an interprofessional team.

The following year, I researched several DNP programs, examining their websites and any additional promotional materials. I spoke with program directors and, through personal networking efforts, reached out to graduates from several programs to learn more about their DNP education experience. I then identified the program(s) that would best meet my educational needs. This important pre-work before applying to DNP programs was critical for me and will be for you too. The decision to pursue doctoral study—at any point in one's career—requires a clear purpose (your why), strong commitment, and deep internal motivation. Education at any level is an investment, and what you get out of it will be largely based on what you put into it. Therefore, learning as much as you can about the program of study and its alignment with your professional goals is critical. Equally important is finding the right program to support your success and the professional transformation that comes with doctoral study.

Mentors

For the first few years of my career, I was fortunate to have several experienced staff nurse mentors. Since that time, however, I have not had specific individuals who have guided my career path. That being said, over the years I have sought advice from many individuals who have expanded my thinking and others who have generously shared their expertise and insights. Nursing is a profession that offers many unanticipated opportunities. Being receptive to new possibilities can be fostered by observing role models and reaching out to them and others for advice and guidance. One of the benefits of seeking additional education is the network of faculty and peers you establish, which serves as an invaluable resource throughout your career.

Milestones

Several important milestones have influenced the trajectory of my career. During my sophomore year in college, my mother was diagnosed with metastatic lung cancer. I was faced with the difficult choice of returning home to be with my mother and family or remaining in school. With my mother's encouragement, I stayed in school commuting home to New York every other weekend to be with her. This personal experience instilled a deeper commitment to my chosen career by providing a firsthand appreciation for the importance of nurses in the lives of patients and their families when they are most vulnerable. My education also provided a refuge from the immense personal pain of watching my mother die, powerless to change the outcome but determined to ameliorate her suffering by using my nursing knowledge to advocate for adequate pain management and palliative care. My mother died 6 weeks before I graduated from college. As the selected graduation speaker for the school of nursing, I dedicated my remarks to my mother, whose support and belief in me had sustained me in college and left me with a strong desire to be present in the lives of others facing critical illness.

The pursuit of graduate education was another important milestone. Additional education expands one's expertise as well as provides the opportunity for critical self-reflection. During my master's program, my network of interprofessional colleagues grew significantly, and I was immersed in a vibrant academic nursing environment with leading nursing researchers and trailblazers. It was during this time that I became aware that advancing the discipline of nursing through education, leadership, and scholarship was a vital dimension of professional nursing practice. This provided the foundation for my future leadership roles and nursing professional development activities in my area of specialization. It also laid the foundation for future doctoral education.

Receiving a doctorate in nursing practice was the most impactful professional milestone of my nursing career. The famous expression, "Luck is what happens when preparation meets opportunity," aptly describes the professional opportunities that followed the completion of my DNP program. Six months after graduation, I relocated to Rochester, New York and began teaching in the DNP program of a school of nursing that was part of an academic health center. Six months later, I became the director of the DNP program director and the following year I was asked to serve as interim associate dean for education and student affairs. After serving in an interim capacity for one academic year, I was appointed as the permanent associate dean and have led the education mission in that role for the past 7 years and been the DNP program director for the past 8 years. Serving in these two leadership roles has brought tremendous professional satisfaction and fulfillment. My professional lens has shifted in recent years from a focus on individual achievement to advancing the profession of nursing by preparing the next generation of nurses.

Barriers and Strategies to Navigate Them

Encountering barriers is part of the human condition. I have learned that when I face barriers, whether individual or in my role as an academic leader, my first response is to reflect on the situation. It may seem counterintuitive to take a pause as opposed to pushing through obstacles. Certainly, perseverance and tenacity are necessary for success. However, reflection is a powerful tool that helps you examine the motivation for your actions as well as your understanding of the source (situation/individual/system) of the resistance. Reassessing and inviting other perspectives when facing obstacles are critical to overcoming barriers or finding alternative or incremental steps to achieve your goals. I have also learned that facing organizational or structural barriers is part of challenging the status quo. New ideas rarely emerge from looking in the rearview mirror. Using the same approach of critical self-reflection, environmental assessment, and leveraging others is essential for implementing organizational change, fostering innovative thinking, and generating novel solutions for practice problems.

Current Focus

As an academic nursing leader, my current focus is on creating transformational academic programs to prepare graduates for 21st-century healthcare. Implementing competency-based education throughout undergraduate and graduate nursing programs is a key priority. Another critical area is leveraging education technology to create reimagined learning experiences and environments that reflect the complexity and interdependencies of contemporary healthcare. Recognizing nurses as knowledge workers living in a digital age, it is critical that nursing education, at every level, incorporate digital innovation to prepare students as systems thinkers and lifelong learners.

Another important focus of my current professional work emerges from a deep commitment to advancing DNP education and promoting DNP practice. Completing ongoing evaluation of the DNP curriculum ensures that our graduates are well prepared as practice leaders and clinical scholars. Specific areas of DNP program innovation that I am currently focusing on are building an integrated Health Systems Science curriculum in a seamless post-baccalaureate DNP curriculum and expanding DNP coursework on the philosophical and theoretical foundations of nursing in the area of practice knowledge development.

Along with curriculum development, I actively support DNP practice by engaging with local health system leaders and promoting the specialized knowledge and skills that DNP-prepared nurses bring to the practice environment. Guiding DNP students to develop scholarly projects that reflect the strategic priorities of their practice setting is a powerful way to demonstrate the value of DNP preparation. Advocacy for DNP practice also includes meeting with state-level policymakers and regulatory agencies to eliminate barriers to DNP education and practice.

Finally, disseminating scholarly work related to my specific areas of interest including academic innovation and DNP education is an important professional responsibility. This can be achieved through publication in print/online journals, presentations, and other outlets. Dissemination is an important professional responsibility. Contributing to the ever-growing body of nursing knowledge can be useful to others as well as advance the national dialogue on emerging issues and opportunities.

Future Goals

My future goals are rooted in a professional obligation to strengthen the capacity of our profession to improve the health of our country. This call to action is detailed in the two Future of Nursing reports (2011, 2021) sponsored by the National Academy of Medicine (formerly The Institute of Medicine) and published over the past two decades. I am eager to accelerate academic innovation leading to the development and dissemination of transformational teaching/learning practices in nursing and interprofessional education. These new educational approaches will prepare nurses for new roles and responsibilities in improving healthcare quality, promoting health and wellness for individuals and communities, and championing health equity. I will also continue my DNP advocacy efforts on the education, policy, and scholarly fronts in pursuit of the realized potential of the practice doctorate in nursing to positively impact the delivery and outcomes of healthcare and advance the nursing profession.

Greatest Source of Satisfaction in Your Work

I have always enjoyed the process of bringing a common vision to fruition. This requires a "beginning with the end in mind" approach—simultaneously balancing the details and incremental steps of a project while clearly remaining focused on the end goal. I have the privilege to engage in this type of work every day. Working with DNP students on designing scholarly projects, forging new academic-practice partnerships, building academic programs responsive to changing workforce needs, and leading a strategic plan for 21st-century nursing education are examples of my daily work that allow me to work synergistically with students and multidisciplinary colleagues.

Words of Wisdom to Nurses Considering Earning a Doctorate

When I meet with prospective DNP students, I emphasize that this is a very unique time for the nursing profession. As the largest segment of the healthcare workforce, nurses individually and collectively are well positioned to lead healthcare transformation. This bold vision, presented over a decade ago by the Institute of Medicine's landmark report (2011), has only gained urgency in the wake of a global pandemic. Doctoral education provides additional knowledge and skills for practicing leadership and changing agency. Creating innovative solutions for challenging healthcare problems, seeing opportunities to fill care gaps or improve healthcare quality exemplify the many ways in which doctoral education is professionally empowering. I urge prospective students to look at the scholarly projects of graduates from several DNP programs to appreciate the system-level changes that are resulting from nurses' doctoral work.

Doctoral preparation also increases an individual's sphere of professional influence. The impact of scholarly work just described is one way to achieve this. Additional DNP coursework in areas such as health policy, healthcare finance, informatics, quality and safety, systems leadership and change management, provides a strong foundation for clinical, executive, and emerging leadership and professional roles. Simply stated, nurses who hold doctoral degrees possess a valuable and versatile skill set to respond to the rapidly changing and highly complex healthcare landscape. Moreover, students repeatedly describe the personal transformation that occurs during doctoral education, which can lead to a professional awakening and new professional opportunities.

Finally, I encourage students to contextualize the introduction of the practice doctorate in nursing in 2006 as an exciting opportunity to be nursing trailblazers and standard bearers as first wave DNPs. As a nascent degree without an expected professional trajectory following graduation, DNP graduates can forge new professional paths and redefine existing roles, which expands nursing's impact and reach. In a real way, the promise of the practice doctorate in nursing is in the hands of today's graduates. While this realization may be daunting, it underscores the unprecedented opportunity to be on the frontier of redefined 21st-century nursing practice during a time when the need for nurses has never been greater.

Bibliography

Institute of Medicine (US) Committee on the Robert Wood Johnson Foundation Initiative on the Future of Nursing, at the Institute of Medicine. *The Future of Nursing: Leading Change, Advancing Health.* Washington, DC: National Academies Press; 2011.

National Academies of Sciences, Engineering, and Medicine; National Academy of Medicine; Committee on the Future of Nursing 2020–2030; Flaubert JL, Le Menestrel S, Williams DR, et al., eds. *The Future of Nursing 2020–2030: Charting a Path to Achieve Health Equity.* Washington, DC: National Academies Press; 2021.

CHAPTER 26

The Military Nurse Narratives

David Bradley, DNP, APRN, AGCNS-BC, CNOR ▪
Jose A. Rodriguez, DNP, JM, RN, APRN, CCNS, CNOR

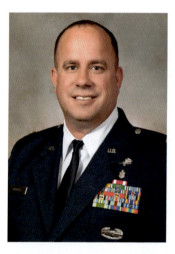

David Bradley, DNP, APRN, AGCNS-BC, CNOR

Lessons Learned #1: Have a Goal—A Goal Without a Plan Is Just a Dream

The views expressed in the presentation are those of the authors and do not necessarily reflect the official policy or position of the Uniformed Services University, the Department of Defense, or the United States Government.

I have always admired Abraham Lincoln because he never quit. He had a goal to save the union. "Lincoln did not feel compelled to justify or explain why the discrepancy existed; he simply acknowledged the situation and expressed his empathy through his few words. His convictions on the topic of slavery and equality were strong. But he acknowledged the challenges and the steps required to achieve his ultimate goal and continued trying even after many roadblocks. He knew that starting the next step would bring about progress toward his goal." (https://alderkoten.com/listening-first-a-lesson-from-lincoln/)

A lifelong goal was to earn my nursing degree and go as far as possible. Eventually, I achieved that goal and received my Doctor of Nursing Practice (DNP). It took me 26 years. The following is the story of my journey from enlisted army medic to Lt. Colonel United States Air Force (USAF) and the challenges I navigated to make my nursing goal a reality.

In high school, my mom would wake me up to help with her college math so she could meet the requirements for applying to nursing school. Though she never went to nursing school, she encouraged me to use my brains to help others. Funds were limited in my household, and my parents barely made ends meet. The financial resources for my college would need to come from elsewhere. The military offered the G.I. Bill, and this was my ticket to pay for college. I enlisted and entered the medical field as a combat medic. I was an Emergency Medical Technician (EMT) trained to tend to soldiers under fire. For a young man who wasn't afforded opportunities to travel in my youth, the travel of the military was heart-opening. After training at Fort Sam, Houston, I was stationed at Fort Irwin, California, for my first duty station. At Fort Irwin, I was a field medic for Foxtrot Troop of the Opposing Force (OPFOR). In other words, I was their medical support when the tank platoon rolled out to do simulated desert warfare. If anyone was injured, I stabilized them and got them to the hospital via helicopter.

Lessons Learned #2: Get Someone to Keep You Accountable, so the Work Gets Done in a Timely Manner

I'm a success today because I had a friend who believed in me, and I didn't have the heart to let him down.

—ABRAHAM LINCOLN

I was in the field for 17 days out of every month. While covered in dust in the desert, I thought of what I would be learning when I got into school and worked in a hospital. I worked hard to find time to complete a prerequisite online course because completing courses with my schedule was brutal. The courses I did find were concentrated courses. I tried to take two at once but withdrew because it was too much. I could only manage one course at a time. One of my friends, Mikey, encouraged me to keep at it. Start one course, finish it, and move on to the next one.

One day Mikey walked up to me and said, "Hey, let's go out for this Green to Gold Scholarship. If we get it, it's a full ride at a college of our choice where tuition and books are included; sometimes lodging. All we need to do is fill out the packet and get leadership support." I saw this opportunity to pursue higher healthcare education and, after some prayer, went for it! Mikey and I worked on our packets together. Wouldn't you know it, we both got picked up to go to school.

We have two ears and one mouth, and I worked hard at using them in proportion. This was critical during nursing school. I clearly remember listening to one of my favorite faculty, a retired Colonel, who shared with the class that he used the military to pay for his doctoral degree. Knowing that was a possibility fired me up! I had to figure out how to make that happen for me. He became a mentor from that moment on. He often shared stories of caring for service members during the day and studying in the evening and on weekends. He gave it to me in real world perspective: obtaining a doctoral degree would take time and knowing when to seize the available opportunities. With his continued direction and the support of friends, I earned my Baccalaureate degree in Nursing in 2003.

In the following 10 years, I transferred to the United States Air Force and earned a master's degree as an Adult-Gerontology Clinical Nurse Specialist. The Navy, Air Force, and Army provide for those who desire to obtain their advanced nursing degree as Certified Registered Nurse Anesthitists (CRNA), Family Nurse Practitioners (FNP), Psychiatric Mental Health Nurse Practitioners (PMHNP), and

Adult-Gerontology Clinical Nurse Specialists (AGCNS). Do your research and decide what works best for you and your family. Be willing to wait.

Lessons Learned #3: Surround Yourself With Others Who Are Encouraging

Graduate school was no joke. I developed a nervous tick from all the stress. But the beauty of it was that we were all in the same boat, and I found a group of encouraging and tenacious peers that helped me see it through. We made it a point to have families interact with each other because we were going through the same journey. We celebrated each other's successes and encouraged each other when we were down. Fellowship increases camaraderie and provides a network you can rely on if you or your family needs assistance during this tough academic season. I keep in contact with these colleagues and families to this day!

I felt grateful that the military provided me an opportunity to get a master's degree and go to a nationally recognized school. The networking opportunity is phenomenal. To this day, I reach out to the faculty to mentor me as an advanced practice nurse and as an officer.

Lessons Learned #4: Mentors Keep You Going When You Want to Quit and Show You How to Overcome Mountains When, in Reality, They Are Molehills

One of the mountains I faced was realizing many of my peers were graduating with their DNPs, but the Air Force only agreed to pay for my master's degree as an AGCNS. I witnessed many of my colleagues stay one extra year and graduate with a terminal degree. Not in my case. That hurt and made me bitter. My wife was unhappy that I was not content and challenged me to get over it and continue going after my dream of having my DNP. The caveat was that I had to do so in a way that would not impact our budget. I prayed about that and asked my mentors for wisdom.

Lessons Learned #5: You Will Make Time for What Is a Priority

REALITY AFTER GRADUATING WITH A MASTER'S DEGREE

I was a recent graduate and had to start a new job as a perioperative clinical nurse specialist in a Level 1 Trauma center. We found out our son had autism and had to go through a lot of rehabilitation. I was expected to sit for my certification test as a CNS, so I had to study many late nights. I was also expected to complete professional military training (promotion requirement), which took away my weekends for a year. My wife and I wanted to expand our family, so we were deep in the throes of learning the foster system; completing the required training to be certified, having a 3-month-old to take care of, having our house pristine for multiple unannounced visits, biological parent visits, and going to court. I tell you this to let you know what I was dealing with when I decided to start my DNP journey.

My Personal Plan to Promote Success

The first step I took was to talk to others who had earned their DNP and to others who were in school actively pursuing it. Next, I wanted to see what schools they recommended and what to expect. What was the lift? How hard would this be on my family and on fulfilling my work commitments? Once I had these details, I found a way for the military to pay for my continued education, using my CNS certification to sign up for a bonus. This substantial bonus came at the price of committing 4 more years to the military. My wife and I were okay with this because we had already communicated our family goal to be in the military for at least 20 years (to get the retirement). Knowing how much the bonus would cover, I compared the costs of different DNP programs. Affordability was not the only reason. I wanted an accredited program that my respected colleagues spoke highly of and were successful in.

> *Upon the subject of education, not presuming to dictate any plan or system respecting it, I can only say that I view it as the most important subject which we as a people can be engaged in.*
>
> —ABRAHAM LINCOLN

My DNP program was online, and several of faculty members in my current employment were alumni and willing to write recommendation letters. A friend who was 1 year ahead of me in my master's program was enrolled in the program and was willing to help me navigate the system regarding admission paperwork. I reached out to others, who knew my level of clinical expertise, also willing to write letters of recommendation.

You might ask, "Who can I reach out to?" I strongly encourage you to keep in contact with those who took the time to invest in you from previous life experiences. I had great success reaching out to leadership or colleagues from work or school faculty (Box 26.1).

Another important step includes back-planning to ensure you have enough time to address the administrative parts, especially writing the essay and completing the application. I knew an essay would be required, so I made sure I did not procrastinate. I put my best effort into putting words on paper to knock out a rough draft. I took the rough draft and went to individuals who would provide the brutally honest feedback needed. Boy, I cannot deny it hurt to see all the red ink, but I knew the intent was to improve the quality of my writing. I asked these individuals to read the essay prompt to ensure I addressed what was being asked. If I did not, I asked how they would address the critical areas of concern. Going back and forth

> **BOX 26.1 ■ Example Letter of Outreach**
>
> Good morning Dr. XX/Ma'am/Sir,
>   I hope this email finds you well. I have submitted your name to the *University of I CAN DO THIS* for a letter of recommendation. You will receive an email from *The University of I CAN DO THIS* Graduate School about instructions on how to submit an online recommendation letter (sometimes, the notification emails may arrive in the Junk Mail folder). The deadline to have this done is DATE, XXXX. For reference, I have attached my current CV. Thank you very much for your time and consideration. Have a blessed day!
>   Very respectfully,
>   David F. Bradley Jr.

with revisions took at least three to six weeks. All this effort was made to ensure that my response was substantial, concise, and written in an academic tone.

Give me six hours to chop down a tree, and I will spend the first four sharpening the ax.
—ABRAHAM LINCOLN

I found the application lengthy and overwhelming at first. But then I remembered that you can't eat an elephant all at once; you must do it in chunks. I put together a checklist that addressed all the parts and scheduled when I needed to complete them prior to the deadline. By doing this, my stress level was manageable, and I knew I was making progress.

Don't be afraid to look for a mentor change. Not all mentoring assignments work as they should. Perhaps a reference on changing mentors or preceptors. Try this source when your are considering changing mentors: https://www.togetherplatform.com/blog/should-you-change-your-mentor.

How to Make a Smooth Switch

Making a smooth transition between mentors takes a bit of work and finesse. You must be tactful but direct with the mentor you are leaving behind. They may not have been a good fit as a mentor, but you don't want to burn the bridge. They may still be a key contact at some other point in your career. Here are a few ways to switch mentors.

1. Write down the reason that the mentorship is not working out for you. Don't forget to add the steps you took to resolve the problems and the outcomes of your actions. Be tactful and professional in your comments.
2. Identify a new mentor match. This step depends on how your organization handles the mentor-mentee matching process. Mentoring software is often one of the best ways to ensure you get the right match. The software offers perimeters set by the mentoring program manager to cultivate suitable matches among mentors and mentees. Using these algorithms also saves time during the matching and introduction process.

3. Plan a professional goodbye. Even though things didn't work out between you and your mentor, it is important not to part ways on bad terms. Oftentimes, they can turn out to be a good resource in the future. Be professional and polite.

4. Practice gratitude. Even if the mentoring experience was not a good fit for you, it would still have served as a learning opportunity. Consider looking at the positives that you gained from it. Perhaps you can acknowledge that your goals need to be further refined. Or recognize that you gained some new confidence in standing up for yourself by recognizing you needed to find another mentor and doing something about it.

Communication: Keep your preceptor and mentor informed of your progress regularly, work ahead, answer discussion questions early, and schedule out carved time to address the complex assignments. This helped me plan with my family what time spent doing schoolwork would mean.

Keep your family informed of your progress. I did most of my schoolwork after putting the kids to bed. If I had an assignment that needed more time than expected, I would spend Saturday doing that, and Sunday would be devoted to family. Taking the time to decide on paid dividends. I had no issues making important family events and meeting my school deadlines.

Jose A. Rodriguez, DNP, JM, RN, APRN, CCNS, CNOR

Lessons Learned #7: Pick a Project That Is Relevant and Feasible to Do in a Short TimeFrame

To accomplish this, check your ego at the door and bring a humble attitude as you meet with your mentor for guidance. This is hard to do, but it's worth it. For my project to be completed in time, I was told I needed to "focus on the eyelash of a gnat." I was guided on the premise that I could take on the more significant projects once I graduated and obtained those three sexy letters behind my name (DNP). Each time I met with my mentor, I was challenged to consider the relevance behind my project and the implementation plan to complete it on time. I often walked away frustrated but determined to get it right. I am grateful I listened and was open to constructive feedback. I saw peers not graduate on time due to the magnitude of their projects. I also noticed that some never published their projects because they picked a topic that was not welcomed by any journal.

I am deeply grateful for my family, colleagues, and mentors who supported the journey. Please take these lessons I learned along the way to enlighten you along your doctoral degree journey. Hang in there and finish strong. We all believe in you.

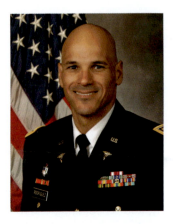

The views expressed in the presentation are those of the authors and do not necessarily reflect the official policy or position of the Uniformed Services University, the Department of Defense, or the United States Government

Since I can remember, I have always taken unique approaches to address life's challenges and make critical decisions. "Cookie cutter" solutions are rarely my first choice, and I always try to find answers that are not just effective but also efficient. I know I can't find all the answers in textbooks and that life experiences are essential when making important choices. The combination of knowledge and lessons learned has allowed me to choose the best path I believe will take me to my desired destination.

Early Career in the Service

I decided to pause my college studies and join the U.S. Army as a logistician. It was an unexpected decision and one my parents did not see coming. For me, it just felt right. Although having a source of income and college aid were reasons to join the military to help my parents, these were not the main reasons I joined. The truth is that I was not doing well or enjoying college life. I felt there was no purpose, and the worst part was that I did not know what to do. I was not motivated and had the feeling that something was missing. I was disappointed and, to some level, depressed for not performing and meeting my parents' expectations.

I was always considered a smart kid. During my high school years, I excelled in all my courses and graduated with a 3.95 GPA. I made sure to stay on track and meet any requirements to be accepted into any college program. I built a very competitive record, and like many of my classmates, it did not take much effort to enter the premed program at the University of Puerto Rico. I remember being excited about joining the program. My parents and my friends were excited too. My mom is a registered nurse, and her dedication to helping people inspired me to consider a healthcare career. But the excitement did not last long and, 5 months later, I found myself questioning my decisions and whether "living within the lines" was the right choice. One way or another, I knew I needed to find an answer.

I was born and raised in Puerto Rico, where family and friends expect you to go to school, graduate, find a job, get married, and have a family, all in that order, or as the famous singer John Mayer says in one of his songs, "they love to tell you to stay inside the lines." I knew the answer I was looking for was not in the books, and for some odd reason, I believed the U.S. Army had the answer. Unfortunately, my family thought the U.S. Army was a choice "outside the lines." I was not afraid of not following the so-called right track, and so I married my wife Alexandra and began my military career. However, my decision was tied to one condition that I set for myself: I would go back to college and not rest until I achieved the highest level of education. Looking back, I know now that I had no idea what I was saying, and perhaps I just said it to make myself feel okay with my decision to get married and join the military.

Moving to the mainland was not easy. I missed my family, and my wife missed hers. Homesickness hit us hard, but we knew it was the best decision for us. The language barrier was significant, and I understood if I wanted to grow personally and professionally, I needed to work to overcome the language barrier. A few months after arriving in Fort Hood, Texas, I decided to go back to college. Suddenly, I saw a purpose for going back to college. I felt motivated and excited to learn. I had no excuses this time. I had financial support from the military and, most importantly, the support of my wife. It was the beginning of my educational journey and perhaps the best decision of my life after marrying my wife.

Navigating Barriers

Balancing work, family, and college was not an easy task. It was challenging to find the time and energy to study, especially after a long workday. But I was motivated and had the support not only of my supervisors but also of my wife, which was and still is a crucial part of my success. After arriving at Fort Hood, I was continuously enrolled in college courses, focusing on introductory classes and science courses for the next 3 years. I decided not to enroll in any specific program. Instead, I wanted to prepare for something bigger while growing professionally and learning the English language. My initial efforts and sacrifices yielded great results right before ending my first military tour. I joined the Non-Commissioned Officer ranks after being promoted to Sergeant just 2 years after arriving in Fort Hood.

Milestones

After 3 years in Texas, I requested an overseas assignment as a condition to extend my contract in the military. I arrived in Hanau, Germany, and was assigned to an aviation support unit. Being overseas did not stop me from taking college courses, and I continued to enroll and complete courses online. The courses were helping me master the English language, and I improved my communication skills at work. I felt effective and productive and was no longer afraid or worried about language as a barrier; that wall had finally come down.

I was happy with my job and new unit. I had the privilege of collaborating and making friends with people from other specialties and learning from aviation experts. It was amazing to be near to all kinds of aircraft and see them perform daily. Likewise, it was also motivating to see many of my friends growing professionally and moving through the ranks. Every month someone in the unit was getting promoted, and I could not wait for my turn. Not having an aviation specialty made it harder to get promoted, and I knew I had to work hard to jump to the next rank.

Friends continued to get promoted as I waited. I was starting to get frustrated and doubting myself once again. I did all I could to get promoted, but my specialty was overstrength, and the open positions for the next rank were limited. I was not going to wait for a promotion that might never happen and needed help figuring out my next move. Perhaps an advisor, mentor, or coach could help me find an alternate path or show me the way. Ironically, the person I was looking for came to me without my asking or searching. This person became a great friend of my wife and myself and showed me a path that I had seen as impossible until then.

As a young sergeant, I remember looking up to the officers in my unit and dreaming about becoming one of them. With almost 5 years in the U.S. Army, I understood the many benefits commissioned officers enjoyed compared to non-commissioned officers. But without a bachelor's degree, I could only dream about becoming one of them. I understood that earning a bachelor's degree would not earn me a commission, but it was essential to becoming an officer.

I realized I needed to focus on a specific program to earn a bachelor's degree. I was not sure what program to complete, and the fact that I was overseas made it challenging to enroll in any science program. The clock was ticking, and my patience was running low. One day, my Staff Sergeant approached me with the key to the door that would lead to my dream of becoming a commissioned officer. He introduced me to nursing.

The key opened the door to participation in the Army Enlisted Commissioning Program (AECP), which was designed to allow any enlisted member to complete a nursing program in a school of choice while on active duty. Upon completing the program and successfully passing the boards, the enlisted soldier would be commissioned as an officer in the Army Nurse Corps. I knew this was my best chance at achieving my dream of earning a bachelor's degree and becoming an officer in the U.S. Army.

The path was long and full of obstacles. The most complex challenge was to find and become accepted into an accelerated nursing program (AECP). Because the AECP was a 2-year program, I was required to have completed enough basic college courses to finish the nursing program within 2 years. I realized then that all the long nights I spent studying for all the college courses since I arrived in Fort Hood and all the sacrifices made were about to pay off. I took 30 days of leave and flew to Puerto Rico. I was committed to finding a nursing program, applying, and being accepted before leaving the island and returning to Germany. It was not easy to complete the applications and interviews in just 30 days, but I did it. I left the island confident I would come back in the following summer to start the program.

After 30 days in Puerto Rico, I was eager to go back to Germany to build and submit the AECP application packet. I needed several letters of recommendation, personal documents, and the acceptance letter from the nursing school to complete the packet. Before I left Puerto Rico, the Dean of the School of Nursing told me that, if accepted, I should have a letter of acceptance upon my arrival in Germany. The anxiety was killing me, and I could not wait to go to the post office to pick up the mail and look for the letter.

Entry to Nursing Practice

The day after I returned to Germany, I received my letter of acceptance into the nursing program of the Interamerican University of Puerto Rico. To say I was excited is an understatement. It was "go" time. I had to take an official photo, make appointments to get recommendation letters, and request official transcripts, among other actions. I had great support from my family, friends, and colleagues. There were also a few "naysayers" who thought what I was trying to accomplish was impossible. But my confidence was at an all-time high, and I could not wait to hear the selection board's decision. When the selection board sent notice of my selection, the US was at war, and Operation Iraqi Freedom almost changed my plans. But very soon, I was back in Puerto Rico, starting nursing school.

Since the first day of nursing school, I fell in love with nursing education and the profession. I was like a sponge, soaking every piece of knowledge and experience from all my courses and clinical rotations. It was not easy, but this was a lifetime opportunity, and I needed to deliver. Organization, motivation, and resiliency were key factors while going to nursing school. Family support was crucial. Without my wife's support, I wouldn't be able to be the person I am today. Nursing school challenged me in so many ways. I discovered many skills and talents that I did not know I had, making me a better student, professional, father, and husband. It was a great experience and one I will never forget. I found my path by not following the "right track" others had defined for me, and I was ready to continue my journey as a nurse.

I graduated from nursing school, passed my nursing boards, and officially became a registered nurse. My first assignment was as a medical-surgical nurse in Moncrief Army Community Hospital in Fort Jackson, SC. Although it was a small medical facility, I acquired a significant amount of nursing experience and knowledge there. Like any novice, I made mistakes. Resiliency and great mentors were essential to move beyond those mistakes. Learning from these mentors helped me improve my critical thinking skills, practice, and, consequently, patient outcomes. For the first time in my military career, I was happy to go to work every morning.

While assigned to Fort Jackson, I became intrigued with surgical services and the role of a perioperative registered nurse. I loved the role and the high pace in the operating room. I wanted it, but had to do my homework to make sure that was the specialization I wanted. I spent time shadowing nurses in the operating room and asked a lot of questions. Every day spent in the operating room helped me realize that I wanted to be an operating room nurse. I also spent time in the psychiatric unit and the emergency room. Still, I felt great in the operating room, so I decided to request and enroll in the perioperative nursing course.

My assignment in Fort Jackson was short. Sixteen months after my arrival, I moved to Fort Sam Houston, TX, to complete the perioperative nursing course. During my training, I discovered that perioperative nursing was another world. There was a lot to learn about multiple surgical specialties associated with a significant number of processes, procedures, and specialized equipment. Again, coaching and mentorship helped me develop new nursing skills and improve others. It was a challenging learning environment, but one I came to love. In November 2007, I graduated from the Army Perioperative Course, and Carl Darnall Army Medical Center in Fort Hood, TX, was my first assignment as a perioperative nurse, the first of many experiences in the perioperative field. I spent the next 7 years learning everything I could about perioperative nursing in different locations, including one that I would never forget.

When I joined the military, I knew one day I would have to leave my family to support our country during times of war, peacekeeping, or humanitarian missions. It would not be honest to say that I was looking forward to that moment. But I was ready to take care of those who put their lives in danger so my family and others could be free. I departed for Iraq in support of Operation Iraqi Freedom. What I experienced while deployed changed me as a person and as a provider. Nothing could prepare me for what I saw every day in the operating room. Although I eventually got used to seeing people coming in lifeless or with fatal injuries, it took a lot of reflection and resilience to overcome the psychological stress and trauma I experienced during the first few weeks.

Milestones

Being thousands of miles away from my family in a hostile environment was difficult, but I would deploy again in a heartbeat. My passion for perioperative care grew tremendously while caring for soldiers and civilians in Iraq. I felt the urge to know more about perioperative nursing and how to improve it. Upon my return from Iraq, I became a Certified Perioperative Registered Nurse, and while studying for that certification, I thought about pursuing graduate education. The decision to pursue a graduate degree and become an advanced practice nurse triggered my academic addiction. It was also the beginning of that promise I made to myself when I joined the military in 1997—to achieve the highest education level.

During my tour in Fort Irwin, CA, from 2010 to 2012, I applied and got accepted to the Uniformed Services University of the Health Science (USUHS), Clinical Nurse Specialist Program. Academically, this master's program was the most challenging program I have ever done and the most rewarding. I completed the program in May of 2014, and it was yet another highlight and professional achievement in my career as a nurse.

Becoming an expert in perioperative care has allowed me to contribute to the practice of nursing and improve surgical outcomes. Being a Clinical Nurse Specialist has enabled me to operate at a higher level while developing and enhancing my clinical and leadership skills. I am thankful to the team at Womack Army Medical Center (WAMC), N.C., for the opportunity to share my knowledge and passion for 3 years as their Perioperative Clinical Nurse Specialist from 2014 to 2017. Together, we were able to improve the surgical services we provided while learning from each other.

Decision to Pursue Graduate Education

As a famous Spanish saying goes, *I always believe that I am an apprentice of everything and a master of nothing*, I was not done learning. Graduating from USUHS was just another step toward fulfilling my promise, and I was motivated to continue my academic journey toward a terminal degree. I decided to enroll in a DNP program at the University of Alabama in 2015 while assigned to WAMC. Meeting good mentors throughout my career, the support of my leadership, and a strong family continuously supported and encouraged my goal of completing a DNP. The 4-year DNP program felt like eight, and after many long nights and sacrifices, I stayed true to myself and fulfilled my promise to complete the program on time.

Earning a doctorate was a dream come true. I am the first in my family to achieve this level of education, and I am beyond happy. I am proud for not giving up when many people doubted me and with many obstacles along the way. Immediately after graduation, I received opportunities that I only used to dream of, such as teaching at a nursing school. I am proud to be part of and privileged to teach at the Uniformed Services University, Graduate School of Nursing in Bethesda, MD. I have met many friends and leaders who have contributed to my development as an educator and person. Teaching at USU has been a wonderful experience and one I will never forget.

Current Focus

Teaching at USU has challenged me to be more adaptable and creative. Transitioning from a clinical setting to an academic environment is not easy, and one must be open to criticism and learn. I am grateful and lucky to have a great team that encourages me to be better every day. I am proud to be part of an organization that invests in its members by providing many opportunities to develop personally and professionally to become better healthcare professionals and educators. It is why, as a faculty, I give 110% every time I step into the classroom.

To that end, and as the singer John Meyer says in one of his songs, "I believe the best of me is still hiding up my sleeve." So, once again, I found myself enrolling in yet another master's degree program. Since I became an advanced practice nurse, my focus has been infection control, prevention, and compliance. I believed that completing a Juris Master's in healthcare compliance could better prepare me to identify and solve healthcare compliance issues. In 2019, motivated by my boss, I decided to start the program at Liberty University.

Law school was complex and significantly different than nursing school. The academic language and writing were different, and readings were hard to digest. I used many learning strategies I acquired while enrolled at USU and the University of Alabama, which made tests and assignments much more manageable. Overall it was a challenging but rewarding program, which I completed and was conferred the degree of Juris Master. The best part of my experience was that as I acquired new knowledge, which I transferred directly to my students in the classroom since healthcare compliance is so relevant to the role of the Clinical Nurse Specialist.

Future Goals

My educational journey has been magnificent. But for now, I am putting a pause on enrolling in school but certainly not to learning. I want to dedicate more time to applying the knowledge I acquired to improving perioperative nursing practices and patient outcomes. My mission is to develop highly reliable organizations over the next few years. I believe there is a tremendous need to translate evidence into practice in many nursing specialties. There is so much to learn about published research focused on those objectives. My passion for nursing and helping others keep me going at work. The satisfaction of being an instrument for healing the sick and treating the wounded that I proudly do every day is invaluable, especially for the men and women who protect this country.

Words of Wisdom

I end my narrative with these thoughts:
1. Do not be afraid of living "outside the lines."
2. Books do not have all the answers.
3. Believe in yourself and surround yourself with people who care about and support you.
4. Find a mentor or coach that can be there for you in times of need.
5. Finally, do not forget your family. School and work will always be there, waiting. Spend time with those you love because family is the final piece of every one of your puzzles.

CHAPTER 27

The Systems Executive Narrative

Angelo Venditti, DNP, MBA, RN

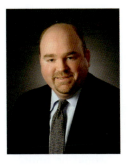

Entry to Practice

I never really wanted to be a nurse; after all, I was an athlete in high school, a manly man interested in sports, firefighting, and high-adrenaline activities like rapelling. Nursing never crossed my mind through high school; what I did know was that I wanted to care for others in some way, and I always thought I would do that as a paramedic or firefighter. I just didn't see nursing as exciting enough for me, and honestly I didn't see it as a profession where men fit in. On the other hand, I grew up spending a lot of time with my grandmother, who was a nurse and I always found interest in the stories she would tell and the work that she did.

The night of my senior year high school football banquet, after wrapping up an undefeated season as national champions, for some reason I was extremely thirsty; by the time the banquet was over I had drunk over seven pitchers of soda, and on my 1.5-mile drive home I had to stop and get a drink at a convenience store. The next day I went to see my primary care physician, who ordered a series of blood tests. It was clear I had a bladder infection, right? Wrong! I was diagnosed with Type I, insulin-dependent diabetes. This new diagnosis caused me to lose a significant amount of weight, which I assumed was the post-football season weight drop that often occurred. Needless to say, the weight loss and complexity of this new diagnosis shifted my focus from playing football in college to managing my newfound lifestyle and looking for what was next for me.

I am sure we can all relate. There are certain experiences and certain people that we cross paths with that change our perspective on life. When I was diagnosed with diabetes and in the hospital, I met a nurse named Maureen (not her real name) who I will never forget. She was an outstanding educator, she was fun, and it was evident from the moment you met her that she was in charge. I don't think I consciously recognized the impact she had on me becoming a nurse until much later. Suffice it to say that she is one of the influences that steered me toward nursing. As I grappled with filling my time in the hospital, a close friend brought me a paramedic book because I had expressed interest in learning more about pre-hospital work.

I started reading and spent the next week in the hospital immersed in this textbook. This was a dramatic turn of events for me. I was a "C" student at best and never really read much due to my struggles with reading comprehension, but I was hooked and knew then that I wanted to be a paramedic and firefighter. To make a long story short, I got out of the hospital and enrolled in paramedic school, preparing for a big move to a city to be a professional firefighter. After paramedic school, I accepted a local position and began applying for professional firefighting jobs. I learned very quickly that it was difficult, if not impossible, to land a firefighting job with a type I diabetes diagnosis. I needed plan B, and my parents convinced me to go to nursing school. I enrolled in our community college nursing program and, as they say, the rest is history.

I approached my first opportunity in nursing knowing that I *only* wanted to work in the Emergency Department (ED). My long-term goal was to become a flight nurse. I knew that becoming a flight nurse would be highly competitive and require joining a long waitlist of the best and brightest in the field. I stumbled along the way when I didn't pass my state licensing exam the first time, forcing me to move into a nursing assistant role on an orthopedic medical/surgical unit. My experience there was both enlightening and difficult. I was one of the few males on the floor, and everyone counted on me for heavy lifting. I knew that this was not a long-term plan for me and luckily, my time there would be limited. I passed my state exam and looked to quickly move onto the next department I could call home.

Unfortunately, the ED did not have any open positions. Imagine a time when the ED did not have any openings. I decided to take a position in adult intensive care. Now this was not an easy decision because I was steadfast, believing I was an ED nurse through and through, and I *did not* see the intensive care unit (ICU) in my future. In hindsight, this was one of the greatest experiences of my life. To say that I learned a lot is an understatement. I am talking about the clinical, technical, and most importantly the leadership and human skills that I learned during my time in the ICU. The experiences you encounter as a nurse in a busy ICU are experiences that you will never forget. This is where I developed the ability to have crucial conversations, troubleshoot life-threatening issues, and triage many high-risk challenges. Because the environment demanded a team-based approach, I developed relationships that would transform into lifelong friendships, mentors, and confidants.

These great mentors influenced my decision to pursue advanced degrees. Initially, because I wanted to be a flight nurse, I never thought that getting a Bachelor of Science in Nursing (BSN) was required, and so I was not all that interested in education. When I realized that I wanted to move into leadership, I knew that higher education would be required. I began to feel an internal drive to educate myself. Maybe it was wanting to feel like I belonged, or perhaps it was my competitiveness that compelled me to take the next step and enroll in a registered nurse (RN) to BSN program. I was surrounded by great mentors who were willing to share their stories to help build my confidence. The decision to pursue a degree while working full time and raising a family is a scary one.

Today, more than ever, there are a variety of programs that meet the needs of different people. These are all designed so the return to higher education does not have to be so intimidating, and there is probably a program for everyone. When I made my decision, I was thoughtful about cost, time to completion, and the mix of in-person, classroom, and online learning. For me, other considerations were the support my employer offered toward my education and finding a program that would be my partner relating to cost and payment. I was able to find a program that offered an accelerated degree with deferred tuition. As a result, I did not have to pay tuition until I had my grades at the end of the semester and could make payments then. This was a game changer because I was intent on not accumulating debt.

As I previously stated, I was determined not to incur significant, if any, student debt as a result of my college education. I feel I chose wisely and went to our local community college to pursue my paramedic and nursing degrees. I understood that this was likely not my last stop, and I knew that many employers had tuition benefits that I could take advantage of once I was employed full time. Additionally, I wanted a quality education so that I could be confident I was going to be knowledgeable and proficient in caring for patients. To sum up my choice succinctly, I was looking for education with value, low cost, and high quality, something we learn about extensively in healthcare.

Mentors

I have met so many people who have impacted my trajectory along the way that it is difficult to be comprehensive. I was fortunate enough to be brought up in a supportive home, something I have never taken for granted. My two most profound mentors are my parents. My father was a factory worker when I was young, and I can remember him working long days and then going to school to be a police officer in the evenings. This is where I developed my work ethic and loyalty to family. Even after he finished school, he would work two to three jobs to make sure we never went without any of the necessities in life. He was rigid about basic rules like respect, hard work, and family, but at the same time he was not overly critical when I made a mistake. He would require mistakes to be fixed but wasn't overly upset when things didn't go perfectly. To this day, I have the utmost respect for how hard he worked, the values he instilled in our family, and his dedication to his family.

My mother was a beautician and self-employed for as long as I can remember. In a few simple words, she is kind, thoughtful, and understanding. She has always been supportive and is one of the most loving people you will ever meet. I can't tell you the countless freebees she has given over her years to people she knew just needed some level of inspiration at that point in time. She is extremely forgiving, hardworking, and conscientious in everything she does. She takes pride in her work and wants to please people. She is extraordinarily uncomfortable when she believes someone is upset with her and worries a lot about the impression she leaves on others. We like to call my mother "the Mayor" because you can't go anywhere in our town without her talking and often hugging someone. She doesn't do it for show or in a loud way; she just cares about people and would do *anything* to help.

I reflect often on how I was raised, and at this point in my life I am confident that it was the combination of these two individuals that made me the person I am today. I do a lot of introspective thinking and often reflect upon how I believe I have the right balance of the two of my parents, and it serves me well to be in a position of success. I don't say that arrogantly; I say that with the utmost respect and admiration for them.

Additional people guided me on the path I have taken in life. It is rare to have a conversation with me without a football reference being included at some point. I had the privilege to play for one of the best high school football coaches to ever coach the game. He is the second-most winning coach in Pennsylvania history and has earned many state titles and several national titles. More importantly, he was an amazing human being. He lived the way he expected his athletes to live: with faith, family, and football. Many think he taught football, those of us he coached know he taught leadership, perseverance, and teamwork. Our team had no business winning! We are a small town, small kids, and relatively unremarkable. It was because of our coach that boys became men in our town, and it was because of him that men got educated. We can count the number of kids from our town who went on to play in the National Football League (NFL) on one hand. You need a calculator to count the kids who got a college scholarship, and free education. Coach lived to help others, lived for his family, and lived for kids, his team, and his community. Now if that didn't help mold me into who I am today, I don't know what did.

Milestones

There were several significant milestones throughout my career. My entry into nursing leadership, after only practicing for 2 years, was a profound achievement in so many ways. It was huge in that, from a competitive standpoint, I was selected for the position over many others who were clinically more qualified. Being the assistant manager of a very busy trauma ICU at the age of 25 propelled my career. While I can speak of many great experiences as the assistant manager, I think it is critical to point out one significant consequence of my early entry into leadership. As I look back, I am able to lead because I was taught leadership early on by virtue of the influences in my life. At the same time, what I missed were critical experiences as a direct care professional nurse that would have been extremely valuable along my journey. I now often tell people that it was a mistake to jump from the bedside so fast. If I were to give myself advice today, I would tell myself to take the time to learn the intricacies of the profession in order to become a better coach along the way.

Next, achieving my BSN was critical in so many ways. It gave me confidence that I could manage furthering my education while having a career in a very complex and demanding profession. For me, it was the gateway into steady inquiry and gave me a hunger to learn more. Also, pursuing my BSN taught me more about the nursing profession and helped make clear the diversity of roles and the impact that nurses have across the world. Achieving my BSN made me proud to be a professional nurse and gave me the confidence to continue to grow. I think achieving my BSN also gave me closure and commitment toward nursing.

Finally, I couldn't talk about milestones without mentioning my wife. Marrying my wife is by far the greatest milestone of my entire life, both personally and professionally. While being married has improved my personal life, my wife has had a significant impact on my professional trajectory as well. As anyone grows in leadership, it is important to stay grounded, humble, and insightful about the decisions you make and how those decisions impact others. Additionally, it is a mandate that you have a strong support system to help along the way. You will need advice, you will need someone to keep it real, and you will need someone to listen to you when the going gets tough. For me, my support system is my wife, and without her I would have turned out to be a totally different person. I could go on and on about my wife and how special she is, but suffice it to say that she is and always will be my best friend, my trusted advisor, and the greatest influence on my life.

Decision to Pursue Higher Education

I was never a great student, in high school especially, and I often wondered if I was dyslexic because I never had great reading comprehension. As I approached my adult learning journey, this struggle gave me great anxiety, and I definitely lacked self-confidence. Lack of self-confidence and fear of failure almost caused me not even to start college in the first place. I would love to say that after my BSN and MBA, I was all "fixed" as I entered my Doctor of Nursing Practice (DNP), but that is far from true. Throughout my program I struggled with not believing I could actually achieve a doctorate because I was a "C" student and no one in my family had graduated college, let alone achieved a doctorate. I learned along the way that I wasn't alone. In fact, many people fear failure and lack self-confidence as they enter doctorate programs.

Navigating Barriers

For me, I think there were critical variables that I identified that helped tremendously. First, when I decided to pursue my doctorate, I convinced a friend and a colleague to go into the program with me. This created a great support system throughout the program. We traveled to class together, studied together, and reviewed papers for each other. We were able to help each other because we were in it together. Clear and simple, you don't need to go at it alone; bring a friend along for the ride.

Finally, find a routine and stick to it. For me, 9 p.m. every night of the week was when I completed my online posts, replied to posts, and worked on assignments. I worked systematically through each assignment. Writing a 10- to 15-page paper is not easy, but writing a paragraph or two every night is, a little bit at a time. When possible, build working ahead into your routine; even if you don't submit your assignment early, you can still have it done and ready to go. There is no better time to mentally review your presentation than when you are driving to class. Now, you certainly need to pay attention to the road, but you can review what you are going to say, how you are going to say it, and what questions you might encounter while driving. In the end, find what works for you and stick to it.

Current Focus

Today, I continue to be extraordinarily passionate about healthcare. From my point of view, we have a long way to go in terms of providing the level of quality that our patients rightfully deserve. As the Certified Nurse Educator (CNE) for a large academic medical center in Pennsylvania, I feel my focus needs to be on the overall health of our communities and the devastating effects that poor health has on our families. I am also focused on doing better for my own personal health. Our profession is fast-paced and stressful, and the weight of what we do has a tremendous impact on our health.

I focus on two key aspects of the nursing profession. First, I believe we have to continue advocating for nurses and require that organizations put nurses on equal ground with other healthcare professionals. It goes without saying that nurses are advocates and purveyors of patient safety. You simply cannot make healthcare decisions without nurses. The how is very complicated, and I don't have all of the answers, but I can identify the problem, and we know a solution when we see it. Nursing needs to be represented at the highest level of healthcare organizations. Think about it this way: if you work in an organization where the Chief Medical Officer and the Chief Nursing Officer (CNO) are not peers and don't report to the same person, nursing is not in the right place. My focus is on making sure that nursing is optimally positioned allowing nurses to take great care of patients.

The second aspect of the nursing profession I am passionate about is staffing. I remember being young and hearing my grandmother talk about how bad staffing was when she graduated nursing school in 1957. Fast forward to 2001, when I graduated nursing school, and I remember hearing from my preceptors and nurses how bad staffing was. Now, in 2021, we continue to hear about significant staffing challenges. My conviction is that no one outside of nursing is going to fix staffing for nursing. We must find new ways to care for patients because what we have been doing isn't working. I wish I had the silver-bullet solution. We know for certain that safe staffing means better outcomes for our patients. Hoping that we can just hire enough nurses every day that we walk in the facility door is not a strategy for getting us where we need to be. As a nursing profession, it is our responsibility to find the way forward. I'm working hard to find a new way to adequately staff using the data and technology.

Future Goals

I am excited and optimistic about what the future holds for me and for healthcare. It is one of the blessings of being a nurse; you will never have to worry about having an opportunity. I hope to transition into a chief executive officer (CEO) role of a hospital/healthcare system or become a consultant in healthcare. Both of these opportunities present a great opening to be a mentor and help others succeed. I know that I must continue having a positive impact on nurses and patients. You might ask: Why not continue to be a CNO and conclude your career in nursing? My opinion is that besides honey, everything has a shelf life, and if we don't continue to grow and reinvent ourselves, we never reach our true potential.

My whole life traveling through Philadelphia my parents would always take the PA Turnpike to Route 476. I never really knew there was a really cool, vibrant city just on the other side of 476 because we never took that route. When I moved to Philadelphia, I learned that 476 was just a very small slice (<1%) of Philadelphia, and there is a whole city out there just waiting for me to explore it. That is how I approach my career; I am intent on not staying on the same path to the end. My goal will always be the same: I want to help nurses and patients, but I will take a different route from time to time to achieve my goal. That is the beauty of nursing: there are so many routes, so many opportunities, and so many challenges to be explored, and ultimately we are better nurses for our exploration and determination to help others.

The greatest satisfaction in my work is, hands down, helping others. Help comes in many forms, and I pride myself on trying to make small, incremental improvements no matter where I am or what I am doing. I never really set out to change the world because I wouldn't know where to start. I try hard to change one experience at a time because I am confident that these changes will take a lifetime. I love watching quality numbers improve and trend lines improve. Nurses sometimes criticize nurse leaders for "looking at spreadsheets," but I personally translate each of those numbers and data to individual patients.

My best advice for anyone pursuing advanced degrees, regardless of specialty, is that you can dream the impossible but achieving academic success isn't impossible. Use your support system and the resources around you to achieve success. Many people think they are doing it alone or that their circumstances are somehow different from everyone else's. At the end of the day, we are far more the same than you might recognize. Don't get me wrong; this next step in your academic career will be challenging, frustrating, and some days will make you want to "Netflix and chill" so you can forget about the mounting "to-do" list. I believe that approaching education from your point in time is the best approach; in other words, how do you incorporate your projects and learning into your current work-life system? When you realize that what you are learning makes you better, faster, and more proficient at your job, you then start to look at learning and work as one. Much of what you do is applicable to the job you are doing every day; you just have to apply it. Earning a doctorate helps you understand the systems and processes that are in place to make you better at your job. They are truly complimentary.

Pursuing a degree is hard, but being stuck in a position because you don't have the credentials or the tools to be successful is agony. All routes are hard; choose the route that provides the most reward. I have come to realize that education is never wasted, never easy, and never the hardest route.

CHAPTER 28

The Telehealth Nurse Narrative

Carolyn Morcom Rutledge, PhD, FNP-BC, FAAN

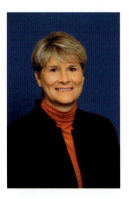

As a teenager, I knew I wanted to pursue a career in healthcare. However, as I explored the available options, I struggled to zero in on one specific field. As the first person in my family to pursue a college education and the oldest child and grandchild, I realized I needed to choose an educational track that would prepare me for a job upon graduation. It finally hit me that nursing was the right career for me. As a nurse, I would not have trouble finding a job. However, more importantly, a career in nursing would provide me with many options. I could be a hospital nurse. I could work in a school. I could be a travel nurse. Being a person who loves new experiences and has a zest for learning, this appealed to me.

Entry to Practice

It was important to me to have a college degree and to demonstrate to my brothers and cousins that they too could pursue higher education. Thus, I chose to enter practice as a Bachelor of Science in Nursing (BSN). I completed 2 years at a women's liberal arts college and then transferred for my junior and senior years to the Medical College. My first job was at a University Children's Hospital, where I cared for terminally ill children. This experience taught me that children are resilient and the source of many miracles we seek in healthcare. I learned about compassion and the importance of working in teams. As I look back on this experience, I realize it set the stage for my beliefs regarding health and healthcare.

Being a military family, we moved frequently, and with each move I started working predominantly on the night shift. My husband and I did not remain at an Army post long enough for me to advance up the ranks as a staff nurse. We spent 6 years in the military and were assigned to mulitple duty stations. As a result, I worked in five different nursing roles. Fortunately, I never had to struggle to find a job. Our longest assignment was 3 years (1982–1985) in West Berlin, Germany, when the wall still surrounded the city preventing access from East Berlin. During the winter, daylight lasted only 5 hours.

Decision to Pursue Higher Education and Advanced Practice

Between working weeks of nights and not seeing the sun, I was feeling trapped. Just when I thought I could not continue, I was approached to serve as an instructor responsible for preparing the soldiers to handle crises in the field. I absolutely loved teaching and empowering these soldiers/students. My experience in Berlin helped me realize that graduate school was in my future. Our next assignment allowed me to be at one location long enough to complete my Master of Science in Nursing (MSN) and become a certified family nurse practitioner. At that time, the role as a nurse practitioner (NP) was relatively new and appealed to me. In fact, my class had only six NP students. My MSN program, which required the completion of a thesis, stimulated my interest in research.

My first position as a NP was in the family practice residency at a medical school. Due to my passion for research and my ability to see patients, I was hired through a Health Resources and Services Administration (HRSA) grant to provide clinical research support. This experience was phenomenal and enabled me to get a broader perspective on healthcare and the importance of research in optimizing healthcare delivery. Within 3 years, I was responsible for writing and administering all the grants in family medicine. My track record of success was significant to the point that the Department of Family Medicine would send me as their representative for writing collaborative grant proposals with other universities. I quickly realized that my success was limited because I did not have a doctoral degree. I realized that without a doctoral degree I would not be able to serve as a principal investigator; and I would not be shown respect by other grant writers. It became clear to me that it was time to advance my career.

I chose to earn a PhD in Health Service Research with a Cognate in Industrial and Organizational Psychology. I found this track to be ideal for my goals. It prepared me as a researcher and gave me insight into the ways various healthcare professions could work collaboratively in a respectful, nonhierarchical model.

Mentors

I have been fortunate to have had many mentors throughout my career. When I was trying to decide on whether to pursue my MSN as an educator or as a NP, I met with the graduate program director, Dr. Helen Yura. She recommended the NP track, emphasizing that more doors would be open to me as an NP and that an NP would also be able to teach. Dr. Yura served as my thesis chair and taught me the importance of theory.

My next mentor was Dr. Jeff Levin, a leading researcher in religion, health, and aging. Dr. Levin encouraged me to pursue my PhD. He helped me learn to write and publish. With his mentoring, I published my thesis and my next four publications. He saw a track for me that I could not visualize for myself at the time. He believed in me when I had doubts. He encouraged me to take the leap required to obtain my PhD.

Milestones

The milestones I marked across my career were numerous. The first was my educator role in Berlin. It was through this experience that I developed my passion for teaching. As a result of that experience, I have had a teaching component in each of my roles since.

My next milestone occurred while conducting the research for my thesis in graduate school. I developed and validated a tool that measures coping of parents of chronically ill children. This was not a typical MSN project. My success in this investigation ignited my drive to seek roles that allowed me to continue to conduct research. Serving as a family NP at the medical school opened another door for me. I was able to develop not only my clinical skills working with a complex patient population but also skills in teaching and conducting research. I became the Director of Research in Family Medicine as well as the Director of the Family Medicine Fellowship program. I still maintain an appointment in the medical school as a professor and collaborate frequently on educational and research endeavors.

My next milestone came with the move from the medical school to the School of Nursing at Old Dominion University. As a faculty member in the School of Nursing, I started one of the first 20 Doctor of Nursing Program (DNP) programs in the country. I have since developed the only Telehealth Center nested in a school of nursing. Most recently, COVID-19 launched me into a role as a national leader in telehealth and telehealth education.

Navigating Barriers

We all encounter barriers. Each one I encountered was solved by pursuing further education. When I realized that I needed to move from a staff nurse role and loved teaching, I sought my master's degree. This opened the doors that had been closed to me as a staff nurse. In seeking to further my role as a researcher and grant writer, I realized that I needed a doctoral degree. This has allowed me to fulfill these dreams.

Current Focus

Currently, I am the Associate Chair of Nursing at Old Dominion University and Co-Director of the Center for Telehealth Innovation, Education, and Research (C-TIER). I also serve as the founding director of the DNP program. My focus as an educator, provider, and researcher has been in care for rural and underserved populations. As such, I empower both students and faculty to achieve their goals. Since 2010, I have focused much attention on training interprofessional teams to collaborate through telehealth. As a result of the COVID-19 pandemic, I have become a national leader in telehealth and telehealth education. C-TIER is the only telehealth center nested in nursing that provides telehealth training to healthcare students, faculties, and providers across the nation.

Future Goals

It is hard to think about future goals when I am so happy with where I am. I would like to continue developing opportunities to refine telehealth and telehealth education. My greatest focus is to develop new models for care that can overcome the limitations of our current healthcare system. At the present time, I am developing six nurse-led student clinics to meet the needs of underserved populations. These clinics provide interprofessional care and maximize the use of telehealth. I have great hopes that such a model will be adopted across the country through more academic/community partnerships.

My greatest fulfillment comes when others express appreciation for the impact that I have had on their lives. Whether it comes from a patient, student, or colleague, it is equally rewarding. I believe that we as nurses hold the key to addressing any healthcare crisis. We must use our voices and our expertise to advocate for change. We must think outside the box and create new models of care. I believe my role is to help others develop/obtain the tools to maximize their impact on healthcare.

Words of Wisdom

It is only through doctoral education that nurses will be able to have a voice in healthcare. We must be sitting at the table with policymakers and leaders. We must collect the data needed to advocate for change. We must speak for the populations in need. We approach healthcare differently from other professions with a focus on a biopsychosocial model. We must use this approach to empower our patients to be full and effective participants in and advocates for their own health. We must seek to raise up our fellow nurses and empower each other as we change healthcare.

CHAPTER 29

The Researcher Nurse Narratives

Ronald Lee Hickman, PhD, RN, ACNP-BC, FNAP, FAAN ■
Tiffany Monique Montgomery, PhD, MSHP, RNC-OB

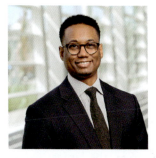

Ronald Lee Hickman, PhD, RN, ACNP-BC, FNAP, FAAN

Your Entry into Practice

As an African American child, growing up in a Rust Belt city in the Midwest, the value of getting an education was viewed as a means of self-determination and opportunity. Television shows like *The Crosby Show* and *A Different World* introduced America and Black communities to the seldom seen Black middle class and fictitious Black Americans who aspired to or held career occupations in medicine, law, or engineering. Little did I know, the Thursday evening ritual of sitting down with my working-class family to watch these Black television shows would inspire my own career aspirations and put me on an unexpected path toward being a nurse scientist.

Through high school, the focus of my academic studies was principally on math and science and my matriculation to Case Western Reserve University as an undergraduate majoring in biological science (pre-medical). For the next 4 years, I continued my journey to becoming a medical doctor by taking biology, chemistry, and other pre-medical courses, as well as eventually taking the Medical College Admission Test (MCAT). Unlike those Black television shows, despite my hard work and perseverance, everything did not go according to plan. Just weeks before graduation, it became apparent that my admission to a medical school was not on the immediate horizon and that I had no alternate career plan. I failed.

Fortunately, a mentor at the time persuaded me to attend a professional networking activity for graduating students. While at this networking event, I was seated at a table with faculty from various health professions. As we introduced ourselves to each other, one of the faculty members leaned over and asked, "Have you ever considered being a nurse?" Reflexively, I answered, "No." For the next few minutes, we continued to converse about the nursing profession and how my interest in science would align with being a nurse scientist. Expecting that we would end our conversation and soon after part ways, I was again, wrong. This persistent faculty member escorted me to the school of nursing and made certain that I applied to its graduate entry program. This chance encounter put me on an unexpected career path in nursing.

My journey of becoming a doctorally prepared nurse scientist was not planned but has been immensely rewarding. In this narrative, I further elaborate on why I became a doctorally prepared nurse scientist, the value of mentorship, the barriers encountered, and the strategies used to navigate my unexpected career path.

Motivation to Become a Nurse

I have been persistently motivated by a desire to maximize my impact on the health and well-being of others. Even before becoming a nurse, I saw, but did not fully appreciate, the impact that nurses working in hospitals and communities have on the well-being of individuals, families, and society at large. Members of the public trust nurses and generally appreciate the contributions of nurses to care delivery. However, nurses often get very little attention in the media and are often portrayed on television and in movies as subordinates to physicians, which lessened my motivation to pursue a career in nursing early on. Just imagine the power of 4 million courageous nurses, the largest workforce of healthcare professionals in the United States, using their authority and power and stepping in to lead our nation's healthcare systems toward higher quality and care that is more compassionate, accessible, inclusive, and effective. All nurses have impact—a declarative statement that has and continues to motivate me.

Using evidence to broaden nursing's impact on the health and well-being of others is the motivation as to why I became a doctorally prepared (PhD) nurse scientist. As a critical care nurse and advanced practice nurse, I was acutely aware that evidence was needed to transform the quality, effectiveness, inclusiveness, and accessibility of care. To be able to ask questions and generate new knowledge to positively change practice and health policy is the motivation that has carried me through my doctoral studies and inspires me to be a leader in advancing nursing research.

Entry to Practice

Having earned a bachelor's degree in biological science, my entry-to-practice began with matriculation into a graduate or master's entry program, a prelicensure program for individuals who have earned a bachelor's or higher degree in a discipline other than nursing. As a graduate entry student, I had the opportunity to work with faculty in critical care settings and join their research teams as a research assistant. In turn, these experiences cemented my aspiration to become a critical care nurse. I worked for several years as a critical care nurse, which laid the foundation for my scientific inquiry and scholarship.

Educational Path

The decision to pursue graduate education occurred simultaneously when I decided to become a nurse. While working as a critical care nurse, I decided to pursue graduate studies as an acute care nurse practitioner student. Even at this early stage of my nursing career, I knew that I wanted to possess advanced clinical knowledge of how to manage critically ill patients. The translation of evidence into practice became more salient, and I enrolled in a Doctor of Nursing Practice (DNP) program. Yet, the skills that I wanted to gain to transform healthcare and generate new knowledge were competencies of graduates of Doctor of Philosophy (PhD) in Nursing programs and not DNP programs. The switch from pursuing a DNP to a PhD was another unexpected change in my educational path, but one that has allowed me to gain the competencies, skills, and knowledge needed to conduct clinical research to improve the care of critically ill patients and their families, as well as influence national research priorities and policy.

The Value of Mentors

The value of mentors is often underappreciated during doctoral education and beyond. *The New York Times* best-selling author Bob Proctor views "a mentor is someone who sees more talent and ability within you, than you see in yourself, and helps bring it out of you." Across my career path, I have had many mentors who have met Proctor's definition. As a cis-gender, African American man, there have not been many opportunities to be mentored by individuals who look like me. Yet, I have been fortunate in that I have mentors who have unselfishly shared their wisdom, created opportunities, and challenged my thinking. When it came to identifying mentors, it was critical that there be reciprocity in terms of respect, authenticity, and shared commitment to advancing science. Other than these qualities, I have been and will continue to be open to mentorship from individuals who meet these fundamental criteria.

Mentors have coached me through my disappointment of not getting into medical school and persuaded me to enter the nursing profession and consider becoming a nurse scientist. These mentors, from a variety of backgrounds and experiences, have all played influential roles in helping me navigate an unexpected career path and become a nurse scientist. Throughout my doctoral studies, and even today, I have had an ensemble of mentors. These mentors have ranged from academic administrators and clinical experts to leaders in business and government. All have shared their perspectives and lessons learned to accelerate my career progression. The key lessons learned include the ability to recognize the talent and drive within individuals, to challenge the realities of situations, to create opportunities that reinforce their importance and impact, and to instill in them a value of mentorship that will continue to produce dividends. Like Sir Isaac Newton has said, "If I have seen further, it is by standing on the shoulders of Giants."

Mentorship during and after your doctoral education should be valued and considered important. As you prepare to begin your doctoral studies, it is important to understand that what you need from your mentors will certainly change as you progress through your program and across career stages. In the first few years of doctoral education, finding mentors who have scientific alignment with your interests and can provide you with opportunities to engage in the research process (e.g., conceptualization of studies to disseminating findings) is paramount. Be open-minded and remember that a single mentor is unlikely able to give you everything you need and assembling a mentor team is an effective approach. Finally, I encourage you to take full advantage of the wisdom and support of those who wish to be a mentor to you. The value of their mentorship is priceless.

Career Path Milestones

As a nurse scientist, I have found that there are several career path milestones. During my doctoral education, the short-term milestones were completing coursework, acquiring research skills related to my scientific area of interest, successfully passing my candidacy exam, and defending my dissertation. Additionally, accomplishing the milestones of providing project management for a large multisite clinical trial, publishing and presenting research, and securing external grant funding for my dissertation research were the career milestones that occurred during my doctoral studies, positioning me for postdoctoral research training and my first faculty post as a tenure-eligible assistant professor.

After completing my doctoral education, another career milestone was attaining a postdoctoral training fellowship, which broadened the focus of my research and helped me launch a program of research focused on behavior change and decision science. During my postdoctoral research fellowship, I achieved several more career milestones, which included submitting numerous first-author publications, obtaining federal and foundation grant funding, and learning how to manage a research team. Thus, my transition to a tenure-eligible assistant professor position was a logical next step and a career milestone that has resulted in promotion and tenure. Altogether, my career milestones have enabled me to amass a record of high-quality research and scholarship, as well as the requisite skills to earn appointment as associate dean for research.

Barriers Encountered and Strategies to Overcome Them

Becoming a nurse scientist was an unexpected career path, and the barriers encountered were not surprising but still unexpected. One undergraduate advisor refused to write a letter of recommendation to nursing explicitly stating that they did not think I was a good fit for nursing. It was difficult for me to untangle if the bias was related to my racial identity as a Black American or my gender identity as a man. These intersecting identities of being Black and a male have posed significant and unique challenges for navigating a career in nursing.

At the bedside, I have experienced racism and gender bias from patients and their families, and even from nurse colleagues. My experience with racism and discrimination as a nurse is not isolated. In the recent report, *Racism's Impact in Nursing*, by the National Commission to Address Racism in Nursing, over 5600 registered nurses (RNs) were surveyed, and among those participants who identified as Black, a majority reported experiencing racist acts from peers (66%) and nurse leaders (70%).

However, racism and bias are not isolated to clinical nursing: in the context of academic nursing, there is individual, structural, and systemic racism that impacts the diversity and inclusiveness of our student, staff, and faculty bodies. It is estimated that in higher education, Black male faculty comprise no more than 1% of the professoriate, based on 2018 report from the National Center for Education Statistics. When considering academic nursing, the number of PhD-prepared Black males are likely to comprise even less than 1% of the nursing professoriate. In line with these data, I have encountered several barriers that should have prevented me from successfully earning a PhD, securing a tenure-eligible faculty position, and serving in an academic leadership role. Yet, despite multilevel barriers, I have gained invaluable insights into how to address or at least attenuate their effects on my career progression.

Undoubtedly, you will encounter challenges. The best strategy as you prepare for your doctoral studies and begin your career as a doctorally prepared nurse is to approach these challenges and obstacles with a *growth mindset*. A growth mindset is a perspective that you already possess an array of abilities that can be further developed by putting in effort and leveraging the resources of others. Using this lens to work through challenges and overcome obstacles helps you reframe these challenges as learning opportunities for your personal and professional growth, and over time, your natural growth promotes resilience. It is evident that talent and ability are sufficient to be successful, but those individuals who can view a challenge through a growth mindset lens are more likely to have sustained success. No matter the challenge or the obstacle, maintaining a growth mindset has been one of the most effective strategies that I have used during my doctoral studies and continues to aid my problem-solving and personal development as a doctorally prepared nurse leader.

Current Focus and Future Goals

Successfully navigating my unexpected career path has afforded me the opportunity to shape nursing research, inform policy, and prepare the next generation of nurses and scientists as a faculty member and associate dean for research. My career path has had many turns, and still I would not have done anything differently. My greatest satisfaction comes from conceptualizing clinical research that addresses a meaningful clinical problem, witnessing my students' learning how to deliver evidence-informed nursing care, and having the ability to provide care to critically ill patients and their families when they are most in need. Additionally, as a doctorally prepared nurse, my impact is manifested at microsystem and macrosystem levels. I serve on national committees, such as the National Academy of Medicine and the American Academy of Nursing, positioning me to shape national research agendas and influence health policy reform—activities that have broadened my impact on public health.

As I look forward, I am inspired by the potential impact of nursing on transforming healthcare delivery in the United States. There are countless ways that I can continue to contribute to transforming our healthcare systems. For the past 5 years, I have enjoyed serving as an associate dean for research and envision continuing to advance my leadership in academic nursing. My aspiration to secure a senior leadership position within a school/college of nursing, or university, aligns with my commitment to helping an organization and its people achieve their goals to positively impact the health of all Americans.

Conclusion

To successfully navigate an unexpected career path and doctoral education, one must be open-minded, embrace uncertainty, maintain a growth mindset, and leverage the support of mentors. Doctoral education was one of the best decisions I have made. It has challenged my way of thinking and being. It has broadened my impact to advance science and ensure that all Americans have access to inclusive, high-quality, and effective healthcare.

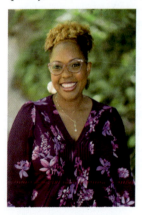

Tiffany Monique Montgomery, PhD, MSHP, RNC-OB

Your Entry to Practice

I first knew that I wanted to become a nurse as a high school freshman. A chance survey in my career development course changed everything for me. I took the assessment as part of a class assignment. We responded to several items related to our personality traits, likes, and dislikes. At the end of the assessment, I learned I was a good fit for a career as a certified nurse-midwife (CNM). I'd never heard the term before this fateful day. I read up on the role and decided that this was what I wanted to do.

Being a midwife made perfect sense to me. I loved pregnant women—I always have, and probably always will. My love for this population goes back to my childhood, when I spent hours looking through a book filled with intrauterine photos of a fetus at various gestations. I would get in trouble for looking at the book because my mother thought it was inappropriate for children, but I was enamored. My awe of obstetrics remains just as strong today as it was back then.

Your Decision to Pursue Higher Education

I decided to become a bachelor's prepared RN with great intentionality. I had a cousin who was a licensed vocational nurse, but I chose not to follow in her footsteps for fear that I would never become an RN if I took a non-traditional route. I pursued a Bachelor of Science in Nursing (BSN) instead of an associate degree (AA) following this same train of thought. I feared that if I didn't enroll in a 4-year university, there was a good chance that I would never earn a degree past an AA. I'd seen this happen to others, and I didn't want to repeat the cycle.

The Educational Path You Chose and the Reasoning Behind That Decision

After earning my BSN, I worked as a Labor and Delivery (L&D) nurse. I enjoyed my time in L&D, but I had a strong desire to become a nurse educator. Two years into my new career, I enrolled in a master's-level nursing education program. In addition to learning all about curriculum development and test design and evaluation, I explored my passion for teen pregnancy prevention programming. The more I learned, the more I wanted to create programs and not just implement them. This led me to consider the impact I could have if I were a nurse researcher. In thinking of how to make a considerable impact on both students and childbearing women, I decided to earn a PhD in nursing.

Upon receiving my PhD, I began an interdisciplinary postdoctoral fellowship focused on health services. I had done some advocacy work with the Association for Women's Health, Obstetric, and Neonatal Nurses (AWHONN), and I wanted to learn more about conducting health policy research. During my time as a fellow, I dug into the world of policy surveillance. In the year after completing the fellowship, I worked as an assistant professor at a small teaching university but realized I missed being heavily engaged in research. In order to gain more experience, I enrolled in an additional postdoctoral fellowship.

My second fellowship was much more traditional than the first. I had an opportunity to work with my research idol, doing important community-engaged work in the West Philadelphia Promise Zone. After two fellowships—a non-traditional fellowship in a School of Medicine and a traditional fellowship in a School of Nursing—I felt ready to apply to a tenure-track position at a research-intensive institution.

Who Were Your Mentors

As a first-generation college student, I couldn't go to most of my friends and family for advice on how to best navigate college. Thus, mentors were an extremely important aspect of my journey through higher education. I needed safe spaces to discuss the issues I was dealing with as the only Black student in most of my classes. I needed to form relationships with people who had been in my position and had successfully completed their degree(s).

Although I was mentored by several of my nursing professors, I wanted to develop relationships with nurses with a shared ethnic background. I sought out mentorship from members of the South Bay Black Nurses Association (SBBNA) and found a welcoming, familiar environment. SBBNA members gave me insight into what it meant to be a Black nurse. They gave me advice when I dealt with microaggressions on campus and in the workplace. They also supported me financially, awarding me with several scholarships and assisted me in my job search. In all, they made sure that I was set up for success. I am forever grateful to the women and men of SBBNA who poured so much of their wisdom, time, and treasure into me.

As a PhD student, I learned the importance of peer mentors, sponsors, and allies. While traditional mentors provided guidance, peer mentors were easy to relate to, sponsors gave me a seat at the preverbal table, and allies were my advocates. Forming these different relationships was critical, especially among those from disciplines other than nursing. I looked for strong support within my program, at other universities in the region, within my nursing organizations, and on social media sites like Twitter. Regardless of how we met and the length of time of our relationship, each of my mentors, sponsors, and allies has served me well.

What Were the Milestones on Your Path

There were many vital milestones on my journey to becoming a PhD-prepared nurse. The first came with my induction into Sigma Theta Tau International Honor Society of Nursing. I joined thousands of nurses worldwide who were acknowledged as being in the top one-third of our prelicensure classes. As one of the few Black nursing students in my class of nearly 100, this meant something special to me. Following graduation, I received the Student Nurse of the Year Award from the National Black Nurses Association (NBNA). My years of service to various on-campus clubs and committees were recognized with the highest honor awarded to a student nurse of NBNA. I could not have been prouder.

At the end of my PhD journey, I was inducted into the Edward A. Bouchet Graduate Honor Society. Dr. Bouchet was the first African American to receive a PhD in physics and the first to graduate from Yale College (now Yale University).

Being in this honor society illuminates my hard work, my commitment to marginalized communities, and my path to impactful scientific discoveries as a nurse researcher. I was also awarded the Courtney H. Lyder Pan African Students and Alumni Association (PANSAA) Diamond Award. PANSAA was the reason I decided to apply to my PhD program over countless others. I knew that being surrounded by other Black students would give me the social capital I needed to succeed. I served as the PANSAA secretary for 5 years. It was a fantastic achievement to see my efforts awarded such a high honor.

In an eerily similar repeat of the event following the completion of my BSN, the summer following the completion of my PhD, I received another critical award from the NBNA. This time, I was among the first cohort of Under 40 awardees within the association. The following summer, I was honored as the Reviewer of the Year by *Nursing for Women's Health*, the AWHONN practice journal. Each of these career milestones encouraged me to continue pressing toward my career goals and reminded me that I was not alone in this journey but surrounded by people and organizations that supported me.

What Barriers Do You Face and What Strategies You Use to Navigate Them

The most significant barrier I faced was limited personal finances. By the time I entered my senior year of high school, my parents were separated. My mother didn't have the money to send me to college, and I knew my father wouldn't be willing to contribute to my education in this way. To prevent an overwhelming amount of debt, I applied to a public state university where tuition was less than $800 per semester. With this low cost and the help of financial aid, my mother could afford tuition, room, and board. I paid for my books and purchased food and clothing with the money I received from my work-study job.

In my junior and senior years, I applied for as many scholarships as I could find. This resulted in enough scholarship money to cover my tuition and living expenses. I was able to quit my job and focus entirely on school and community service. Scholarships also helped me pay for my tuition and living expenses while earning my Master of Science in Nursing (MSN) and PhD degrees. To this day, I have never taken out an educational loan. I have completed four degrees with no debt.

Your Current Focus

My research interests center on sexual and reproductive health disparities, particularly unplanned pregnancy and sexually transmitted disease/illness transmission among vulnerable women. My research aims to identify complex individual, interpersonal, societal, and structural facets predicting risky sexual behavior and to develop interventions and policies to address these issues. I use community engagement methods to mitigate the mistrust of disenfranchised communities, along with innovative technology platforms to penetrate underrepresented and traditionally hard-to-reach populations. I have used quantitative and qualitative methodologies to develop culturally tailored individual and community-level interventions; evaluate women's health policies; and appraise health promotion programs in urban communities.

Whether in the classroom or the field, I am dedicated to the successful enrollment of all nursing students, particularly minority and first-generation students. I have a solid commitment to increasing the number of minority nurses and ensuring increased diversity in nursing education. This inspires me to mentor students and expose them to professional activities early in their nursing education. I do this to help them achieve a rich educational experience and position them as future nurse leaders. Reciprocity is an essential component of my mentoring style, where my mentees and I are teaching and learning concurrently. I regularly speak at high school career days and establish mentoring relationships with those interested in nursing. I work hard to support minority students because I believe our profession is only made better as we enhance the diversity of its workforce.

Your Future Goals

My future career goals are to identify and decrease sexual and reproductive health disparities and diversity, equity, and inclusion (DEI) disparities in nursing. Whether this work occurs in an inpatient, outpatient, or higher education setting is not important to me. My goal is to do the work wherever I may find myself. Ultimately, I want my scholarship to inform clinical practice and public policy affecting women's sexual and reproductive health outcomes.

The Most Significant Source of Satisfaction You Find in Your Work

The most significant source of satisfaction in my work comes from giving people new insight. When someone tells me that I helped them see sexual health disparities or interventions through a new lens, I know that my work was not in vain. The work I do is for my communities of interest; I am not doing this work for personal accolades. I no longer want to see marginalized groups being mistreated by my healthcare providers or the communities in which we live and the systems in which we work. As data on sexual health and nursing DEI shows closing gaps and decreasing disparities, I feel like I am doing my job. When these data support ineffective interventions and care, I am encouraged to work harder. Whenever a student, colleague, or patient tells me that something I've said or done has helped them see the importance of working to end health disparities, I am wholly satisfied. My goal is to create other change agents and not try to do everything on my own.

Any Words of Wisdom to Nurses Considering Earning a Doctorate

My thoughts on doctoral education have changed significantly since earning my PhD. My perception of those with doctorates changed almost as soon as I enrolled in the program. No one earning a doctorate is more intelligent or more prepared than you. Everyone in a doctoral program starts at ground zero. If you want to apply for a doctorate, apply. If you need to apply more than once, that's ok. These programs are small and often receive more applicants than they have space to accept. *Don't let a dream deferred become a dream denied.*

Once you are admitted to the program, avoid letting impostor syndrome creep in. This is especially important for first-generation college graduates and those from racially/ethnically minoritized groups. Don't second-guess the decision of the admissions committee. They didn't make a mistake. You weren't admitted by accident. You are exactly where you are supposed to be, doing exactly what you are supposed to do. Don't isolate yourself. You don't have to go it alone. Many people, both inside and outside of your institution, are willing to mentor you through the program. We will support you, give you tips and tricks, and help you cross the finish line however we can. So, here's an early congratulations, Dr.! You can do this! You will do this!

CHAPTER 30

The Health Disparities Nurse Narrative

Jennifer M. Brown, DNP, MSN, RN

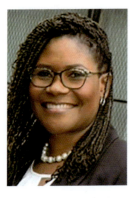

Your Initial Motivation to Become a Nurse

Whenever nurses surround me, I often introduce myself as a third-career nurse, mainly because I do not want to be perceived as inexperienced or a late starter, but even more so because most of my colleagues have been nurses for many years. I tried to value the wealth of my experience acquired over the years, albeit elsewhere. I was 20 years old when I graduated from college with an education degree. The highlight of my classmates' journey was to find high schools and make their mark on society. To my parents' dismay, I was not looking forward to a career in teaching but had set my sights on becoming a flight attendant with the a national airline. This had been my dream ever since I was a child, and I felt I had fulfilled my parents' wishes, and it was now time to embark on mine. Suffice to say, I was an obedient child, and after hearing of all the sacrifices it took to get me through school with no student loan, I acquiesced and decided to give teaching a chance for my mother's sake.

I accepted a job at my alma mater; the principal had a glass desk, and my photograph had earned a coveted place there, so it was a no-brainer that I would have landed my first job there. I did not realize how much the experience would add value to my life. I taught English and literature to ninth graders in my first year. I became very involved in extracurricular activities, created a debate club, and provided free tutoring in Jamaica School Certificate (JSC) exam preparations on the weekends for students who were unable to afford private lessons. I also advocated for the early Caribbean Examination Council (CXC) exam attempt for those students who were outstanding in the subject to complete English in their junior year and focus on passing their more complex subjects in their senior year. The results were great, and over the next 2 years I became course coordinator and prepared senior-level students to sit for the CXC and O-Level Examinations. I was the youngest on staff, but my students and colleagues respected me, and I felt like I belonged. I had found my niche. I enjoyed the experience, and my students achieved significant success in their terminal examinations.

After teaching for 5 years, I had an unusual opportunity to fulfill my dormant dream of being a flight attendant. My friend, who I also worked with, asked me to accompany her to an interview one day. I cannot recall asking what the job was or why she might have been looking elsewhere. I took some students' papers I had to grade to get some work done while I waited. Getting to the location, I realized that the airline (the one I had dreamed of working with) was having a job fair. However, I was not prepared, I had no documents with me, and I enjoyed teaching more than I had anticipated. As I waited, I was disturbed twice to ask if I was waiting to be interviewed, to which I politely replied that I was there with my friend who was being interviewed. The third time I was disturbed was by the Human Resources Director, and she informed me that she would like to interview me for a flight attendant position. To my surprise, not only was I given the job without documents (I was told to bring them the following day), but I was made an offer I could not refuse. I shared this information with my principal (who had heard my flight attendant's story before) as soon as I got to work, only to learn that the airline had already contacted him. He was supportive of me taking the opportunity. He surpassed my expectations when he offered me the option of taking the job on a 3-month trial basis, and he would fill my position temporarily in case I decided to return.

With only 2 months remaining in the school year, I recruited my friend, who had recently graduated with her Master's degree in education, to fill in for me at the high school. For the next 2.5 months, as I embarked on training in my new job, she taught my classes, and I graded all the papers, as well as continued my weekend tutoring obligations. I later decided to remain with the airline, and she went on full time in my place. Over the next 7 years, I enjoyed an incredible journey with the airline, transitioning through various customer service departments, then revenue management, and later becoming Codeshare Coordinator for the airline in less than 5 years. I later relocated to the United States and resigned to focus on being a full-time mom. This sabbatical didn't last long, and I later entered Pharmacy Benefit Management (PBM) as a Customer Service Supervisor. With my work ethic and passion for succeeding, I soon saw outstanding achievements in my position. However, being in an environment with high attrition, it was hard to maintain productivity margins consistently. I realized that I needed to focus on the people and to get my staff to buy in and align themselves to the company's mission for us to be successful. I became very intentional in opportunities to boost employee morale by facilitating professional development activities. Utilizing resources and options available, I encouraged team members to enroll in continuing education, based on areas of interest, and to position themselves for promotion within the company. I motivated and encouraged teamwork by conducting monthly team meetings and job enrichment activities, provided timely feedback on performance and expectations, held monthly recognitions in various categories, including celebrations of birthdays and anniversaries and outstanding achievement on productivity metrics. I encouraged top performers to challenge themselves by seeking promotions within the company and identifying areas of strength in members of my team, even at the expense of losing them to leadership positions in other departments. I achieved a 0% attrition within a year, with consistently outstanding results, and my department was in first place in all performance areas for the next 2 years.

I was offered a promotion and relocated to work in quality assurance, with a challenge to improve the standardization of policies and procedures in preparation for the Utilization Review Accreditation Commission (URAC) visit. As a member of a five-person task force, my responsibility was to create documented work instructions for every process, within both the front-end pharmacy and the fulfillment locations. I worked with each department to identify subject matter experts and spent hours observing employees fulfilling specific job functions to accurately document work instruction. I often traveled to locations working with pharmacists and technicians who spoke very little English. I transitioned all paper processes into workflow and created a place where all standard operating procedures were shared and maintained. I was later asked to facilitate similar improvement at the other two sites in our region. Through an organized task force and weekly meetings, we achieved full implementations for all three facilities. After that project, I continued working with our quality assurance (QA) team and Pharmacists in Charge (PICs) to facilitate audits at all locations, ensuring that I updated procedures every 2 years, and working with sites to ensure that all citations were resolved promptly. while taking on the role of coordinating pharmacists and pharmacy technicians and successfully addressing complaints of poor customer service. In less than 6 months, we were able to restructure the department, create a training manual for consistency in procedures, rotate the entire team through refresher training, and achieve a 24- to 48-hour turnaround time on escalated calls and presidential issues. I was recognized for my contributions to increasing efficiency and productivity. I was awarded the BRAVO Award for outstanding Leadership and Team Development (2007 and 2010) and the STAR Award for Outstanding Leadership and Projects Completion (2010).

Getting close to my 10th anniversary with the company, I started to reflect on my journey and what the future held for me. With increasing parenting responsibilities, nursing for me was a career that would allow me to have a full-time job working only 3 days, and have the remaining 4 days for my family. I completed nursing school part time while still working full time in PBM. I remember forgetting something in my office and having to stop by on my way to clinical one Saturday. I was picked up on surveillance, and the security supervisor asked me if that was me; I then shared that I was in school for the first time. This never affected my job, as I was adept at successfully working on competing priorities. I later finished my program, passed the NCLEX, and stayed on 6 months before taking a nursing position, to oversee my role being transitioned to three different departments and train my successors.

Your Entry to Practice

My educational experience while pursuing my Associates Degree in Nursing (ASN) and later my Registered Nurse to Bachelors of Science in Nursing (RN-BSN) degree helped improve who I am as a person and molded me into the individual I want to continue to become. Working as a nurse, I have learned to take comfort from the small things in life and appreciate the powers of healing that come through caring. Through experience, I have gained new confidence in myself that will ensure that I maintain a commitment to my profession as a nurse and professional. After spending time in many different clinical settings, working in the Progressive Care Unit and later in the Medical Intensive Care Unit (MICU) and seeing the vast area of knowledge that nursing encompasses, I realized that there was so much more I needed to know to be a better and more effective nurse. My drive to prepare myself to provide the highest level of care to my patients has always been the force that keeps propelling me. Being what I considered a late starter in the nursing profession, I had that sense of "playing catch-up" and wanting to make the most of my time to be at the level of expertise and confidence I aspired to achieve in my professional development.

Being a critical care RN, I worked daily to learn new skills and, at the same time, improve the skills I had so that I could respond to patient needs in a timely and confident manner to achieve good outcomes. Not simply for myself but for the unit and the team. I always believe that we accomplish more when we feel empowered with the knowledge and skills necessary to achieve and surpass anticipated expectations—sharing my knowledge. At the same time, recognizing areas where I need to grow has helped me seize opportunities for education and growth while gaining the respect of my peers. This has steadily increased my confidence and comfort in the care I provide and has encouraged me to grow beyond the role of an RN to an area in which I believe I can contribute even more. With recognition from my supervisors, I was always given opportunities to learn new skills and embrace challenges. My leadership abilities were recognized very early in my nursing career, and I was appointed Charge Nurse in my unit. My ability to develop others led to the responsibilities of precepting new nurses and assisting them in gaining confidence in their abilities to change lives through the care they provide. Within 2 years as a nurse, I was recognized for excellence in patient care while working in the MICU. Still wanting to learn more, I later started working per diem in the Critical Care Pool at another area hospital and rotating through different intensive care units (ICUs).

Your Decision to Pursue Higher Education

It became apparent that to have a more influential voice in nursing I needed to continue my development as a professional nurse, which would require advanced education. Throughout my graduate education, I became further involved and aware of changes in the world of nursing. My initial goal then for completing my graduate degree was to build a career as an advanced practice nurse with areas of involvement in providing preventative care and treatment and management of acute and chronic illnesses. I would be able to accomplish this by having advanced clinical skills and providing advanced therapeutic interventions as appropriate while demonstrating a high level of independence, expertise, and professionalism in practice. My focus later shifted to the education of others and the ability to be involved in research efforts, providing outstanding leadership while consulting with peers and members of other disciplines. I felt compelled to make a difference at every level of my life, and this was no different.

Being a clinical adjunct instructor and then full-time nursing instructor at my alma mater again represented a significant aide-mémoire in my life, one that has increased my motivation for sharing my knowledge and assisting in preparing new nurses for the world of work. My philosophy of education centers on my scholastic preparation and the ability to adjust to meet the demands around me successfully. In my chosen profession, it is my relentless drive to equip myself through continued education to be an effective instructor to play an essential role in the development and growth of my students, creating interactions that foster interest and understanding of their individual needs. I became persistent in my efforts to identify my students' varied learning styles and adjust my teaching strategies to complement the pace and depth of their understanding. This approach enhances the learning experience. I work with each semester's results, always making changes in response to feedback on my IDEA/class evaluations/reports and dean evaluations for improved student outcomes.

I felt that having a graduate education should have allowed me to competently advance in areas of education, research, and practice. However, I realized that a doctoral degree would allow me to have a more significant impact on nursing by providing recommendations and solutions to existing problems. Also, a Doctor of Nursing Practice degree would enable me to improve my professional network, leverage support systems, and be more equipped to advance change and increase outcomes. Additionally, adequately preparing our students to excel in critical thinking and possess sound clinical judgment will propel them to the next level in clinical practice.

The Educational Path You Chose and the Reasoning Behind That Decision

My start in academia is somewhat nontraditional, especially among my current peers. As a clinician, I entered graduate school and even pursued my doctorate with an open mind that I could end up working anywhere. My first inclination was to be prepared to work in a hospital setting. Still, I also wanted to remain marketable, with the skill set to compete for positions in academia if that was where the opportunity presented itself. Making the transition from a graduate student to a nursing instructor/assistant professor was very exciting. My path as a clinician was also a bit different. I was fortunate to begin my teaching career with my Masters of Science in Nursing (MSN) while completing the Nurse Educator Track and then continuing to my DNP to fulfill the professional requirement of academia and my self-actualization.

While in graduate school, I had the same academic advisor throughout my program, and this person also doubled as a placement advisor of sorts during my final semester. She knew I hadn't decided between working in nursing education at the hospital or in a faculty role in a nursing program, so she would share opportunities with me as she learned of them. While keeping an open mind, I tried to learn about openings at local universities and hospitals by just searching organizations' websites. She shared with me that I could begin as an adjunct professor (limited fixed-term appointments, usually with a high teaching load but lower salary), or I could work at a hospital as an educator, which would require more experience in that department's processes, especially with my critical care skill set. The ultimate goal was to secure a nursing instructor position (usually for 1 to 3 years), but with a requirement to enroll in a doctoral program to be eligible for the promotion. Most of the universities then had a freeze on tenure track positions, so that was out of the question. During my teaching practicum, I was offered an opportunity to teach in the skills and simulation lab (as an adjunct), and I taught didactic and clinical over the summer.

This was exciting, and I immediately started considering how this could change what happened in my career later. First, I had been in the classroom before, although not at the same level. My first degree was in education, and I had taught high school for 5 years before changing career paths. Secondly, the adjunct faculty position was co-teaching courses that I loved, like Health Assessment, Med-Surg, and teaching critical care clinical to junior nursing students. This was somewhat familiar territory and gave me the chance to learn if this was something I would want to do long term, gain a lot of knowledge and skill so that I could prepare for the full-time position application process. It was also an opportunity for me to work with and teach nursing students, providing my exciting experiences to help them develop critical skills and clinical reasoning. This was also very similar to the hospital setting, should I then opt for the nurse educator role in the hospital.

The tremendous faculty I worked with mentored and showed me how to put together a nursing syllabus and create my PowerPoint presentations. Plus, I was able to get a feel for the courses that I enjoy teaching and shadow other faculty so that I could observe the different methodologies, watch the interactions with students, and create my strategy for what works and what doesn't.

I believe it was by the Fall term that my advisor provided me with two opportunities she had learned from networking: one was as a critical care nurse educator (Professional Development), and the other was a full-time faculty position as a nursing instructor. I went through the application process for the nurse educator role and even completed my presentation to the nursing staff, shadowed, and met with the ICU team. We hit it off, and I received a call from my advisor that the university where I was a student was considering me for a full-time position. I met with the Dean shortly after, and the rest is history.

Who Were Your Mentors?

I am fortunate to have been blessed with more than my fair share of guardian angels, persons who have assisted my development and helped me with decisions at different junctures of my life. They have helped me navigate opportunities, provided guidance, recommended me for job opportunities, provided constructive feedback, and been my supporters, advocators, and friends.

Bonnie Zuckerman, a nursing professor, has been a constant source of encouragement and one of my staunchest supporters, both professionally and on social media. She epitomizes professionalism and has taught me what having patience and resilience can accomplish. She is one of the most selfless, genuine persons I have met in nursing, who wishes the best for her students and "walks the talk." She is one of the first people I usually reach out to whenever I am considering a career/professional move and the first to offer to write my recommendation (validate my credentials/accomplishments).

Dona Molyneaux—I met Dr. Molyneaux while completing my RN-BSN degree. She would later become my professor during the completion of my graduate degree and one of the committee members for my DNP project. With over 40 years of experience in higher education as Director of the Nurse Educator track, as well as similar tenure in clinical practice as Research Director, her repertoire comprises knowledge on both ends of the healthcare spectrum, and she is someone I consider to be among the most valuable resources in healthcare. Suffice to say that she has not only been my preceptor, advisor, and professor but one of my closest colleagues. She has always been the go-to person for vibrant debate on the trends in healthcare, both on the clinical and academic sides, and someone with whom I am always confident of being appreciated for my authentic self.

Diane Breckenridge—I was fortunate to meet Dr. Breckenridge during the summer of my first year of graduate school. I was introduced to her as a research volunteer, by my mentor Dr. Molyneaux, to assist with work she was completing at a neighboring university after being awarded a Nursing Workforce Diversity Grant entitled "Students at Risk, Strategies for Success." The purpose of the grant was to prepare diverse, underrepresented, disadvantaged students for the academic challenges of a baccalaureate nursing program and to retain them in the nursing major. Under her mentorship, I appreciated the role of advocacy and how commitment to the needs of nursing and our community exceeds boundaries of race. I was able to explore the challenges that existed for minority nursing students and share my perspective as a minority on the strategies and implementation of the processes for success. While I have lost contact with Dr. Breckenridge during my evolution in nursing, her words of encouragement, wisdom, and commitment to diversity in nursing continually propel me to do my part to affect change in an area that lacks representation.

Charles "Chuck" Reed—Chuck, to me, is the boss every person should have the opportunity to work with, and I have worked for some fantastic bosses over my time. Before becoming a nurse, I was fortunate to have had a 7-plus-year stint in pharmacy benefit management. Chuck was the Director, Senior Director, and then VP of a Fortune 150 company. It was no coincidence that he was able to rise through the ranks as quickly as he did, but even more impressive was his ability to empower the people around him. A boss who was confident enough to let you know your value to the team, Chuck seized every opportunity to recognize and develop his workforce, always highlighting the strengths of his top performers without missing a chance to develop the others to reach their full potential. A boss who made the most remarkable statement I have ever heard about myself, which inspires me to this day, "Jen, you are cream, and cream always rises to the top." He remains a trusted confidant and friend and someone from whom I always seek counsel regarding any major professional decision I make.

Mary Terhaar—as my education and development continues, Dr. Terhaar has been the mentor I needed during this phase of my professional life. The Chair of my current nursing program, Dr. Terhaar is someone with foresight for the endless possibilities of nursing and a commitment to equip her workforce with the tools and opportunities to have an impact in any area they choose. She has taken the time to appreciate my passion and provided opportunities to help me advance my career. Another advocate for diversity and equitable opportunities in nursing, Dr. Terhaar enjoys authenticity and welcomes different decision-making perspectives. I have been awed by her selflessness and the lengths she will go to help her staff achieve professional success.

Nancy Rothman—I have had the pleasure of working alongside Dr. Rothman as a colleague and on a grant awarded to increase diversity in the nursing workforce by increasing the number of minority nurses in the nursing program at the university we teach. I have found her to be a true champion of the cause of the underrepresented and an advocate for improving healthcare access for people of color. She has guided me as I transition to a new job and has been a great teammate and counsel.

What Were the Milestones on Your Path?

Since being appointed as a full-time instructor in 2016, I have taught at all three levels of the BSN nursing program. Being one of the first two faculty at the start of the Accelerated Bachelors of Science in Nursing program at my previous job required that I present to students the highest level of professionalism while representing the values and mission of the school community, in and out of the classroom. It was also incumbent on us as founding faculty to create a foundation of high standards to position our students and the university for success. Our current accomplishments attest that we have not only achieved success but, through consistent improvements, have maintained it over the years.

With a proven track record of achieving success, I have provided didactic and clinical instructions to students, utilizing my vast experience in critical care nursing to create an environment where students develop the necessary thinking skills to make sound clinical decisions to improve patient outcomes. I continued individually teaching the full complement of classes taught in the first 2 years and accepted the opportunity to co-teach the senior seminar and NCLEX preparatory course when asked. I have exceeded 95% passes for all courses to date. I attributed my outstanding success to my ability to anticipate and communicate issues. I have incorporated current evidence-based teaching and learning strategies by being relentless in my efforts to improve processes for instruction and best practices. I have successfully implemented action plans to prevent a repeat of the issues that could derail students' success.

As Medical-Surgical course coordinator, I exemplified leadership qualities overseeing the clinical component of the Medical-Surgical course, with responsibilities for creating assignments and facilitating adjunct faculty orientation and practice by providing mentoring opportunities and ensuring consistency of content taught and achievement of objectives. I initiated opening and closing meetings for clinical courses in ABSN, which allowed adjunct faculty to meet as a group and address the expectations of the clinical experience to ensure quality preparation. With support and follow-up, we have been able to identify breakdowns in procedures, standardize practices, and empower faculty in their delivery of content and understanding of concepts.

Over the past 5 years, I have been involved in service to the university and the external community. With contributions to outstanding leadership as the VP and then President of Iota Kappa Chapter of Sigma Theta Tau, Faculty Counselor of Student Nurses Association of Pennsylvania for the ABSN campuses, I was facilitating monthly meetings, the election of officers, fundraising events, chaperoning students at regional conventions, and advising in other capacities, in collaboration with our faculty president. I have identified among students, especially those with English as a second language, challenges with mastery of concepts due to the accelerated process, and have created student partnerships for peer tutoring, which has yielded significant results.

I have been an advisor to students both during the program and after graduation, assisting them in transitioning into practice by creating resumes and portfolios, conducting mock interviews, and even identifying opportunities for seminars for those with an interest in specialized nursing. In my ongoing drive to give back to the community, I have partnered with Philadelphia Fight to provide a workshop on topics impacting the community and have participated in education and screenings for diabetes and hypertension for those at risk. I have been involved in clinics providing influenza vaccines and blood pressure and diabetes screenings for many years, and was awarded a certificate of recognition from the state of Pennsylvania for my contributions to the community.

What Barriers Do You Face and What Strategies Do You Use to Navigate Them

YOUR CURRENT FOCUS

I am passionate about nursing education, and I realize that a solid foundation in teaching, service, and scholarship is required for ensuring that our students are equipped to provide the highest quality of nursing care while advancing healthcare. With my doctoral degree, I intend to solidify my scholarship. The DNP program has equipped me with the knowledge to embrace the role of assistant professor with aspirations to attain full professor in the future and commit to my responsibilities while contributing to academia by making a difference and sharing my project. In seeking opportunities in research, I aspire to have publications in both the national and global journals and a presentation at professional conferences, disseminating my work, and making my contributions to nursing. I also plan to share my project at the hospital and university levels, as well as through posters, lectures, and seminar presentations. I am confident that disseminating my work will add to the body of knowledge and bridge the gap between knowledge and practice existing in my area of specialty. In enriching my career while alleviating disparities, my goals include the creation of a course that provides orientation, support, and resources to second-degree students entering the nursing profession, especially those with English as a second language (ESOL), to navigate better the demands of accelerated learning experienced at the ABSN level. This effort mitigates the challenges of learning a new language and a new career unlike any other (which nursing certainly is). With this in mind, I endeavor to incorporate new knowledge in teaching by strengthening the quality of evidence through continued research and clinical practice.

Your Future Goals

One thing that is so amazing about nursing is that there are so many different opportunities for involvement and growth. There are many areas of nursing that I enjoy and hope to pursue in different ways. I still would like to complete a post-master's degree as an Advanced Practice Nurse to prepare to teach at all higher education levels and participate in practice to remain current in nursing trends and disseminate DNP research projects clinically. My goals and aspirations range from creating more accelerated programs at both the BSN and MSN levels to being an administrator of those programs to increase accessibility to nursing and improve the nursing shortage that exists—providing service to members of the adult population in my community and even opening a dialysis facility in an area that is lacking this service. I also plan to use my nursing skills on a global level by becoming involved in short-term mission trips to third-world countries, including my native Jamaica, to impact healthcare in a positive way to give back to schools and communities alike. There are many opportunities available to nurses in the world today. I am excited to continue my career with even more confidence as a nurse and see what options lay ahead.

The Greatest Source of Satisfaction You Find in Your Work

Promoting positive outcomes for those in the classroom and the community through my teaching, scholarship, and service, and providing students with an increased awareness that will create advocates for the populations they serve have been my most significant sources of satisfaction in my work to date.

I am proud of my sustained contributions toward achieving meaningful diversity, inclusion, and belonging for students of color in nursing education and the nursing profession, and of having led two teams in this challenging and essential work, with each advancing a different approach and promising to achieve substantial gains for our discipline. Each has changed the lives of young students from underrepresented minorities by helping them overcome barriers to success in demanding nursing curricula. I am deeply engaged both personally and professionally in this vital endeavor.

As the first in my family to attend college, I have been very intentional in my efforts to create supportive and inclusive experiences in nursing education for students of color and first-generation college students. Because of my passion for this work, I have assisted students from diverse backgrounds in achieving their academic and career goals by being a role model, coach, and mentor, doing my best to inspire students through my accomplishments with the hope of helping them see what their success might look like.

I am very fortunate to be the faculty lead for a $1.5-million grant to create a pipeline for high school students who wish to become nurses. This program provides a bundle of evidence-based strategies to promote academic success of nursing students from underrepresented minorities (URM) and disadvantaged backgrounds (DB). This bundle translates a set of strategies demonstrated to advance academic success and goal attainment among Science Technology Engineering Mathematics and National Collegiate Athletic Association student-athletes to meet the needs of Baccalaureate of Science in Nursing (BSN) students from URM & DB.

The project, conducted in partnership with Temple University Health System (TUHS) and five area high schools, complements the Department of Nursing's commitment to educating a resilient nursing workforce dedicated to this disadvantaged community and serving Philadelphia. Our team is working to mitigate barriers to higher education for students from URM & DB, focusing on five objectives:

1. increase the number of nursing students from URM & DB;
2. increase the number of faculty from URM & DB;
3. promote the academic success of nursing students from URM & DB;
4. overcome financial barriers to nursing education; and
5. create an environment of belonging and inclusion in the nursing department.

In this role, I have been responsible for coordinating learning assessments, tutoring, learning communities, coaching, and mentoring that accompanies full 4-year tuition support for a cohort of students from North Philadelphia high schools. With this project, we have been providing immersion and enrichment experiences for high school students, education about nursing careers for high school guidance counselors, and planning the course work and application materials required for admission to our nursing program. I plan to continue to help build a more inclusive, respectful, and diverse community in which students of color will belong, achieve, and thrive.

Increasing diversity, equity, and inclusion is essential and requires support from all levels, but, most importantly, organizations are at the forefront of nursing and are change agents. As many have argued, there is an "opportunity gap" in higher education. More specifically for me, it is among nursing students, and is not in the students' abilities but in the disparate opportunities they are afforded. Diversity among students and faculty allows for representation and a sense of belonging and inclusion. Speaking up for equity is a recipe for successful outcomes and increases retention. Students are accepted into nursing programs with the required prerequisites, but their circumstances are different, affecting their outcomes. The challenge is for leaders to commit to ensuring sustained efforts in identifying those needs and "leveling the playing field" for everyone. I consider myself a champion of that cause and continue to hope for those opportunities to share my vision and collaborate on creating that change at the highest level of nursing with organizations such as the National League of Nursing Fellow in the Academy of Nurse Educators (ANEF) and the Fellow in the American Academy of Nursing (AAN) (FAAN), to name a couple.

I have engaged with Independence Foundation by participating in a workshop that brings leaders from the community from various organizations providing social services within the Philadelphia community, including board members, CEOs, managers, HR directors, and other leaders, to learn strategies for implementing diversity, equity, and inclusion within their organizations and improve work cultures. I have completed two sessions of 6 weeks of learning each to explore and share plans for sustained initiatives and have signed on the be among the workgroup for ongoing dialogue and to be a resource for other groups new to the DEI initiative.

I have volunteered my time and insight to help form an affiliate group within the nursing department to address implicit bias and other negative behaviors and to create a more inclusive workplace where everyone can be free to be themselves. I believe this work aligns with the mission and goals of the leading organizations in nursing, such as the American Nurses Association (ANA), National League for Nursing (NLN), American Association of Colleges of Nursing (AACN), Sigma, and others, and that by advancing these practices at the college and community level by creating equitable opportunities and increasing awareness among students, and through continued efforts to build our communities by identifying the social determinants of health that exist, my work will continue to promote excellence in nursing education to build a stable and diverse nursing workforce to advance the health of our nation and the global community.

Any Words of Wisdom to Nurses Considering Earning a Doctorate

The October 2010 Institute of Medicine (IOM) report focused on *The Future of Nursing: Leading Change, Advancing Health*. The report made eight recommendations to support efforts to improve the health of the U.S. population through the contributions nurses can make to care delivery. Four of these recommendations address areas such as:

"Nurses should practice to the full extent of their education and training. Nurses should achieve higher levels of education and train through an improved education system that promotes seamless academic progression. Nurses should be full partners, with physicians and other health professionals, in redesigning healthcare in the United States. The nurse should be involved as effective workforce planning and policymaking requires better data collection and information infrastructure."

I agree with these recommendations and concur that a terminal degree in nursing should empower nurses to forge this path and be at the forefront of these efforts as they take our profession forward while improving our nation's health. However, it is imperative to pursue that degree in the area you are most passionate about. I initially thought that a PhD was the "best" route to earn my doctorate. Where I am from, all other doctoral degrees are considered second best and often require defining. Understanding my passion and the work I want to pursue in academia or clinical practice, the DNP route is my best option. Therefore, I encourage future doctoral students to consider their lifelong plan, and if they are inclined to work mainly in research, the PhD may be their route. If they plan to be nurse educators with dreams of creating curriculums, the EdD may be their route. For those interested in teaching and clinical practice, with less focus on research, the DNP is their best bet.

CHAPTER 31

The Practice Nurse Narratives

Vanesa Velez, DNP, RN ■
Nicole Angelique Gonzaga Gomez, DNP, CRNA, APRN, CHSE ■
Sunghee Kim, DNP, ANP-BC, NP-C

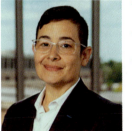

Vanesa Velez, DNP, RN

Your Initial Motivation to Become a Nurse

On January 1, 2000, my best friend's daughter was mede-vacked to a local hospital with chest pain and difficulty breathing. By the end of that first day, she was on extra-corporeal membrane oxygenation (ECMO) and fighting for her life with the help of a world-class medical team. The stars of that team were the nurses. They bathed her, then brushed and braided her hair while talking to her kindly and gently. They took the time to help each of us understand what was happening. They advocated fiercely for what they believed was best for her. They were the ones who noticed she'd had a stroke related to the anticoagulation necessary to run the ECMO pump and insisted she get a computed tomography (CT) scan. They were an impressive balance of brains, heart, and clarity of thought and voice. I wanted to help people the way they'd helped me, so I went to nursing school.

Your Entry to Practice

I entered nursing with an Associate's Degree when I was about 30 years old. I'd studied psych, then had several jobs in the psych field, but felt adrift and without purpose.

Your Decision to Pursue Higher Education

Several years into my nursing career, I found that I was precepting new graduate nurses a lot. Almost half my year was spent teaching nurses new to the unit how to care for our patients. I found that I loved it and wanted to learn more about teaching and learning. I went back to school for my Bachelor of Science in Nursing (BSN).

The Educational Path You Chose and the Reasoning Behind That Decision

First I needed to get my BSN, and chose a local school with a registered nurse (RN) to BSN program that ran in cohorts. I chose a cohort program because I knew the work would be hard, and I wanted to have peers that I could count on for support and to give support in return. I also wanted a program where the faculty would get to know me and I could also get to know them.

Who Were Your Mentors

Mentors have made all the difference in my life and my career. I am grateful for my mentors because they often saw more in me than I saw in myself and pushed me to become the nurse and leader they saw I could be. My first mentor was the nurse manager who hired me out of nursing school. She tucked me under her wing and gave me opportunities to learn and grow. She offered me feedback that was a gift because she showed me how to get out of my own way and cheered for me every step of the way. Other mentors have been faculty who challenged me to think more deeply and to challenge my understanding of nursing, clinical challenges, and my role. A faculty mentor who made a huge difference was my mentor during my master's practicum. She encouraged me to apply for doctoral programs and placed me with a practicum preceptor who, as faculty in a school of nursing, was in a very different role than my role as a unit-based educator. She was a model of professional nursing on the academic side and was so generous with her time and knowledge.

What Were the Milestones on Your Path

Key points on my journey include going back to school for my BSN and attending a workshop for nurses considering doctoral degrees. I would not be where or who I am today without each of those decisions. When I started my BSN, I planned to keep going for my Master of Science in Nursing (MSN), so that first step was a milestone. Talking with the students and doctorally prepared nurses at the workshop helped me see that I could do it and that it was worth trying.

What Barriers You Faced and What Strategies You Used to Navigate Them

Barriers I faced included working full time, parenting a young child, and my own thoughts and beliefs about my capacity. At the start of every semester, I would sit down with my calendar and the syllabus for each course and map out when each assignment and its components were due, and when I would work on them.

I scheduled time for literature reviews, for writing, and for reading. Every part of my day was mapped out to ensure I did what I needed to do. My days included early wake-ups for school work, a full day at work, dinner with my daughter, then back to studying once she was asleep. I didn't attend to the imposter syndrome in any systematic way; when the negative self-talk would start and that small voice inside challenged my ability to be successful, I would put my head down and work harder.

Your Current Focus

I am the director of graduate nursing programs and chief nurse administrator at a local university. My focus is to prepare the next generation of nurses and to inspire them to achieve.

Your Future Goals

Nursing is at a crossroads. My goals at this point are to push the envelope on how we train and prepare nurses for the work ahead.

The Greatest Source of Satisfaction You Find in Your Work

I love being a nurse and take great pride in preparing future nurses to be and give to patients and their families what those nurses were to me so many years ago.

Any Words of Wisdom to Nurses Considering Earning a Doctorate

Do it! I am where I am and who I am because I was willing to take the risk and to walk through every open door. It is hard and it is worth it.

Talk about it! Talk about what you're doing and let your people support you. You'll also be an inspiration to others who may be considering taking the next step.

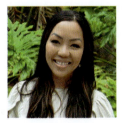

Nicole Angelique Gonzaga Gomez, DNP, CRNA, APRN, CHSE

My Initial Motivation to Become a Nurse

Becoming a nurse in the Filipino culture was so commonplace—in fact, even a stereotype. (The comedian, Jo Koy, has said that the "safest place to be was at one of his comedy shows" because of all the Filipino nurses in the audience.) The ironic thing was that my parents never encouraged the profession of nursing, yet I still chose it anyway. The only nurse on either side of the family was my mother's first cousin, and she was a charge nurse at the Manhattan VA for many years. So, there were not any nurses in my immediate family.

For the longest time I wanted to be a medical doctor, and I wanted to go to schools out of state, but as time got closer to graduating high school, I realized there were so many other professions I was deeply passionate about—eclectic ones even. Around the middle of my sophomore year of high school, I laid out four options for myself: an aeronautical engineer to fly fighter jets and become a pilot; a creative journalist or an editor of a classy newspaper or magazine; a classically trained musician (which has always taken a stronghold in our family with my mother being a classically trained pianist and having earned a degree in music education); or a medical doctor (mostly likely a surgeon). My mother's father was a doctor in the Philippines, so that was always in the back of my mind, and my mother always felt the need to remind my sister and me of that fact. I felt strongly about becoming any one of the four that I laid out for myself, but as a young 16-year-old with a steady boyfriend who went to school only 2 hours away (instead of out of state), staying in-state looked more and more attractive as graduation from high school neared. I chose nursing because it offered a balance between doing what I was passionate about (medical field), working hard, and still having opportunities to live life. I joined my beau a year later at the University of Texas. It was the best decision that declared itself and was my first step in my journey on the path to becoming a nurse.

Entry to Practice

Prior to graduating from nursing school, I flew out to Los Angeles on spring break to look for opportunities in the intensive care unit (ICU). I knew that I wanted to go straight into critical care because of the challenges of a higher-acuity patient population. At the time, there weren't many new graduate-to-ICU positions in California like there were in Texas. I called many hospital systems in Los Angeles, but I came up against a brick wall. Only University of California, Los Angeles (UCLA) offered some ray of hope—a possible pilot new graduate-to-ICU program in their infamous cardiothoracic ICU. I returned home to Austin defeated, but I had my backup plan in place. Over the Easter break, I was interviewed at the Memorial Hermann Hospital for a night position in their shock/trauma ICU. I was elated as I was offered the position on the spot. Six more weeks went by, and graduation day finally arrived. As I was practicing my speech as the Nursing Students' Association President, I received a letter from UCLA inviting me to interview for the inaugural pilot new graduate ICU program. The irony behind that call was that it happened on my graduation day, when I was supposed to give an inspirational speech. I took it as a sign to interview. Long story short, I ended up with the position after I had started my position in the shock/trauma ICU. I knew once I stepped foot on the unit that this ICU was where I belonged. It was a huge turning point in my life, and one I didn't want to pass up. While I don't recommend accepting/resigning from a position after starting orientation, let's just say that it was a large lesson to learn early on in my career.

My Decision to Pursue Higher Education

I always knew that I would go on to graduate school. When I started in the ICU, I worked closely with cardiothoracic acute care nurse practitioners who also "opened" and "closed" for the surgeons during their procedures. *Wow—a Nurse Practitioner (NP) doing surgery.* I never knew that could be a role for an NP while in nursing school. I was fascinated. I remember hearing about the nurse anesthetist profession when I was a sophomore in high school from a close friend of mine who wanted to join the Navy and pursue that career. I loved the science behind anesthesia—even though I didn't really fully understand what it meant to be an anesthesia provider at the time. It sounded "hard" or challenging, so I put that on my list for the future. I even flirted with the idea of travel nursing because I thought it would bring me the best of both worlds—doing what I love while experiencing and living in different places. (One of the new graduates I started with did do just that and eventually went on to the nurse anesthesia school.) Eventually, I settled on the path toward becoming a Certified Registered Nurse Anesthetist (CRNA). I had already submitted my application to Columbia University earlier that May; however, in the wake of the 9/11 attacks, I wanted to go there—be there, live there, and somehow do something more with my career. I was accepted in 2001, and I never looked back. It still amazes me how quickly I pivoted and started on that path 20 years ago. *Time flies.*

My Mentors
THE EYES OF TEXAS: LONGHORN NURSING

When I think about my mentors throughout my career, there have been so many of them, since before graduating high school. I think about my Biology Advanced Placement (AP) instructor from my senior year in high school, my freshman ethics professor, and my senior year nursing clinical instructor. I found out that my faculty mentor passed away recently when I received my *Longhorn Nursing* magazine. There was a book she wanted us to all read: *The 7 Habits of Highly Effective People* by Stephen Covey. She taught with love and compassion in her work and with her students, but there was so much substance and truth to what she would say. She brought a wealth of knowledge about empathy and beneficence that shaped who I was as a nurse at the bedside.

I also have to mention a nursing student in the class ahead of me who paved the way for me to follow in her footsteps to be our Nursing Students' Association President and a Junior Fellows Research scholar. I looked up to her and observed how she approached things. Some of my biggest milestones during my undergraduate studies are owed to her. When I delivered our class speech at graduation,

I felt accomplished. It was a huge milestone for not only me but also my family. After working in the same shock/trauma ICU in Houston where I (almost) started, she went on to University of Alabama Birmingham for her PhD. We keep in touch to this day and send Christmas cards every year.

Milestones

BECOMING A NURSE IN THE CARDIOTHORACIC ICU

All the UCLA cardiothoracic unit nurses were my mentors in the beginning of my nursing career. (I have to chuckle a little here because they all scared us.) All of them were tough; I had to grow up fast. "There is no crying in ICU nursing". Although Tom Hanks's character from *A League of Their Own* was not our nurse manager, the average number of years of experience for the nurses was probably close to seven. We had adult, pediatric, and neonatal cardiothoracic surgical patients, so my first 2 years were spent learning about the adult population. After proving myself, leadership decided I was ready to take on the congenital heart surgical patients. I was up for the challenge, and soon enough I was taking care of 3-kg neonates after a Stage I Norwood repair for hypoplastic left heart syndrome.

It was exciting (and stressful); it was emotional and mentally taxing as well. I had my first death, my first postmortem, my first everything. Some of these nurses watched us grow up before their very eyes and take on leadership roles. Soon, I was precepting and making the schedule, and set to take charge. Taking on more responsibility and being one of the "pedi" trained were huge accomplishments, but the itch was always there to keep going. *What else can I do and accomplish?* I was the first to leave for Nurse Anesthesia school, and then a few more of us new graduates left a year or two later (and later on, our doctoral degrees). Then, a funny thing happened on the way to the Doctor of Nursing Practice Degree: Those very same nurses eventually went back to pursue their own graduate and doctoral degrees. *Our mentors looked at all of us as mentors.* When they started their journeys, they stated that *we had inspired them* to keep going. It was touching to see how life had come full circle. I keep in touch with a few of the fellow "new graduate" ICU nurses (four of whom are CRNAs, and one a Doctor of Nurse Anesthesia Practice -(DNAP).

THE CITY THAT NEVER SLEEPS

In Nurse Anesthesia school, my first rotation was in the city, and it was a pain to get to work in the morning (three trains and a bus), but the hospital was nice, and the operating room (OR) started later at 0830. It was the only hospital that had operating rooms with windows. My first CRNA preceptor was so instrumental in guiding me during those first 3 months of nurse anesthesia residency. The content in the program was front-loaded, so when clinical rotations began, we were truly in a residency program. We received a stipend like physician residents, and we worked 4 days a week, all hours of the day, until our cases were finished. Occasionally, we were sent home if the case was set to go on for several more hours and we had to be back the next day.

My preceptor was the right combination of tough love and warmth. She was an avid reader, so she recommended a lot of "non-anesthesia" books to make my commutes back and forth more tolerable. I read *a lot* during those days. One day that summer, I took the train back into the city while reading *The House of Sand and Fog*. As I exited the subway, all the streetlights were out, and people were running around. The 2003 blackout had just begun. People were worrying about looting and violence, and I was worrying about making it to clinical the next day. Needless to say, we were all excused from clinicals, but my preceptor found my worry and stress when we all finally returned to work quite amusing. *You can't sweat the small stuff, kiddo.* (I did read *Tuesdays with Morrie*, and she recommended it.) Everything with her was about balance. It was important that I understood the relationship between work and play, self-care, and rest—especially in my personal life. I was a week shy of 26 years old when I started the program, and I had a lot yet to learn not only about anesthesia but also *life*. But I did not know it back then.

After 2 years (the degree was a master's degree back then), I graduated and started working at one of my rotation sites: a large urban academic medical center. Graduating from an Ivy League school was huge; I wanted my parents to be proud, and education in our culture is very important. Passing my board exam (and getting 96%, *yes—we used to receive percentages*) and starting my CRNA career was also a milestone. I had never studied and worked so hard in my life. To this day, I will always say that Nurse Anesthesia school was the most challenging and taxing of all my degrees.

Many mentors, both CRNAs and attending anesthesiologists alike, helped shape the beginning of my CRNA career. The anesthesia department's culture was inclusive, diverse, and progressive—all ahead of its time. There were new graduates who started with me *(the Fab Four of '04)* and there were seasoned CRNAs who had worked for over 15 years or even with the inventor of the *Laryngeal Mask Airway Device* in London. *(Wayne was like a Jamaican father to all of us. Rest in peace.)* I felt supported and encouraged to spread my wings, tackle any case, and do any procedure within my scope of practice. I started my obstetric (OB), pediatric, and cardiac specialties, and I am grateful to many of them who are still practicing there to this day.

WELCOME TO MIAMI, BIENVENIDO A MIAMI

After 2 years, I made the decision to move to South Florida for a career opportunity. I became an OB CRNA, one who specializes in OB anesthesia, and it was a new position at the hospital that I was working for at the time.

Leaving the medical center was tough, but many factors (including financial) influenced my decision. It was a great opportunity, new city to experience, and I was ready for the next phase of my career. Again, I found many mentors when I first landed in Miami, and they, too, helped grow my experience in the OB anesthesia specialty as well as the busy tempo of private practice anesthesia groups. So many people have touched the path of my nursing career and continue to do so currently.

THE ROAD TO THE DOCTOR OF NURSING PRACTICE

Several years later, when I decided to go back and earn my doctoral degree, I had mulled over the idea of going to medical school. So much of my early childhood had been wanting to become a doctor *(or because of my Filipino mother)*, but as I grew up, I knew nursing offered the right blend of the things that I was looking for in a career. I had come to a fork in the road. I had been working in Miami as an OB CRNA, and I became the Chief OB CRNA shortly thereafter. I spoke with several colleagues/mentors—my chief of anesthesia, my (soon-to-be) Doctor of Nursing Practice (DNP) site advisor, all of my CRNA colleagues, and friends. I knew later in my career that I wanted to teach, yet I wasn't certain if the time was right.

Many times in my life, when forks in the road popped up, the right decision would declare itself. After researching a few programs, I applied to three. I had gotten an early decision in November, but I wanted to wait to see all my options. In February, I got a call, so I flew up for a night to interview the next day. The right decision had declared itself. I learned "outside of my silo" from our fantastic program director, and I have used much of her teaching style and readings in my classroom today. My DNP faculty advisor was also instrumental and mentored me in a way that I also mentor my DNP mentees. She was the right fit for me. She held me to deadlines, and we met every beginning of the semester to nail down our schedules. *Respect* was an important characteristic in our mentor–mentee relationship. (*As the rubber hits the road, respect was always the center of all things.*) Graduating from the DNP program at my top-choice university was a huge accomplishment for not only myself but also my family. If I had not been so blessed by so many rich and instrumental mentors over my long career in nursing and my education leading up to my career, I would not be where I am today—as the Associate Program Director and Assistant Professor in a DNP Nurse Anesthesia Program.

Barriers I Faced and the Strategies I Used to Navigate Them

Going back to school is a financial decision of sorts: One must make the decision on *whether the struggle is worth the investment*. And by that time I had been working in a career that afforded options. My schedule was 2 weeks on, 1 week off. My fellow OB "angels" helped work out the schedule for the weeks during the semester I had to be at school. I was also in a better position financially after moving to Miami, and I had also gotten my financial plan and goals aligned. However, doctoral education was not inexpensive, and I could have chosen to stay locally and not spend as much time/money on commute twice a semester. My heart was set on going to a new city, a hallowed institution, and to be different. I was the only CRNA in my cohort.

Suffice to say, I have put myself through all my degrees. There was not much in the way of financial grants or scholarships for Asian/Pacific Islanders in the 1980s, 1990s, or even early 2000s. I received merit scholarships while in nursing school, but there was not much for nurse anesthesia residents (except our stipends each semester). Diversity, equity, and inclusion was just blossoming, and mostly African-American and Hispanic/Latino cultures had the many opportunities. I had saved some money but still applied for school loans much like I had done in the past, and I worked past those barriers. *The struggle was worth the investment.*

My Current Focus

My current focus: Growing the future generations of our profession. *100%*. After graduating, I took some time to think on what the next step was—*yet again*. I often questioned, *Why couldn't I just be content? Was I ready to teach?* (As Twyla Tharp said, *I had to knit…*). I had gained an adjunct faculty title and was guest lecturing at the University of Miami since 2012, but I still wasn't sure if I was ready to leave the clinical setting for an academic teaching position. It wasn't until Spring 2017 that an opportunity came knocking. One of the faculty was starting her PhD studies, and teaching was stretching things a bit too thin. She had asked me if I was still thinking about teaching. With a family and studies to think about, it was the right time for her to step away. I stepped into a part-time position that summer. I taught eight credits and worked part time clinically. I learned a lot during that year, and I realized that "straddling the fence" with teaching and being in the OR wasn't sustainable for my schedule (not to mention being engaged and planning a wedding). I made the transition to full-time faculty in the summer of 2018.

My Future Goals

My goal at the beginning of my academic teaching career was *to be a good teacher*. All these years I have learned *to do*; now I had to learn *to teach*. I have since expanded on those goals to include facilitating, disseminating, and assisting in publishing my doctoral advisees' projects. I have gained my Certified Healthcare Simulation Educator (CHSE) and have done work with mixed-reality and expanding to virtual reality in simulation for skills and high-acuity/low-frequency case scenarios. Peer mentorship in nurse anesthesia and in simulation-based education is important to me, as is OB anesthesia education and research. Though the pandemic has brought international medical mission trips to a halt, slowly but surely, trips are restarting with organizations across the globe. I have been a medical volunteer with the Healing Hands Foundation since 2010, and I hope the foundation plans on resuming missions next year. I have taken three doctoral nurse anesthesia students to Guatemala in the past, and I hope to continue in the future.

Since being appointed to Associate Program Director, I had to sell my shares in a medical aesthetics spa that I co-owned for 4 years as my schedule and life took a different turn. I had learned a lot in running a business with my partner, but she has taken the reins and fully taken off (and is a successful family nurse practitioner [FNP], might I add). I would not have had the guts to start the business without the knowledge I gained during my doctoral studies. I plan to finish my 200-hour yoga teaching training this year and incorporate that work into my classroom—the importance of self-care, well-being, and mental health. I have been practicing yoga for the better part of 16 years, and it has helped me maintain that balance Maggie spoke about so long ago.

My Greatest Source of Satisfaction

One of the greatest sources of satisfaction and reward in teaching at the doctoral level is seeing people grow, flourish, and evolve. I teach a review course that begins at the start of students' third year in the DNP Nurse Anesthesia Program. I have worked on self-study modules with a focus for students to self-reflect: *To know who you are and who you will become as a future, doctoral-prepared CRNA will be your greatest asset moving forward.* It is one of the most eye-opening moments for me as a professor to read a 15-minute set of assignments throughout the course because I learn a little bit more about each of them.

Sunghee Kim, DNP, ANP-BC, NP-C

Words of Wisdom

Find what makes you tick. Nothing is worth doing if you don't have a passion for it. Life is unfortunately too short to be wasting time doing something that doesn't get you up in the morning. The pandemic has woken many with career changes or retirements. I know that I can't do this career forever—I am in clinical 1 day a week, and I still get excited about doing cases, doing anesthesia, precepting a future CRNA. I smile when I see the lightbulbs go off in students' eyes. I remember thinking while in my DNP program: *Besides teaching, what else can I do with my doctoral degree?* Well, folks, I started a medical aesthetics business (that I still consult and advise), I have been asked to be a subject matter expert (SME) for virtual-reality applications for simulation teaching and design, and I have been asked to consult on medical legal cases regarding anesthesia or related issues. Earning your doctorate opens not only doors but windows, chimneys, side doors—you name it. There is an unlimited version of yourself just waiting to be discovered.

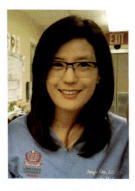

I am so honored to receive this opportunity to talk about my nursing career, a long journey that has culminated in my current position as a Doctor of Nursing Practice (DNP) in the Emergency Department at an academic medical center. I hope to share my story with others who have made the decision to pursue a doctorate degree in their nursing career.

I felt deeply nervous and terrified every time I attended my classes during the DNP program—a fear that stayed with me until the final day. At the same time, I can confidently say that the program was one of the most unforgettable and valuable experiences of my life. My advice is to not be discouraged or irresolute about your choice to pursue the highest nursing degree.

I can say with confidence that you are more than capable of completing this degree. I know that because I survived the Master's and DNP degrees as an adult immigrant. To this day, I struggle with my second language (English), even though I passed the TOEFL (Test of English as a Foreign Language) multiple times. On top of that, when I was attending the DNP program, I was raising two kids, managing family obligations, including taking care of my mother, who was suffering from chronic medical conditions in South Korea, and keeping on top of my urgent care work as an NP. Since my family was based in California, I would fly from the west coast to Maryland for school on a regular basis. But with the help of my mentors, family, and friends, I made it through. This is not to say it was easy: between these commitments and the challenging assignments and the Capstone/Scholarly project, there was not quite enough time for sleeping during those 2 years.

Despite the challenges, pursuing the DNP was certainly rewarding. The highlight for me was publishing my quality improvement Capstone/Scholarly project in a peer-reviewed journal.[1] In general, it was an invaluable time to learn more about myself and advance my professional career.

My Initial Motivation to Become a Nurse

I was born and raised in Seoul, South Korea. When I was young, my mother had a lot of medical and mental problems and was frequently hospitalized. I distinctly remember the smell of the hospital, the medical equipment, and the nurses and doctors who took care of my mother. As a result, I was exposed at an early age to various healthcare professionals and settings, which led me to choose the nursing route without hesitation. In my opinion, what nurses do represents the full scope of human interaction. I very much appreciate the sublime beauty that is nursing and nurse care.

Ever since I started my career as a Registered Nurse (RN) in the Intensive Care Unit (ICU) at a university medical center in South Korea, I have always tried to be thoughtful and compassionate in my interactions with patients. Nursing is in many ways an intimate form of human interaction, and my experiences regularly led me to confront the deepest parts of the human experience and to think about the meaning of our lives and our deaths. These reflections helped motivate me to be a better nurse for my patients and to build a wide range of skills to meet the diversity of patient and family needs.

My clinical experience as an RN spans multiple ICUs at several university-based hospitals where I have worked, including the medical intensive care unit (MICU), the respiratory intensive care unit (RICU), and the cardiac intensive care unit (CICU).

As I continued working in the ICU and witnessed many more patients suffering from critical conditions and living with tremendous pain, I yearned for more knowledge as a healthcare professional, which led me to consider pursuing a higher degree in nursing in South Korea. However, in South Korea, the Master of Science of Nursing (MSN) meant taking one of two paths: either the academic track that focused on teaching with little time spent in the clinic; or the clinical nurse track that lacked the autonomy to make diagnoses or order prescriptions. As I was preparing to take the TOEFL to qualify for the MSN in South Korea, I happened to learn about the role of the NP in the US healthcare system. As soon as I heard of it, my intuition told me that this path would better align with my dream to learn and practice with more advanced knowledge in nursing. That, among other factors, prompted me to expand my horizons toward the United States.

Milestones

In 2000, I moved to the United States, where my first job was to be the charge RN at a skilled nursing facility in Kansas City. There, I struggled to learn the responsibilities of my role as an RN in a nursing home, a healthcare setting that was not common in South Korea at the time. My second position in the United States was that of an RN in the MICU/RICU in Cedars Sinai Medical Center in Los Angeles. Fortunately, my time in that role was an enlightening experience, and I learned many critical care nursing skills that eventually helped me secure an RN role in the coronary intensive care unit (CICU) at Loma Linda University Medical Center.

After attaining the CICU RN role, I worked my way up to the charge nurse. Once I became accustomed to the charge role, I decided it was finally time to move on to the next step, to pursue the master's degree, which I had been thinking about ever since I moved to the United States. At the time, the MSN program was an important professional stepping-stone to the DNP, so I started there. I was convinced that my past experiences and heartfelt commitment to patients would enable me to succeed in the program. Among the various MSN programs, I was initially drawn to Nurse Anesthesia because of my ICU experiences. However, Loma Linda University did not have that program back in 2006.

So, instead, I applied to the adult nurse practitioner (ANP) program and graduated in 2009.

After graduation, one of my mentors, who worked in occupational medicine at a community medical center, helped me find a work experience quickly. I was lucky to have a mentor who appreciated my passion and gave me the opportunity to advance my career and expand my horizons. I learned that it is very important to express your enthusiasm for the paths that interest you during your clinical rotations. In my case, my passion and enthusiasm helped show me the right path.

My first NP role was as a clinician in the urgent care at a local medical group in 2009. Then I moved to the urgent care of Loma Linda University Healthcare in 2012. Once I got used to working at the urgent care and became more comfortable in my new role as an NP, I felt motivated to pursue another, higher academic challenge. This led me to apply to the DNP degree from Johns Hopkins University School of Nursing (JHUSON).

Educational Path

In 2014, I audaciously decided to apply to one of the top-rated DNP programs in the United States. I was convinced that earning the DNP degree would be the highest achievement of my career and allow me to grow to become a leader in my field. I was working as an NP in one of the busiest urgent care centers in the area and regularly met not only with patients with common urgent care problems but also with patients with more serious conditions. Practicing as an NP in urgent care (UC) required strong clinical knowledge along with critical thinking and multitasking skills. But the more I honed my skills as an NP at the UC, the more my dream of becoming a DNP grew. I realized that it was an important goal for me to reach the apex of my profession in my life. I just was not sure when to make the attempt. But I knew that I firmly believed in the DNP degree and thought that it would portray my profession positively to patients and to my colleagues, including the physicians and the staff. I was the first person who earned the DNP degree in the urgent care in 2014, which meant that I had to explain my title and role to my colleagues and patients. Nowadays, I notice more and more NPs who aspire to the DNP, and our title and role do not need to be explained as frequently.

For me, being an expert NP means being able to apply evidence-based practice in my care and to serve as a leader for creating better patient care outcomes in clinical settings. Part of that is motivating other NPs and students to seek and translate clinical research into real clinical practice. In short, my role is to be a leader, motivator, and clinical educator in my clinical field.

My Mentors

During my career, I was fortunate to meet many pivotal mentors. In particular, I would like to thank my mentors from the DNP program for inspiring me to improve my project throughout the process. An incisive remark from my mentors helped me at every stage, from defining the problem I wanted to address to presenting my final project on the final day of the program. Eventually, I was able to publish my quality improvement project for the sickle cell disease population in a peer-reviewed academic journal.

Completing the DNP program remains in many ways the pinnacle of my professional career. It taught me that if I wanted to make a difference as a leader, my power to do so would have to come from my knowledge and competence. The DNP, not just the final degree but also the unforgettable journey of the program itself, has been so formative and significant in my life and has helped me mature personally and professionally in many ways. I am especially grateful to the DNP program and my mentors for encouraging me to connect my project to community issues or problems that we face and to integrate all learning experiences.

Barriers I Faced and the Strategies I Used to Navigate Them

For me, the most significant barrier was that I wasn't born and raised in the United States, making English my second language. I used four to six dictionaries to make the sentences to express my thoughts and ideas, which was challenging and time-consuming. Often, I had to stay up all night to submit the assignments on time.

Another barrier was balancing studying with work and family obligations. I tried my best to balance my work schedule with my study schedule, including trips to the school, but it wasn't easy. Without the support of my family, I wouldn't have graduated from the program. As a mother and a wife, I had many responsibilities that I could not sacrifice, which meant reducing my sleep hours to find time for the assignments. Cultivating time management skills and communicating my questions regularly with mentors were crucial to my success in the program. I always reviewed the syllabus of each class ahead of time to prepare questions and make sure I understood the directions.

My Current Focus

My current title is a DNP and assistant professor in the emergency department at Loma Linda University Medical Center. Since starting my role, I have kept trying to expand my knowledge and become an experienced DNP who is a valuable asset to the healthcare team.

Your Future Goals

I would like to give case presentations at NP conferences to share my experience and some of the interesting clinical cases I have managed. More generally, I would like to serve as a guide and preceptor to novice NPs, PAs, or students in my clinical setting. I am as motivated and committed as ever to my profession, and I want to be an excellent DNP who has earned the respect of patients, staff, and colleagues.

My Greatest Source of Satisfaction

I love challenges, achievement, and recognition—all of these factors motivate me to work efficiently and effectively. I have been lucky to work with several high-functioning teams during my career. The faculty who taught me and their commitment, passion, and teaching methods remain a source of inspiration. Another thing that motivates me is the fact that more and more patients, staff, colleagues, and administrators are recognizing the role of the DNP in a positive way.

Words of Wisdom to Nurses Considering Earning a Doctorate

"Push yourself! You can achieve more than you think!"

"Be bold and calm, keep your nerve!"

CHAPTER 32

The Psychiatric Mental Health Clinician Narrative

Susan Painter, DNP, APRN, PMHCNS-BC

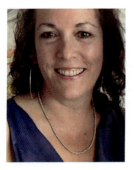

Motivation to Become a Nurse

I envisioned myself being a nurse for as long as I can remember. I was the youngest of four children born to parents who were raised in rural Appalachian communities in Southern West Virginia. My mother was 24 years of age when I was born, which left her with four children under the age of four, including me, subsequently I was born on my eldest sibling's fourth birthday. My mother shared with me (once I was old enough to understand) that she had her "tubes tied" after my youngest brother was delivered 18 months prior to my birth. She would remind me of this story at various times throughout my nursing education when I felt too tired or conflicted over continuing my educational career. "Quitting is not who you are" she would say. "You overcame the obstacle of arriving on this earth when you were medically deterred...you were determined then, and you are determined now." End of conversation.

Both my parents were incredibly bright people, and my mother often said her biggest regret was not having the opportunity to attend university. Her own mother was diagnosed with terminal cancer when she was in high school and quite sadly died when my mother was just 19 years old.

My biological father was a Navy veteran who suffered from chronic mental illness and alcoholism. I am certain the effects of being a veteran escalated his addiction and concurrent mental illness once he was discharged from service. The effects of "secondary trauma" for children being raised in the early 1960s was not even a term that had yet been coined. During this time, if a married woman contacted the police for emergency assistance at home, they were told "*he's your husband*," and the police would leave and move on to other, more important matters. It was not customary to discuss "family issues" such as these outside the home, and children struggled through childhood most often without support from a society that was then accepting of the privilege of men being the provider and the head of the household. I learned a great deal from the imprint these experiences left on me. The positive swing on histories such as these is that I learned to observe behaviors and eventually gained insight into reading nonverbal behaviors of others, all of which is keen in one's development of communication skills in becoming a psychiatric nurse. I have often said my best education came from my childhood experiences, as I learned to understand empathy, compassion, and stigma as well as the life lessons that accompanied them.

Your Entry to Practice

The metropolitan public school system in which I attended high school went on strike during my junior and senior years. My class graduated in the middle of the summer. I had a research project in my senior year that entailed writing a biography of someone we admired from history. I chose Florence Nightingale and was inspired by her contributions to the nursing profession and the monumental changes that she made throughout her life and career. One of my high school teachers nicknamed me "Flo" because he said I was so incredibly animated when I spoke about her life. Feeling enlightened by her insight, my passion for nursing changed from a flame to a fire. Although I had always dreamed I would be a nurse someday, this was the point in time when I began to realize that I could not see myself doing anything else in my life.

Although I was a bright child and excelled in school, I also carried some cognitive blocks from those earlier childhood traumas that impaired my ability to learn and obtain certain subjects. I was never the student who was strong in standardized testing. Understanding people and having compassion for others were my strongest social and personal strengths, but these were not measured or honored on entrance exams. Therefore, my American College Test (ACT) scores were lower than my school allowed, and my acceptance into a nursing diploma school was on a probationary basis only. My writing and math skills were not as strong as they needed to be, so I was asked to attend two remedial courses at the local university to strengthen these scores. I was successful in both classes that summer. My family did not have the money to support me through nursing school; fortunately, I was able to attend through a scholarship for dependents of impaired veterans. The program was sadly dropped from government funding the year I graduated as a nurse.

My mother had the words "*Look out world here comes Susie*" inscribed in icing across my cake. Up until that time I was the first child to graduate from any form of higher education in my family.

It was shortly after this momentous occasion that I learned serendipitously that my mother (without my knowledge) had sent a "thank you" card along with my graduation picture to her obstetrician, sharing her joy and excitement to thank him for the mistake he made two decades earlier.

Decision to Pursue Higher Education

I had transitioned to the South, beginning my career in Georgia. During the first decade of my career, I worked as a charge nurse on an inpatient child and adolescent unit in a large city. By this time, I was married and had my first child, and the impact of the pressure of early adulthood was also being experienced.

I was experiencing a lot of transference during my first few years in practice and was forced to face and reflect on my own developmental years as I was engaged with children who had similar experiences that I too had lived. I remember learning terms such as "underprivileged children," "at-risk youth," "barriers to care," and "disparities in services" that gave me pause. I realized early into my career that those terms defined me as well. Interestingly, I never felt underprivileged and actually considered myself privileged to have lived the childhood experiences that helped frame and mold me as a human being, a nurse, and a mother. "At risk" to me seemed foreign as well, as my experiences deeply imprinted an understanding of the human experience that I knew all too well on a very deep and visceral level.

I began to feel a sense of boredom with my current level of practice and did some investigating into options for pursuing more freedom in practice. I was fortunate enough to work at a mental health facility where a large percentage of the staff I worked with were pursuing higher education. This was incredibly motivating for me, as I found knowledge and new experience both challenging and exciting. Because I had attended a diploma school, I needed to decide whether to complete a Bachelor of Science in Nursing (BSN) program or another option in psychiatry. At the time I was not aware of the psychiatric Clinical Nurse Specialist (CNS) programs, and therefore I subsequently enrolled in a psychology program at Georgia State University. During my time in this BA program, I learned about the CNS option with a subspecialty in child and adolescent psychiatric nursing. I soon transferred into this graduate student role, as my heart always brought me back to nursing. This program connected my entry level into nursing with my ideals regarding graduate education. Bridging the gap in my education in this manner just made perfect sense to me at that time in my career. Personally, I felt that I had deep insight and understanding of the effects of trauma on children, and it was time to step out and integrate these two paths.

Shortly after my acceptance and admission, I learned of a Health Resources and Services Administration (HRSA) grant through the university that supported psychiatric graduate nursing students progressing into advanced practice, and I was able to land a seat in this program. My graduate program was fully funded, which was an unexpected gift. I completed my Master of Science in Nursing (MSN) after a few of life's detours in the summer of 1995.

I graduated on a Saturday and opened a private practice for "underprivileged" kids the following Monday. I continued to teach at my alma mater and began my career as a consulting psychiatric liaison and advanced practice registered nurse (APRN) across the state. During this time, CNS requirements for certification boards called for 2 years or 500 hours of supervised experience before sitting for the exam. I obtained my Psychiatric Mental Health CNS-Board Certification

(PMHCNS-BC) in early 1997. I was content for some time with that level of practice, until I was not.

Early in my career I had worked with children and adolescents at various summer camps and participated in community-building events with this population. I found this work resonated with my future work in the field helping traumatized children heal. I sensed that, knowing my own history, I could ensure a safe place for children to land and find the support needed to overcome trauma and heal. I recalled a few times during my childhood when I visited my dad in the veterans' hospital and another psychiatric facility when he detoxed or came in after a relapse of some form. Both these sites were frightening for a young child, in part because staff did not approach me to calm my fears. I internalized that I must be strong and handle this situation. Looking back at those times I realized it would have helped to have a nurse validate my fears or, at the very least, acknowledge that I was even in the room.

I had so many wonderful mentors along the way throughout my career path, some of whom probably did not even realize their impact. One of the things I learned early on was to only take advice about my career from someone I respected and wanted to emulate in some manner. I had two incredible professors in the first graduate school I attended. Both were certainly memorable. One of them was my advisor and had a sense of humor that was so delightful; she clearly never took herself too seriously, which was so helpful to me at the time. Another faculty member at that university was influential because of her research and work in forensics, particularly her research on Munchausen syndrome, which I found incredibly fascinating and which clearly expanded my psychiatric experiences and education into forensics later in my own career.

Another advanced practice colleague taught me about Pesso Boyden Psychomotor work, challenged my biases, and supported my growth as a person, not just as a professional. He did amazing work with adolescents. I mirrored his presence in developing an honest rapport and transparency with patients. He made it all look like so much fun and showed me how to maintain one's own recovery program as well as the importance of taking the time to recover from whatever our issues in life may be. He lived the life of setting limits and boundaries and accepting responsibility for oneself. This experience transformed my life.

Milestones

In the early part of my career, I was raising my daughter. I kept telling myself to stay interesting and challenged myself to rise above and evolve as a human-emotionally, spiritually, and intellectually. I often said I wanted to ensure I stayed informed so that students would pull from my knowledge and add to their own experiences and find delight in their career paths. I would say the greatest opportunities in the field came from the freedom to make my own schedule and work when I wanted to work. My family always came first, and obtaining an advanced degree and staying open to the endless possibilities of freedom to create my own reality ensured that my family remained first. I had my own struggles along the way of course. Divorce slowed my academic career, along with bouts of my own mental health challenges. There were certainly periods in my life that I thought it best to pause and step back for a moment as life presented me with opportunities to heal so that I could be fully present for myself and others.

Barriers I Faced and Strategies I Used to Navigate Them

I hit a few roadblocks in my professional life as I lost my job a few times due to downsizing and reprogramming that happened quite often during the 1980s and 1990s at mental health sites. Although this made life a bit unpredictable, it did allow me the opportunities to reprogram and take a moment and once again head back to school. I was fortunate to obtain all my degrees while working at a university that covered my tuition or supported me through grant money, so I did not have to take on much student debt. Working for teaching hospitals and being an academic is certainly one way to find financial support, and in all my work experiences I have been supported by colleagues to continue my education. I believe this is paramount to a successful career.

My Current Focus

My current focus as I round home plate is to continue to educate and train nurses to be their highest and their best, and to develop competencies at the highest level of their degree. I joke about retirement, but I cannot truly imagine what that would be like because I am still not ready to pass the torch completely. I do, however, feel I am an expert in the field at this point in my career, and I find myself sharing my knowledge and experience in ways that will influence the future of nursing across various specialties of practice. I try and instill hope in my students and encourage them to carry on and continue to challenge the course of nursing for future generations through their voice and in their practice.

My Future Goals

I am aware of my current desire to leave some type of nursing legacy to support my decades in the field. I am a coauthor on a developing manuscript regarding Psychiatric Consultation Liaison practice for APRNs. I believe this is the best way to share my expertise with future generations of NPs who find their joy in consultation. I feel my career has been somewhat of an outlier, as I never felt a "shift job" was a match to my core personality. It is difficult to take in 8 straight hours a day of vicarious trauma stories, so I found it best to always break up my working day in a way that honors my truth on how much I can take in. Each one of us needs to determine what our limit of carrying other people's pain will be. My roles in advanced practice have been numerous and constantly evolving throughout my career. I have worked in private practice and academia and have been both an executive director and a clinical director of substance use facilities. I believe I have covered most of the territory we can encounter in advanced practice. Almost always I had at least two jobs at a time: one in academia and one in practice. It's just how I operate.

I want to continue to push each of us to demonstrate the importance of self-care to all nurses, across all levels and specialties of practice. It is so important to make you, your family, and those closest to you your top priority. We are not responsible for the changes others need to make, but we are responsible to ensure we are in a solid headspace to do the work we do. We are mirrors for all to see. Let us make the best of it. One of my favorite sayings that I heard a long time ago is "only go as fast as the slowest part of you can go," and when you are going too fast, slow down, and when you are going too slow, speed up.

I have tried to carry this through to all aspects of my life and career.

Most recently, I opened a painting studio in the community where I was raised, which serves as a place to connect and create for all ages across the life span. I do not charge for others to come in and paint. I just ask that they give back to the community in time and talent. This is my fifth year in the community, and the healing for some who enter there has been palpable. I believe it is imperative to give back and enjoy the process as well.

Greatest Source of Satisfaction in My Work

I find deep satisfaction in growing as a person, a mother, and a friend. Working with children and adolescents has given me additional tools to integrate in my personal life and assisted me in raising emotionally healthy children. By working in the field of psychiatry I have learned to communicate more effectively. I have seen firsthand the glory of telling the truth and telling it fast, and I have seen the devastating effects of secret-keeping. All of my clients have been mirrors for me and have taught me things I will carry throughout the rest of my life. I cannot say I have always made the best decisions for my highest self. But working in the mental health field has certainly allowed me to consider choices that benefit rather than cripple me, and inscribed in me the importance of letting go and letting things just be.

Words of Wisdom to Nurses Considering Earning a Doctorate

My philosophy throughout my nursing career has been to ensure that we take care of ourselves first and foremost. I have learned to understand the moments when I too did not take my own advice. There will always be a need for support and guidance with our patients. But if we do not care for ourselves, we will get lost and bury ourselves in the lives of others. Our families need us to be fully present. Mirroring positive life experiences and living a healthy lifestyle for ourselves must be on the forefront. According to the American Nurses Association ethical guidelines, "The nurse owes the same duty to self as others including the responsibility to promote health & safety, preserve wholeness of character & integrity, maintain competence, and continue personal & professional growth" (American Nurses Association, Code of Ethics for Nurses With Interpretive Statements, nursingworld.org 2015).

My best advice is that you:

- Do it for yourself and only you.
- Do it when you are ready and when it works best for you.
- Do it even if no one else wants you to, do it for yourself (even if it means one course a semester).
- Take your time. Choose your graduate work projects wisely. Ensure your project will be something that will help you grow. Choose a project you love because you will spend a few years with the work.
- Make sure you are manifesting your own truth and not someone else's.

A Toolkit for Preparation for Doctoral Study

CHAPTER 33

Tools for the Journey

Laura A. Taylor, PhD, RN, ANEF, FAAN
Mary F. Terhaar, RN, PhD, ANEF, FAAN

We change our tools, and then our tools change us.
—Jeff Bezos

Each contributor to this book has explained a specific dimension of preparedness for doctoral education. In some chapters, the content is quite discrete, and in others, you have found intersection and connectivity. Many of the authors have introduced references to tools that can help you on your journey.

This section of the book presents a compendium of useful tools, either by providing a link through which you can access that tool or by providing the tool itself. We have assembled some tools you might find helpful as you organize and prioritize your thinking. Others you will find useful as you prioritize the characteristics of the programs you are considering. A few will help you put your time to its best use and maintain balance in life to help you achieve wholeness and happiness by keeping your eyes on the big picture of your life and your progress toward your goals. Some can help you ensure that you put your most constructive time to its best use. These can help you remove the gremlins that suck time into unimportant or, even worse, unhelpful uses. Others can help you prepare for standardized testing, plan your finances, build a budget, improve your writing, and increase your confidence in what you write. Finally, we offer a tool and some resources to help you prepare for your interview.

We have not built these items but have searched for useful ones to help you on your journey and we have experience putting them to good use. Try them out. We hope you will find them useful on your journey. Learn these tools now, use them now, count on them for life.

Your Journal

Your first assignment is to get yourself a nice journal in which you can track your thoughts and experiences over this year of preparation. Take time to reflect on both your progress and what you have learned along the way. Write about how you used the tools and what you learned about yourself in the process. Date your entries. On days when you are struggling, go back and review your entries. It will help you see your progress, reflect on sticking points, identify when and where you might want to speak with your mentor, and help you continue to move ahead. This journal will be the first of the tools you create on your journey.

Evaluating Readiness

The Robert Wood Johnson Foundation has developed a resource to guide you through a self-assessment process. This guide provides prompts to which you respond using an online survey format. Questions focus on your perceptions of the impact of obtaining a doctoral degree, and your connection with the richness of the education that will be provided in each program. Once completed, you will have had a very deep and thorough conversation with yourself about your priorities, interests, and motivation which will help you progress to your goals and avoid errors that can cost you time, money, and energy. Follow this link to the RWJ tool: https://www.surveymonkey.com/r/DoctoralReadinessAssessmentDANStudent Assessment.

Setting and Achieving Goals

Setting manageable goals and then organizing your time and efforts precisely to achieve those outcomes are important especially when working toward a stretch goal like gaining admission to your program of choice, earning the degree you seek, and continuing on your professional journey.

Search "Goal Setting" and you will find a great many tools for project management. You do not need these just yet. You will also find a plethora of consulting groups that provide an assortment of tools you can purchase. Most of these are quite attractive and have high production value. Not all of them will provide the structure you need.

We want to connect you to some of the tools that are of good quality and can be used for free. You will want to look at several of these and find a resource that is helpful without making unnecessary work. We encourage you to choose tools that invite you to provide details so your plan can be implemented and tracked. We suggest you review the tools available at the following sites to get started:
- https://www.smartsheet.com/goal-tracking-setting-templates
- https://www.developgoodhabits.com/goal-setting-worksheet/
- https://minimalistfocus.com/the-ultimate-goal-setting-worksheet-to-keep-track-of-your-progress/

Saying "No, Thank You"

Saying no is not something many of us have learned to do. It is important to understand that failing to say "No, Thank You" to distractions can result in your accepting too many responsibilities which seriously erodes the time and energy you have to achieve the things that are important to you.

We suggest you visit the following links if you would like to learn more about the importance of saying "*No, thank you,*" and the ways to do so respectfully and effectively.

- https://www.inc.com/jonathan-alpert/7-ways-to-say-no-to-someone-and-not-feel-bad-about-it.html
- https://hbr.org/video/6200580690001/how-to-say-no-at-work

Maintaining Balance and Enjoying Your Journey

Achieving balance between work, school, family, faith, service, community, and fun requires attention and intention just like all your other goals. We provide two tools you may find helpful as you seek to maintain balance or at least not lose sight of the big picture. We encourage you to consider and perhaps try using *The Work/Play/ Love/Health Balance Sheet* and the *Odyssey Planning Worksheet.*

Work, Play, Love, Health Dashboard

The *Work, Play, Love, Health* (WPLH) Dashboard (Burnett and Evans) is similar to the dashboard in your car. Much like the dashboard in your car that helps you keep an eye on the important things like the amount of gas in your tank, and whether you have enough windshield wiper fluid so that you can clean the windshield effectively and see the road and horizon ahead of you, the "*WPLH*" Dashboard helps you keep an eye on the major facets of your life. It can help you see if you are on time and on the correct route. It can help you "*fill up*" when you need to so you can achieve your goals.

Like Maslow's Hierarchy, you want to recognize "*Health*" as the foundation because the rest of the engine won't work if you are not healthy. You want to build *Work, Play, and Love* on top of the base of health and self-care. Remember that everyone's dashboard will be different and may be different over time as well. A "Perfect Balance" is NOT A REASONABLE GOAL. Yet, just like checking the "gas gauge" in your car, when the light goes on and your engine pings when you press ignition, take pause and address the indicator light. Something may not be right. "Knowing the current status of your health/work/play/love dashboard gives you a framework and some data about yourself, all in one place" (p. 25). This tool is presented in Fig. 33.1. The two links that follow take you to sites that emphasize health as the foundation for all success. You will want to consider both the tool and the philosophical grounding for it.

- https://designingyour.life/wp-content/uploads/2016/08/DYL_WORK-PLAY-LOVE-HEALTH.pdf
- https://lifedesignlog.com/personalizing-the-love-play-work-health-dashboard-for-university-students/

Work-Play-Love-Health balance worksheet

Current

Work 0 ▦▦▦▦ FULL
Play 0 ▦▦▦▦ FULL
Love 0 ▦▦▦▦ FULL
Health 0 ▦▦▦▦ FULL

• If you could make one incremental adjustment, what would it be? Redraw your improved dashboard.

Revised

Work 0 ▦▦▦▦ FULL
Play 0 ▦▦▦▦ FULL
Love 0 ▦▦▦▦ FULL
Health 0 ▦▦▦▦ FULL

• What would you get if you could attain this revised level of balance? How would life (really) change for you?

• What incremental change could you attempt to move in this direction? What would it take for you to live this way for two weeks?

Fig. 33.1 The Work/Play/Love/Health Balance Sheet. https://designingyour.life/wp-content/uploads/2016/08/DYL_WORK-PLAY-LOVE-HEALTH.pdf; https://lifedesignlog.com/personalizing-the-love-play-work-health-dashboard-for-university-students/.)

Odyssey Planning Worksheet

We also encourage you to try *The Odyssey Planning Worksheet* (Fig. 33.2). Burnett and Evans have created an *Odyssey Planning* tool because they assert that the best way to plan your life is to plan in parallel for the variety of choices ahead. Although the tool is called a plan, "it supports a process for designing your way forward in life on a journey into the future influenced by your own hopes, goals, helpers, lovers, antagonists, unknowns, and serendipities all unfolding over time in ways we both intend at the start and weave together as we go" (p. 92). The *Odyssey Planner* helps you create a minimum of three plans for the future, spanning the next five years. You can even make Odyssey plans for different parts of your life: your career, your family, your fun and play.

Life Plan 1 centers on how you would achieve what you already have in mind. It is the plan for the life goals you already envision. Creating this plan is a good idea and deserves your thoughtful attention.

Life Plan 2 begins to organize your thinking around what you would do if Plan 1 was suddenly gone. For example, what might you do if you are not admitted to your first-choice program, if the school or program you wish to attend closes, if the available funding doesn't come up to the level you anticipated, or if your partner and family need to relocate. In each of these scenarios, doing nothing is not an option. Plan 2 helps you wrap your brain around what you might do. Think this through. It takes some creativity.

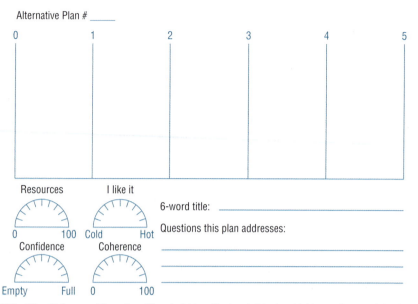

Fig. 33.2 The Odyssey Planning Sheet. (https://schoolofdesignthinking.echos.cc/blog/2018/01/starting-the-year-just-right/.)

Life Plan 3 is the fantasy plan. It details the path you would take, the things you would do, or the life you would live if money or image were of no consequence. If you knew that money was totally free flowing or the world wouldn't laugh at you or think less of you for doing it, what would you do? Allow some of this to be a little wild.

For each of these lives you will want to include:

1. A visual/graphical timeline. Include personal and noncareer events as well—do you want to be married, train to run an ultramarathon, or take an adventure and travel to see the Royal Edinburgh Military Tattoo?
2. A six-word title for each option describing the essence of this alternative.
3. Two or three questions that this alternative is asking. A good designer asks questions to test assumptions and reveal new insights. In each potential timeline, you will investigate different possibilities and learn different things about yourself and the world. What kinds of things will you want to test and explore in each alternative's version of your life?
4. *A dashboard* where you can gauge:
   a. Resources (time, money, skill, contacts—you need to pull off your plan)
   b. Likeability (hot or cold gut feeling about your plan)
   c. Confidence (confident or pretty uncertain about pulling this off?)
   d. Coherence (Does the plan makes sense? Is it consistent with your worldview?)

Key Contacts Directory

This tool is simple, but very useful. As you begin this journey you want to build a list of all your contacts. Whether you choose to keep your contacts electronically or the old-fashioned way using a notebook, you want to keep track of the people you speak with, how to reach them, the people to whom they refer you, and any other information you consider relevant. It can be challenging to remember everyone, but doing so will be helpful along the way. This will be a living document that you will maintain as you proceed in your preparations. You will likely choose to edit and maintain a similar record as you progress in your program. An example of such a list or directory is presented in Fig. 33.3.

Program Selection Decision Matrix

You will want to develop a decision support tool to help you keep track of the most important considerations in your year of preparation. The simplest way is to build an Excel spreadsheet. We suggest that you populate the x-axis with the names of the schools you are considering and use the columns to track the data you learn about them. Within this document you may want to add workbooks for other related decisions. These resources will be unique to you and the variables you consider to be important. An example of such a Decision Matrix is provided in Fig. 33.4.

	A	B	C	D	E	F	G	H	I	J
	CONTACT	CREDENTIALS	AFFILLIATION	ROLE	EMAIL	PHONE	ROLE	DATE OF LAST CONTACT	DATE FOR PLANNED FOLLOW-UP	NOTES
2	Laura Taylor	PhD, AGCNS, ANEF, FAAN	Uniformed Services University of Health Sciences	Professor						
3	Mary Terhaar	PhD, RN, ANEF, FAAN	Temple University	Professor						
4										
5										
6										
7										
8										
9										
10										
11										
12										
13										
14										

Fig. 33.3   Contacts Directory.

	A	B	C	D	E	F	G	H	I	J	K	L	M	N	O	P	Q	R	S	T	U
1	UNIVERSITY	PhD	BS2PHD	DNP	BS2DNP	RESEARCH STATUS	RANK	# STUDENTS	# FACULTY	LOCATION	PROGRAM LENGTH	% COMPLETION	TA OPPORT UNITIES	RA OPPORT UNITIES	NFLP	SCHOLA R-SHIPS	FT	PT	ON-LINE	F2F	RESPONS-IVENESS
2																					
3																					
4																					
5																					
6																					
7																					
8																					
9																					
10																					

Fig. 33.4   Program Selection Decision and Selection Matrix.

Four-Quadrant Time Management Grid

Covey's easy-to-use 4-Quadrant Time Management Grid is a tool that is practical and transformative. Use it to help you track time use and management. The data gathered by using this tool for just 1 week will enable you to dedicate your time to achieve your goals. It will help you understand where you are using time well and where it is squandered. It will help you understand the gaps in your use of time and where you manage your time poorly (Covey, 2003; Rohn, 2014).

We encourage you to make seven copies of this chart and commit to tracking where and how you spend your time for one full week. Track your time use in relation to the four quadrants identified in the tool. You will then track and qualify your time use by recording activities and efforts according to their urgency (Oxford dictionary defines urgent as "requiring swift action") and importance (Oxford dictionary defines importance a being of great significance or value).

Tracking your time this way enables you to reflect on your patterns and manage your time effectively. This knowledge can help you to pivot effectively when it is important to do so. The four quadrants are summarized by Covey as follows:

Quadrant 1 (Q-1): Urgent and Important. Crises and emergencies are categorized here. Interestingly, spending too much time in Q-1 increases the likelihood of getting stuck in Q-1. The most effective people respond to opportunities to do what's important instead of reacting to urgent problems.

Quadrant 2 (Q-2): Not urgent, but important. Q-2 is where effective people focus their time and energy. Q-2 includes activities that could easily be put off for their lack of apparent urgency but will significantly benefit your life long term if you invest the time in them. Like pursuing your doctoral degree! Do not fail to prioritize yourself and your doctoral education. When things come up, it is easier to determine what's important and what isn't once you've defined your goals and personal mission statement.

Quadrant 3 (Q-3): Urgent, but not important. You are likely unaware that these situations are unimportant because of the "urgency" placed on the action by someone else's implied importance. This might include emails and meetings that could have been accomplished through an email. When labeling and defining the contents of Q-3, you can see how others' goals and values guide your efforts rather than your own.

Quadrant 4 (Q-4): Neither urgent nor important. You may do things in Quadrant 4 purely for enjoyment or confusion about what's truly important. Quadrants 3 and 4 are irresponsible uses of your time, and effective people tend to avoid these activities. The most common of these today would be the time vortex of social media and binge streaming of the next new television show. Awareness of the size of your Q-4 offers critical insights into the time spent achieving your goal.

The Four-Quadrant Time Management tool is presented in Fig. 33.5.

Quadrant 1: Urgent and important	**Quadrant 2**: Not urgent but important
Quadrant 3: Urgent but not important	**Quadrant 4**: Not urgent and not important

Fig. 33.5   Four Quadrants of Time. (Covey, S., Seven Habits of Highly Effective People, 1989.)

Graduate Record Exams Preparations

Graduate Record Exams (GREs) are still required for admission to some doctoral programs across the country. So, after you have outlined the assets and liabilities of the programs you are considering in your Decision Matrix, you may want to complete one of these programs or use one of these preparation resources to help you confidently tackle the GREs.

There are many options for test prep support, and several websites summarize the outcomes and consumer experiences reported by learners who used various prep resources. These data can be helpful as you select the prep course that best meets your needs and expectations. You will want to browse through these sites and see which meets your needs. Several examples are provided in the links below.

- https://top10prepcourses.com
- https://www.bestcolleges.com/blog/best-online-gre-prep-courses/

Financial Planning

Chapter 9 is chock-full of smart approaches to help you tackle the cost of the education you seek. The Decision Matrix provided earlier in this compendium can be used to help you rank your options. Many of the variables you listed in that matrix will become important considerations as you assess your best options financially. It is important not to simply look at tuition when you think of cost. The tool in Fig. 33.6 will help you anticipate and plan for the actual costs of the programs. You will need to know the length of the program, the tuition (cost per credit and total credits) as well as related expenses like lab fees, tests, uniforms, books, technology, site fees, and travel in order to project the total costs. This information will help you determine the debt load you may carry which will most likely factor into your decisions. The figure below provides a reference to help track this information and understand your expenses.

Program & Degree	Ranking	Fit with career goals	Fit with faculty	Total credits	Cost per credit	Years to completion	Completion rate	Fees	Total tuition	Scholarships available	Ta & ra opportunities	Additional costs	Other considerations

Fig. 33.6   Program Expenses Worksheet.

The U.S. federal government and the U.S. Department of Education maintain an online resource that you can use to help you choose a loan repayment option that best meets your needs and goals. It explains how financial aid works, the types of aid available, and helps you understand the aid for which you are eligible. It provides the information you need to calculate the duration of the loan you would carry and the amount due for each payment. The Financial Aid Calculator is available at the link below:

- https://studentaid.gov/loan-simulator/

Budgeting

Understanding and managing your income and expenses is a life skill that will help you achieve your goals, including earning your doctorate. Mapping out a budget will prepare you to handle your current and future expenses. It can also help you anticipate and manage the high, irregular costs you are likely to incur along the way (car repairs, travel, veterinarian bills, large appliances that go on the blitz). Box 33.1 provides an overview of strategies to create a budget, evaluate your financial readiness, and make a plan to manage your money to meet your goals.

- https://www.forbes.com/advisor/student-loans/build-a-college-budget/
- https://www.forbes.com/advisor/student-loans/build-a-college-budget/
- https://goodbudget.com/
- https://www.hughcalc.org/coffee.cgi
- https://www.youneedabudget.com/

The skills you build now in preparation for this doctoral journey will set you up for a lifetime of financial accomplishment. Once you know what expenses to expect and what money you'll have coming in, you can build your action plan. In Chapter 9, we introduce the many financial options available.

BOX 33.1 ■ How to Build Your Budget

Financial Assets

1. Calculate your total savings (*consider all sources*)
   - Consider all sources (savings accounts, bonds, education accounts, and gift accounts)
   - Make a list with the amount for each source
   - The sum of these is your total savings
   - Consider how much of your savings you are willing to access over your school years

Income

2. Calculate your monthly income, which is the sum of the following (*consider all sources*)
   - The amount of your earned income (from all employment)
   - Contributions from family members (spouse, partner, parents)
   - Child support
   - Teaching Assistant income
   - Research Assistant income
   - Other sources of income (rental from roommates, other income)
   - This is your monthly income
   - That money is how much you must spend each year. Many find it more helpful to divide that amount by semester or by month.
3. Calculate your school-related annual income, which is the sum of the following (*consider all sources*)
   - Scholarships
   - Fellowships
   - Grants
   - Loan disbursements
   - Tuition benefits from your employer
   - This is your school-related annual income
4. Calculate total annual income. (sum of #2 and #3)

Expenses

5. List and quantify all school-related expenses for the year (make note of those that will be covered by aid, scholarships, or other means)
   - Tuition
   - Books
   - Uniforms
   - Lab fees
   - Course fees
   - Technology
   - Study abroad experiences
   - Program specific requirements
6. List and quantify all other monthly living expenses
   - Rent (or mortgage)
   - Car payments
   - Other transportation
   - Groceries
   - Phone
   - Insurance
   - Memberships (gym, social, etc)
   - Clothes
   - Gasoline
   - Eating and drinking out
   - Entertainment (concerts, movies, etc.)

Continued

BOX 33.1 ■ How to Build Your Budget—cont'd

- Gifts
- Activities
- Discretionary spending
- Emergency expenses that you budget to cover, just in case
7. Calculate your living expenses for the year
   - Sum of your monthly expenses for 12 months
   - Be sure to add in any other annual expenses (health-related, vacation, etc.)
8. Calculate the sum of your annual expenses (school-related #4 + living expenses #7)
9. Subtract your total annual expenses from your total annual income
   - Is your total annual income sufficient to cover your total annual expenses?
   - If your answer is YES, that is amazing!
   - If your answer is NO, that means you need to plan carefully.
10. Identify opportunities to reduce spending
   - Look for areas where you can cut back
   - Even small adjustments can pay off over four or more years of school
   - Cook your own meals to reduce expenses for restaurants
   - Ride share to reduce gas expenses
   - Rent textbooks instead of buying them, or purchase secondhand
   - Downgrade your cell phone plan
   - Use the gym on campus
   - Make your own coffee
   - Pack your lunch
11. Keep your eyes on the prize!
   - When creating your budget for college student life, make sure you focus on your educational and financial goals. For example, you may want to study abroad for a semester or buy a car once you graduate. To make your goals a reality, set aside a little money each month so that you'll have the cash you need.
12. Do it all again …… regularly.
   - After creating a budget, make sure you check it often. It's a good idea to review your budget weekly or monthly to help you stay on track. By making it a habit, you can minimize excess spending and stay within your limits. If you stray, you can get back on track. Once you see that you are good at managing your budget, it becomes very rewarding to do just that.

Purdue Online Writing Lab

The Purdue University Online Writing Lab (OWL) is the go-to resource for scholars across the country who are looking for tools to help them produce well written papers and satisfy American Psychological Association (APA) requirements. It is free, accessible, and very user friendly.

- https://owl.purdue.edu/

Grammarly

Grammarly is a cloud-based resource that offers both free or fee-driven resources to assist you to ensure your grammar, punctuation, and overall quality of writing is accurate, error-free, and engaging.

- http://Grammarly.com

Writing Confidence and Skill

You will find there are a great many user-friendly resources available online to help you take your writing, and your confidence, from good to great. *Coursera* (coursera. org) is a U.S.-based Massive Open Online Course resource (MOOC). Coursera works with universities and organizations around the world to offer online courses, certifications, and even degrees. We suggest you explore the offerings and find those that best meet your personal needs. The following are a few links you might find interesting and useful.

- Good With Words: Writing and Editing Specialization
  https://www.coursera.org/specializations/good-with-words
- Grammar and Punctuation
  https://www.coursera.org/learn/grammar-punctuation
- Writing Your World: Finding Yourself in the Academic Space
  https://www.coursera.org/learn/writing-your-world
- Getting Started with Essay Writing
  https://www.coursera.org/learn/getting-started-with-essay-writing
- Edu.com/writing tools: https://edubirdie.com/writing-tools

Strengths, Weaknesses, Opportunities and Threats: SWOT

SWOT and WOOP are exceptionally useful in structuring your responsiveness to the challenges that will arise during your doctoral journey.

A SWOT Analysis is a tool that can help you analyze what you do well now and devise strategies for a successful future. SWOT invites you to reflect honestly in order to better understand yourself and what you bring to doctoral education, as well as what you want to improve or strengthen. Areas where you have *strengths* become areas to emphasize in your application. Areas where you are *weak* become areas where you might need support, coaching, or effort. You can expect to be asked about these strengths and weaknesses during your interviews. So, a thoughtful conversation based on your own self-assessment will be most helpful during that process. Fig. 33.7 provides a tool you can use to organize your thoughts for your SWOT.

- SWOT Analysis: Understanding Your Business, Informing Your Strategy
  https://www.mindtools.com/pages/article/newTMC_05.htm

Wishes, Outcomes, Obstacles, Plan: WOOP

Much like SWOT, WOOP provides you with an integrative, visual representation of your self-reflection. In this tool you will capture your thoughts about "Mental Contrasting." The first step is to identify your wish for the future and align the reality of your current situation with how your position fits into this wish and the

Strengths	Weaknesses
Opportunities	Threats

Fig. 33.7 Swot. SWOT Analysis: Understanding Your Business, Informing Your Strategy (https://www.mindtools.com/pages/article/newTMC_05.htm.)

outcome you seek. Being honest about likely obstacles will help you create a plan for when they occur (and they will).

We provide a guide to completing your *mental contrasting exercise* in Table 33.1.

The results of this activity will yield your WOOP. We provide a simple tool you can use in Fig. 33.8. You will also find that many easy-to-fill-in tools are available, and we provide links to those below. An app you can build and carry with you on your smart device is also available (Table 14.2). And resources are available to help you create a WOOP approach for your wellbeing and life outside this doctoral journey.

- WOOP App: Wish-Outcome-Obstacles-Plan:
  https://apps.apple.com/us/app/woopapp/id790247988
- WOOP
  My Life https://woopmylife.org/en/home

Interviewing

Nearly every doctoral program in nursing, whether large or small, conducts some form of an interview before accepting a student for admission. The importance of interviews cannot be overstated. You will have already submitted your application which will likely have included your vitae, personal statement, goals, transcripts, and letters of recommendation. The interview is your opportunity to display your professionalism and etiquette in front of the program's admissions committee and other critical faculty you will be working with throughout your education across the next 3 to 5 to 7 years. Table 33.2 lists interview preparation tools.

TABLE 33.1 ■ **Mental Contrasting**

W—Wish	Identify your wish for the future: Describe in 3–6 words.	Apply to a doctoral program.
O—Outcome	The most significant benefit that will result from this wish. Again 3–6 words here.	Submit application by Fall Due Date.
O—Obstacle	Obstacles to achieving this wish. Be realistic; earning a doctorate includes time management, addressing lack of motivation, and preparing for the loss of financial support. Be open and list as many as you can.	Time management is not my strength. I frequently doubt my own knowledge and get down on myself; I think "I don't belong in a doctoral program so I shouldn't even apply."
P—Plan	Make a plan to address the obstacles, not if, but when, they occur. Make this plan so that you are not reactive in your approach when this obstacle arises.	Carve out 30 minutes before usual wake-up time 3 days a week. Use the "If then Rule: If I spend 30 minutes on the application, I can watch one episode of my favorite streaming show." When I feel like an "imposter" send email/text to Mentor and peers who are just ahead of me in school. Seek advice.

Shout it Out! WOOP WOOP!

Modified from https://mindfulambition.net/woop/.

Wishes	Obstacles
Outcomes	**Plan**

Fig. 33.8 Woop. WOOP App: Wish-Outcome-Obstacles-Plan: https://apps.apple.com/us/app/woopapp/id790247988. WOOP: My Life: https://woopmylife.org/en/home.

You can find multiple resources online to help prepare for this interview.
- Interview Research and Preparation
  https://www.coursera.org/learn/interview-preparation
- Successful Interviewing
  https://www.coursera.org/learn/successful-interviewing

TABLE 33.2 ■ **Interview Prep Tool**

	Prep Activity	**Notes**
1.	Review CV or Resume	*Be prepared to provide a high-level summary of your career.*
2.	Review Personal Essay	*What did you emphasize in your essay?* Why was that important to you? What do you want the committee to understand about your narrative?
3.	Identify strengths	*Which items make you unique?* Which items connect to the mission of the program? How are you well suited to the program?
4.	Identify your weaknesses	*Where are you weak?* How will doctoral study mitigate those weaknesses? If there is an area that stands out as problematic, be prepared to speak to it, honestly.
5.	Review program materials	*Why do you want to be educated in this program?* Why do you seek this degree option?
6.	Prepare your questions	*What do you need to know that you couldn't learn from the website?*